METHODS IN MOLECULAR BIOLOGY

Series Editor
**John M. Walker
School of Life and Medical Sciences
University of Hertfordshire
Hatfield, Hertfordshire, AL10 9AB, UK**

For further volumes:
http://www.springer.com/series/7651

Cancer Bioinformatics

Edited by

Alexander Krasnitz

*Simons Center for Quantitative Biology, Cold Spring Harbor Laboratory,
Cold Spring Harbor, NY, USA*

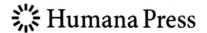

Editor
Alexander Krasnitz
Simons Center for Quantitative Biology
Cold Spring Harbor Laboratory
Cold Spring Harbor, NY, USA

ISSN 1064-3745   ISSN 1940-6029 (electronic)
Methods in Molecular Biology
ISBN 978-1-4939-9404-5   ISBN 978-1-4939-8868-6 (eBook)
https://doi.org/10.1007/978-1-4939-8868-6

© Springer Science+Business Media, LLC, part of Springer Nature 2019, corrected publication 2019
Softcover re-print of the Hardcover 1st edition 2019
This work is subject to copyright. All rights are reserved by the Publisher, whether the whole or part of the material is concerned, specifically the rights of translation, reprinting, reuse of illustrations, recitation, broadcasting, reproduction on microfilms or in any other physical way, and transmission or information storage and retrieval, electronic adaptation, computer software, or by similar or dissimilar methodology now known or hereafter developed.
The use of general descriptive names, registered names, trademarks, service marks, etc. in this publication does not imply, even in the absence of a specific statement, that such names are exempt from the relevant protective laws and regulations and therefore free for general use.
The publisher, the authors, and the editors are safe to assume that the advice and information in this book are believed to be true and accurate at the date of publication. Neither the publisher nor the authors or the editors give a warranty, express or implied, with respect to the material contained herein or for any errors or omissions that may have been made. The publisher remains neutral with regard to jurisdictional claims in published maps and institutional affiliations.

This Humana Press imprint is published by the registered company Springer Science+Business Media, LLC part of Springer Nature.
The registered company address is: 233 Spring Street, New York, NY 10013, U.S.A.

Preface

Modern cancer research, both basic and translational, routinely generates massive amounts of digital data and increasingly relies on computing for their interpretation. These data come from a variety of sources, among them next-generation sequencing of tumor DNA and RNA, epigenomics, imaging, and pathological evaluation. It is expected that in the near future data-driven methods will become an integral part of clinical practice in oncology, leading to earlier detection, more accurate diagnosis, and better-informed management of the disease.

With this development in mind, the present volume covers a wide variety of cancer-related methods and tools for data analysis and interpretation, reflecting the state of the art in cancer informatics. The volume is designed to attract broad readership, ranging from active researchers in computational biology and bioinformatics developers, to research and clinical oncologists who require bioinformatics support, to anticancer drug developers wishing to rationalize their search for new compounds.

Cold Spring Harbor, NY, USA *Alexander Krasnitz*

Contents

Preface v
Contributors ix

1 A Primer for Access to Repositories of Cancer-Related Genomic Big Data 1
   John Torcivia-Rodriguez, Hayley Dingerdissen, Ting-Chia Chang, and Raja Mazumder

2 Building Portable and Reproducible Cancer Informatics Workflows: An RNA Sequencing Case Study 39
   Gaurav Kaushik and Brandi Davis-Dusenbery

3 Computational Analysis of Structural Variation in Cancer Genomes 65
   Matthew Hayes

4 CORE: A Software Tool for Delineating Regions of Recurrent DNA Copy Number Alteration in Cancer 85
   Guoli Sun and Alexander Krasnitz

5 Identification of Mutated Cancer Driver Genes in Unpaired RNA-Seq Samples 95
   David Mosen-Ansorena

6 A Computational Protocol for Detecting Somatic Mutations by Integrating DNA and RNA Sequencing 109
   Matthew D. Wilkerson

7 Allele-Specific Expression Analysis in Cancer Using Next-Generation Sequencing Data 125
   Alessandro Romanel

8 Computational Analysis of lncRNA Function in Cancer 139
   Xu Zhang and Tsui-Ting Ho

9 Computational Methods for Identification of T Cell Neoepitopes in Tumors 157
   Vanessa Isabell Jurtz and Lars Rønn Olsen

10 Computational and Statistical Analysis of Array-Based DNA Methylation Data 173
    Jessica Nordlund, Christofer Bäcklin, and Amanda Raine

11 Computational Methods for Subtyping of Tumors and Their Applications for Deciphering Tumor Heterogeneity 193
    Shihua Zhang

12 Statistically Supported Identification of Tumor Subtypes 209
    Guoli Sun and Alexander Krasnitz

13 Computational Methods for Analysis of Tumor Clonality
   and Evolutionary History... 217
   Gerald Goh, Nicholas McGranahan, and Gareth A. Wilson

14 Predictive Modeling of Anti-Cancer Drug Sensitivity from Genetic
   Characterizations 227
   Raziur Rahman and Ranadip Pal

15 In Silico Oncology Drug Repositioning and Polypharmacology 243
   Feixiong Cheng

16 Modeling Growth of Tumors and Their Spreading Behavior
   Using Mathematical Functions 263
   *Bertin Hoffmann, Thorsten Frenzel, Rüdiger Schmitz,
   Udo Schumacher, and Gero Wedemann*

Correction to: Computational Analysis of Structural Variation in
Cancer Genomes... C1

Index 279

Contributors

CHRISTOFER BÄCKLIN • *Department of Medical Sciences, Uppsala University, Uppsala, Sweden*

TING-CHIA CHANG • *Department of Biochemistry and Molecular Medicine, George Washington University, Washington, DC, USA*

FEIXIONG CHENG • *Center for Complex Networks Research, Northeastern University, Boston, MA, USA*

BRANDI DAVIS-DUSENBERY • *Seven Bridges Genomics, Cambridge, MA, USA*

HAYLEY DINGERDISSEN • *Department of Biochemistry and Molecular Medicine, George Washington University, Washington, DC, USA*

THORSTEN FRENZEL • *Institute for Anatomy and Experimental Morphology, University Cancer Center Hamburg-Eppendorf, Hamburg, Germany*

GERALD GOH • *Cancer Research UK Lung Cancer Centre of Excellence, University College London Cancer Institute, London, UK; Genome Institute of Singapore, Singapore, Singapore*

MATTHEW HAYES • *Computer Science, Xavier University of Louisiana, New Orleans, LA, USA*

TSUI-TING HO • *Cancer Institute, Department of Radiation Oncology, University of Mississippi Medical Center, Jackson, MS, USA*

BERTIN HOFFMANN • *Competence Center Bioinformatics, Institute for Applied Computer Science, University of Applied Sciences Stralsund, Stralsund, Germany*

VANESSA ISABELL JURTZ • *Department of Bio and Health Informatics, Technical University of Denmark, Lyngby, Denmark*

GAURAV KAUSHIK • *Foundation Medicine, Cambridge, MA, USA*

ALEXANDER KRASNITZ • *Simons Center for Quantitative Biology, Cold Spring Harbor Laboratory, Cold Spring Harbor, NY, USA*

RAJA MAZUMDER • *Department of Biochemistry and Molecular Medicine, George Washington University, Washington, DC, USA*

NICHOLAS MCGRANAHAN • *Cancer Research UK Lung Cancer Centre of Excellence, University College London Cancer Institute, London, UK*

DAVID MOSEN-ANSORENA • *Department of Biostatistics, Harvard T.H. Chan School of Public Health, Boston, MA, USA; Department of Biostatistics and Computational Biology, Dana-Farber Cancer Institute, Boston, MA, USA*

JESSICA NORDLUND • *Department of Medical Sciences and Science for Life Laboratory, Uppsala University, Uppsala, Sweden*

LARS RØNN OLSEN • *Department of Bio and Health Informatics, Technical University of Denmark, Lyngby, Denmark*

RANADIP PAL • *Electrical and Computer Engineering, Texas Tech University, Lubbock, TX, USA*

RAZIUR RAHMAN • *Electrical and Computer Engineering, Texas Tech University, Lubbock, TX, USA*

AMANDA RAINE • *Department of Medical Sciences and Science for Life Laboratory, Uppsala University, Uppsala, Sweden*

ALESSANDRO ROMANEL • *Centre for Integrative Biology (CIBIO), University of Trento, Trento, Italy*

RÜDIGER SCHMITZ • *Institute for Anatomy and Experimental Morphology, University Cancer Center Hamburg-Eppendorf, Hamburg, Germany*

UDO SCHUMACHER • *Institute for Anatomy and Experimental Morphology, University Cancer Center Hamburg-Eppendorf, Hamburg, Germany*

GUOLI SUN • *Intuit Inc., Mountain View, CA, USA*

JOHN TORCIVIA-RODRIGUEZ • *Department of Biochemistry and Molecular Medicine, George Washington University, Washington, DC, USA*

GERO WEDEMANN • *Competence Center Bioinformatics, Institute for Applied Computer Science, University of Applied Sciences Stralsund, Stralsund, Germany*

MATTHEW D. WILKERSON • *The American Genome Center, Collaboration Health Initiative Research Program, Department of Anatomy, Physiology and Genetics, Uniformed Services University, Bethesda, MD, USA*

GARETH A. WILSON • *Cancer Research UK Lung Cancer Centre of Excellence, University College London Cancer Institute, London, UK; Translational Cancer Therapeutics Laboratory, The Francis Crick Institute, London, UK*

SHIHUA ZHANG • *National Center for Mathematics and Interdisciplinary Sciences, Academy of Mathematics and Systems Science, Chinese Academy of Sciences, Beijing, China*

XU ZHANG • *Center of Clinical and Translational Sciences and Department of Internal Medicine, The University of Texas Health Science Center at Houston, Houston, TX, USA*

Chapter 1

A Primer for Access to Repositories of Cancer-Related Genomic Big Data

John Torcivia-Rodriguez, Hayley Dingerdissen, Ting-Chia Chang, and Raja Mazumder

Abstract

The use of large datasets has become ubiquitous in biomedical sciences. Researchers in the field of cancer genomics have, in recent years, generated large volumes of data from their experiments. Those responsible for production of this data often analyze a narrow subset of this data based on the research question they are trying to address: this is the case whether or not they are acting independently or in conjunction with a large-scale cancer genomics project. The reality of this situation creates the opportunity for other researchers to repurpose this data for different hypotheses if the data is made easily and freely available. New insights in biology resulting from more researchers having access to data they otherwise would be unable to generate on their own are a boon for the field. The following chapter reviews several cancer genomics-related databases and outlines the type of data they contain, as well as the methods required to access each database. While this list is not comprehensive, it should provide a basis for cancer researchers to begin exploring some of the many large datasets that are available to them.

Key words Cancer resources, Genomics databases, Cancer ontology, Cancer genomics

1 Introduction

Every day a rapidly increasing amount of biological and biomedical data is generated due to high-throughput sequencing (HTS) methods being used to explore genomics and proteomics hypotheses. These methodologies allow for the capture of large amounts of data relevant to a target or set of targets of interest for the researcher then to further analyze. This data and the related analysis are usually then deposited in a database and/or published in a journal. Because of the scale and expanse of the data generated, the data can often be used to answer questions far beyond the original research hypothesis making general availability of this data important for the research community. Several consortiums have been developed to moderate access to such data due to potential privacy issues, allowing either general access to the entire dataset if these issues are not relevant or controlled access to some subset thereof if they are. Recent years have seen an increase in the volume of data in these repositories, accompanied by an increase in the appearance of specialized repositories leading to fragmentation of valuable data. This has created a system where important and sometimes even related data is stored in many different places. Further exacerbating the problem is the fact that most of these repositories have unique rules and methods for access to said data and they often adhere to different nomenclatures, standards, and ontologies.

There have been attempts to ease the resulting frustration of accessing data by combining data in secondary, experiment-independent repositories and synchronizing data contents between such repositories. For example, the National Center for Biotechnology Information (NCBI), the European Bioinformatics Institute (EBI), and the DNA Data Bank of Japan (DDBJ) exchange data on a regular basis as part of the International Nucleotide Sequence Database Collaboration (INSDC) [1]. While significant, these efforts have not been transformative for the field, so there still remain many distinct and partially redundant specialized data centers. There have also been efforts to create unified cancer genomics resources, such as the Cancer Genomics Resource List [2], which focus on clinical applications of cancer screening tests but have limited consideration for the management of, or access to, and use of primary data [3].

Here, we summarize a subset of current (as of 2017) important cancer data-related repositories by describing the information they contain as well as how to access them. Where appropriate, we have provided images to help the user access the services by recognizing they are in the correct location and template source code for quick retrieval of data (for systems that allow this application program interface (API) access). This chapter is not meant to be exhaustive but rather to aid the reader in understanding both the current landscape of available cancer genomics resources and the overarching principles of accessing and navigating data in these resources.

Please note, whenever Linux is referenced in this chapter, it is referring to a Debian distribution of the operating system, such as the popular Ubuntu distribution. Other distributions can be used but may require minor changes to the information provided here. Additionally, when statistics are given for datasets in this chapter, these numbers are accurate as of November 2017 unless a different date is specified. The statistics reported were taken directly from databases as published on their access portals and not calculated by the authors. These are provided where available to give the user an idea of the scope of the data and to better inform their decision-making.

Throughout this chapter, there are terminal commands or other types of commands you will enter into the computer. These commands are differentiated from the surrounding text by using a different font—`this is an example of a code command`. This should be helpful in determining what needs to be entered directly into the terminal. Also, commands may have parts offset by "< >." This indicates that the placeholder text in that space should be replaced with specific information unique to the user as explained in the surrounding text. For example, the command `cd <downloads directory>` (which navigates you to a new directory) would be `cd Downloads` for a user that wants to navigate to a directory called "Downloads" from their current directory. Readers of this chapter may find it useful to go through a command line interface tutorial before reading further to better understand how to access these databases.

2 Databases and How to Access Them

There are many different databases that contain cancer-related data: while the scope of these individual repositories has been described elsewhere [3], the following chapter aims to give a quick introduction to some highly used cancer genomics-related databases broken down with respect to the different types of datasets available. Some datasets provide a single type of information (microarray data, HTS, etc.), while others store many different types of data. Figure 1 describes the different types of data that may be accessed in the repositories covered in this chapter.

In general, accessing any data repository will consist of the following steps:

1. Navigate to remote database via HTTP or FTP.
2. Determine which datasets you would like to download.
3. Determine access rights required.
4. If you do not have access credentials, apply for them.
5. If the number of desired records is small, you may generally download directly through the web or FTP interface.
6. If the number of desired records is large, you will likely have to download through a batch download submission process. This can sometimes be facilitated through a web portal but frequently requires command line access.
7. If needed, unpack the data.

The remaining sections include descriptions and access protocols for a number of resources (containing both raw sequence data and processed information), cancer-specific terms, and upcoming projects. Please *see* Table 1 for the full list of databases and resources explored in the following chapter. These repositories and databases are highly accessed in the field and represent a sample of the diverse methods required to access cancer-related data.

		HTS					Processed Data									Ontology		
		TCGA	TARGET	CCLE	ICGC	SRA	COSMIC	BioMuta	BioXpress	ClinVar	LNCipedia	IntOGen	EGA	UniProt	cBioPortal	NCI Thesaurus	OMIM	Disease Ontology
DNA Sequencing	Whole genome	X	X		X	X								X				
	Whole exome	X	X	X	X	X								X				
RNA Sequencing	RNA-seq	X	X		X	X												
	miRNA-seq	X	X		X	X												
Processed	Alignments	X			X	X												
	Single-nucleotide variations						X	X	X			X						
	Amino acid variations							X										
	Gene fusion mutations						X											
	Copy number variations	X	X	X	X		X								X			
	Non coding variations						X											
	Pharmacological profiling			X														
	lncRNAs										X							
	Gene mutations													X	X			
Expression	Gene/mRNA expression	X	X	X			X								X			
	Exon expression	X																
	Protein expression	X													X			
	Expression changes								X									
Epigenetics	Methylation	X	X		X		X								X			
	Epigenetic information (General)													X				
	Clinical information/data	X		X										X	X			
	Cell line annotations			X														
	Oncomap mutations			X														
Annotations	Disease associations (incl. cancer)						X	X		X								
	SNV associated genes							X										
	SNV associated proteins							X										
	Driver gene mutations											X						
	Interacting therapeutic agents											X						
	Phenotype data												X					
	Protein Annotations													X				
	Classification data						X											
Other	Microsatellite instability	X																
	Images	X																
	Negative Datasets						X											
	Data Visualization														X			
	Disease Ontology Categories															X	X	X

Fig. 1 Matrix of the data resources listed in this chapter as well as the general types of data that are found at each resource. Entries marked with an "X" have data of the associated type in the repository

Accessing a database is often difficult and time-consuming; however, many tools have been developed to automate the workflow of retrieving and computing on genomic data. Tools and platforms such as the High-performance Integrated Virtual Environment (HIVE) [4] and Galaxy [5–7] are able to retrieve publicly available data from a number of different sources and allow a user to perform a series of computations on the data for further analysis. There are many additional tools that can be discovered through a simple Internet search.

2.1 Genomic Resources

2.1.1 High-Throughput Sequencing Data

TCGA

The Cancer Genome Atlas (TCGA) project [8] provides a unified platform where researchers can search, download, and apply further analysis to the wealth of data generated by the TCGA consortium. TCGA can be accessed by navigating to http://cancergenome.nih.gov/ in any modern web browser (Opera, Mozilla's Firefox, Google's Chrome, Apple's Safari, Microsoft's Edge, etc.). Some TCGA data, such as HTS and patient-specific information, is access-controlled and was previously made available solely through CGHub [9], a meta-repository for data across projects intended to provide researchers with adequate sample sizes to obtain

Table 1
Index of data repositories examined as well as their hierarchy

Genetic resources	
High-throughput sequencing data	
The Cancer Genome Atlas (TCGA)	http://cancergenome.nih.gov/
Therapeutically Applicable Research to Generate Effective Treatments (TARGET)	https://ocg.cancer.gov/programs/target/
Cancer Cell Line Encyclopedia (CCLE)	https://portals.broadinstitute.org/ccle
International Cancer Genome Consortium (ICGC)	https://icgc.org/
Sequence Read Archive (SRA)	http://www.ncbi.nlm.nih.gov/sra
Processed genomic data	
Catalogue of Somatic Mutations in Cancer (COSMIC)	http://cancer.sanger.ac.uk/cosmic
BioMuta	https://hive.biochemistry.gwu.edu/tools/biomuta/index.php
BioXpress	https://hive.biochemistry.gwu.edu/tools/bioxpress/index.php
ClinVar	http://www.ncbi.nlm.nih.gov/clinvar/
LNCipedia	http://www.lncipedia.org/
Integrative Onco Genomics (IntOGen)	https://www.intogen.org/
European Genome-phenome Archive	https://www.ebi.ac.uk/ega/
UniProt	http://www.uniprot.org/
cBioPortal	http://www.cbioportal.org/
Cancer Terms	
NCI Thesaurus	https://ncit.nci.nih.gov/ncitbrowser/
OMIM	http://www.ncbi.nlm.nih.gov/omim/
Disease Ontology	http://disease-ontology.org/

statistical power (*see* below for access instructions). Currently, all restricted data is now available through the NCI Genomic Data Commons (GDC). Publicly available data, however, is accessible directly through the data portal.

The GDC data portal allows you to filter based on certain search criteria (*see* Figs. 2 and 3). As you select your filters on the left side of the portal, the data will dynamically refresh showing you both graphical and table information on the right side of the screen. Data from here can be added to the site's "cart" which will allow you to download directly through the website.

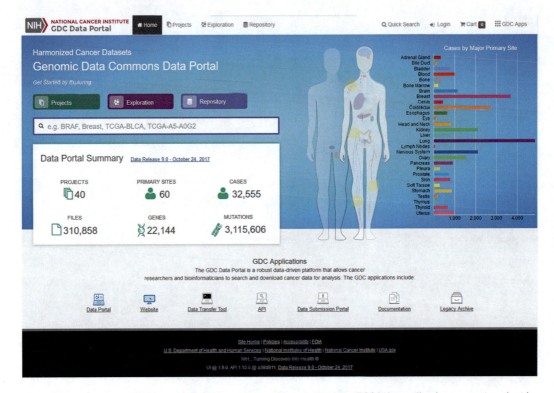

Fig. 2 TCGA data portal. This screenshot shows the entry portal into the TCGA data, allowing a user to select by project or repository, or otherwise explore the data. This entry site also allows for searching directly by gene or TCGA id. In addition, this landing page has the data portal summary statistics prominently displayed

Data from several cancer types are available through TCGA (*see* Table 2), and the number of cases available per type ranges from 36 to 1098 cases.

It should be noted that GDC also provides access, in the same way, to legacy data. Legacy data is the original data referenced against human genome build 19, nonharmonized, and is not actively being maintained beyond being provided for researcher's use. Access to this data can be found at https://portal.gdc.cancer.gov/legacy-archive/search/f or can be found by searching for TCGA Legacy Archive.

TCGA Access

Access to TCGA is split into two "Access Data Tiers." The first tier is the open access data tier. The data in this tier is considered public and is not specific to any individual. There is no registration process required to access this data. You can download this data directly through the Data Portal hosted in GDC (the repository for TCGA data).

To request access to the second tier of data, or protected data, perform the following:

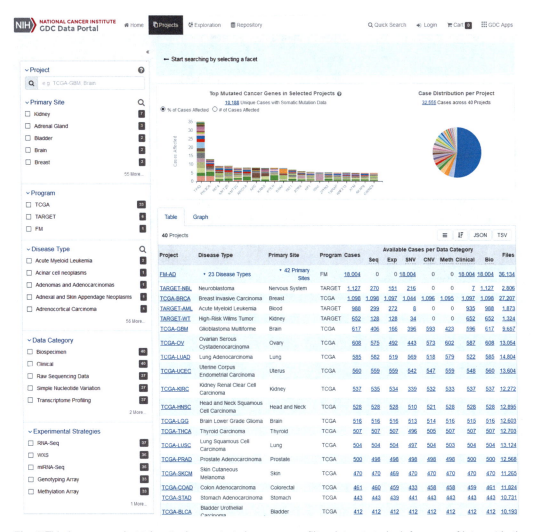

Fig. 3 This is a screenshot taken to demonstrate how you can filter datasets to look for ones of interest in the GDC Data Portal which includes TCGA data. Filters are applied on the left side of the screen and specific data files and visualizations are shown on the right side of the screen

1. Through the Database of Genotypes and Phenotypes (dbGaP), there is an electronic Data Access Request (DAR) form. Navigate to this page https://dbgap.ncbi.nlm.nih.gov/aa/wga.cgi?login=&page=login, and click on the link on the right-hand side of the page that reads "Log In." The instructions are included on that page, but most importantly you will need either an eRA Commons account or an NIH Login account.

2. Each dataset that you apply for can contain specific requirements (such as local approval to use). Any such requirement should be listed on the dbGaP study page. You should make yourself aware of any particular dataset requirements for your

Table 2
Cancer types available in TCGA along with their TCGA abbreviations

TCGA cancer types			
ACC	Adrenocortical carcinoma	LUSC	Lung squamous cell carcinoma
BLCA	Bladder urothelial carcinoma	MESO	Mesothelioma
BRCA	Breast invasive carcinoma	OV	Ovarian serous cystadenocarcinoma
CESC	Cervical squamous cell carcinoma and endocervical adenocarcinoma	RAAD	Pancreatic adenocarcinoma
CHOL	Cholangiocarcinoma	PCPG	Pheochromocytoma and paraganglioma
COAD	Colon adenocarcinoma	PRAD	Prostate adenocarcinoma
DLBC	Lymphoid neoplasm diffuse large B-cell lymphoma	READ	Rectum adenocarcinoma
ESCA	Esophageal carcinoma	SARC	Sarcoma
GBM	Glioblastoma multiforme	SKCM	Skin cutaneous melanoma
HNSC	Head and neck squamous cell carcinoma	STAD	Stomach adenocarcinoma
KICH	Kidney chromophobe renal cell carcinoma	TGCT	Testicular germ cell tumors
KIRC	Kidney renal clear cell carcinoma	THCA	Thyroid carcinoma
KIRP	Kidney renal papillary cell carcinoma	THYM	Thymoma
LAML	Acute myeloid leukemia	UCEC	Uterine corpus endometrial carcinoma
LGG	Brain lower grade glioma	UCS	Uterine carcinosarcoma
LIHC	Liver hepatocellular carcinoma	UVM	Uveal melanoma
LUAD	Lung adenocarcinoma		

data of interest to avoid any penalties or legal repercussions. All access expires and is subject to re-approval at periodic intervals.

3. Once logged into the dbGaP DAR system, you will click on the "My Projects" tab, if it is not already highlighted. Next, click on the "Create New Research Project" button (*see* Fig. 4). You will be brought to a general "instructions page on creating a project" in order to request data. Remember that any approval for data requests applies only to this specific project: you will need to request permission for the data each time you plan on using it for a new project.

4. The instructions page for creating a new project lists several pieces of information you will need before you can create your project: the listed requirements must be collected prior to requesting your data. Once you have collected this information, select the "Begin New Research Project" at the bottom of the page.

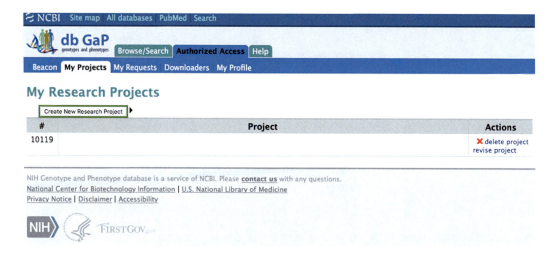

Fig. 4 Where to click to generate a new project in the dbGaP system

5. You will then fill out the form, beginning with your chosen datasets. The dbGaP system contains data from several projects, but here you can filter by project to include only TCGA data.

6. You then complete the project request by entering in the appropriate information over the next few pages of the form. Under the research project tab of the form, you will create a password for the data in the project. All other items on the form should be readily answerable with the information gathered above.

7. Once you have submitted the research project, you will need to complete the TCGA Data Use Certification (DUC): instructions for this step will be provided by dbGaP. You will be issued a National Cancer Institute (NCI) username and password that will be required to download any data through the data portal.

8. After approval has been granted, you will be able to directly log into the Data Portal in GDC to either download restricted access data in the same way you can with publicly accessible or to retrieve a security token that can be used to programmatically access the data (*see* Fig. 5, download section outlined in red).

Once your request for data access has been processed, you can download the data in several different ways. If you are interested in downloading a small set of either publicly accessible data or restricted access data, the visual Data Portal hosted on GDC (*see* Figs. 2 and 3) is the easiest method. You can filter for the data of interest and then add to a cart, allowing you to download all at once. The user-friendly interface has quite a few options available and should be explored thoroughly to see if the data you are

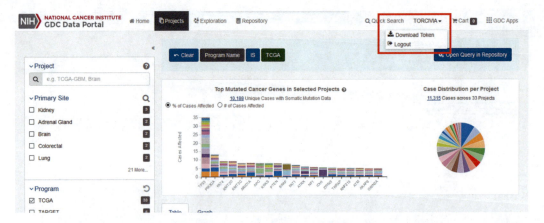

Fig. 5 This screenshot shows where the security token can be downloaded from (highlighted in the red box). The user name will appear when logged in and allow a Download Token option. This token is downloaded in text format and may be copied and pasted into an appropriate command line argument or file as needed

interested in is available. As you find data you would like, you can add it to your "cart" in the same way you would on any modern commercial website. Once you navigate to the cart (in the upper right corner of the website), you will have the option to re-evaluate the data you've selected to remove any you are no longer interested in, download metadata about the data you're interested in, or download the data (or manifest) directly. Downloading directly is easy for smaller sets of data. The manifest can be used for accessing the data through the download tool (*see* below for more information on this).

If you are interested in large quantities of data, it is more robust to access the data through either the GDC API (https://gdc.cancer.gov/developers/gdc-application-programming-interface-api) or through the GDC Data Transfer Tool (https://gdc.cancer.gov/access-data/gdc-data-transfer-tool). The use of the GDC API is beyond the scope of this chapter, but it can be used by computer programmers to allow their programs to communicate directly with GDC. End users of the data will likely opt for the GDC Data Transfer Tool to avoid writing their own access program from scratch.

The GDC Data Transfer Tool is a high-performance downloader that is useful when large amounts of data need to be retrieved from GDC. Downloads of the data tool as well as instructions on how to use can be found at https://gdc.cancer.gov/access-data/gdc-data-transfer-tool. Linux (Ubuntu), Windows, and Mac OS (OSX) are currently supported. The source code is additionally made available on GitHub at https://github.com/NCI-GDC/gdc-client for researchers interested in building the tool for other platforms. If you have downloaded the executable (binary) version of the tool, you should now have an executable called gdc-client

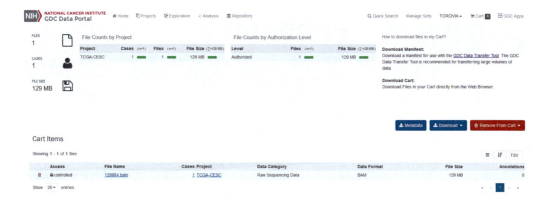

Fig. 6 This is a screenshot of the download page in the GDC Data Portal. In this example a single file is selected, and downloading of the file itself, the metadata, or the manifest for the file(s) is provided on the right side of the screen

(or gdc-client.exe for Windows) available in whichever folder on your computer you extracted the download to.

Basic use of the tool is relatively straightforward. You begin by selecting the data files you are interested in using the interface in the same way as you would with noncontrolled data. However, when you navigate to the cart and select the Download option, you will be given the sub-option of downloading the manifest. The manifest specifies all the data that you have moved into your card and will be downloaded as a text file (*see* Fig. 6). This is what is used to specify to the robust downloading tool which files you are interested in retrieving. You will also need the security token (explained above, *see* Fig. 5) which you can download from the same site to use the GDC data transfer tool.

Given the gdc-client.exe tool, the manifest file, and the security token, you can now use the gdc-client to download the files of interest. In the example in Fig. 6, a single file has been selected. Multiple files could be selected and will work accordingly.

To access the gdc-client.exe built in help for downloading files, execute the following in Windows:

```
gdc-client.exe download --help
```

Or the following in Linux/Mac OS:

```
gdc-client download --help
```

Both will give a list of the various different parameters that can be specified for downloads. The specifics of each of these are outside of the scope of this chapter, but basic use is as follows (with gdc-client replacing gdc-client.exe if you are using Linux/Mac OS instead of Windows).

```
gdc-client download --token-file <security_token_file> --man-
ifest <manifest_file>
```

The --token-file flag specifies the security token, and the name of the security token file downloaded should follow this flag. The --manifest flag specifies the manifest file which was downloaded from the interface instead of the data directly. The file name should be specified here after the flag. Relative or absolute paths can be used for both the token and the manifest files. This command should be executed from where the gdc-client executable program is at on your computer, or otherwise an advanced user can set up universal access to it via an internal PATH variable. Once this command is executed, a directory for each entry will be created and named with the file's UUID. When downloading multiple files, it is helpful to keep a spreadsheet mapping each of the UUIDs to each file in human readable terms.

TARGET

TARGET [10], or Therapeutically Applicable Research To Generate Effective Treatments, aims to be a comprehensive resource focused on the molecular changes that cause childhood cancers. *See* Fig. 1 for data types that are available through TARGET.

Specific data that is available can be found on the TARGET Data Matrix at https://target.nci.nih.gov/dataMatrix/. This Data Matrix operates as TARGET's web portal for publically accessible data. A sample is included for acute lymphoblastic leukemia in Fig. 7. *See* Subheading 2.1.1.3 for how to download data.

TARGET Access

To access TARGET you should complete the same steps above as for TCGA, except that in **step 7** you will agree to TARGET's DUC and **step 8** will not apply. If approved, you will be granted access to TARGET's data for 1 year. In order to renew access at the end of

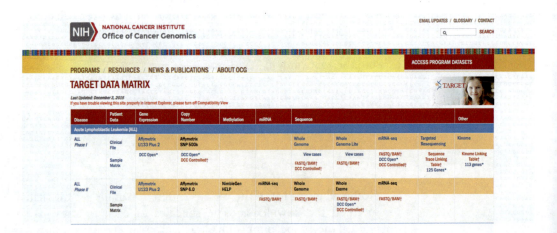

Fig. 7 TARGET data matrix which includes the types of cancers in the repository as well as the specific data available for each

that period, you will be required to send a progress report to the NCI Data Access Committee (the committee that approved the electronic form submitted through dbGaP). You will receive a reminder about this condition approximately 1 month prior to your access expiration date.

To download the data, simply go to the TARGET Data Matrix (*see* Fig. 7) at https://target.nci.nih.gov/dataMatrix/ and click on the data in which you are interested. You will be redirected to a new page where you can directly download your data by clicking on the link. Here you will also be able to find dataset IDs for controlled data which you can then use to search and retrieve in dbGaP under the appropriate study/consent group field. Some controlled datasets will directly prompt you for the NCI username and password generated by the dbGaP system (as described for TCGA data above), and others will take you to the Sequence Read Archive (SRA) for access to the data. *See* the section below on accessing data through SRA in this case.

CCLE

The Cancer Cell Line Encyclopedia (CCLE) [11, 12] project conducts both genetic and pharmacologic characterizations of human cancer models. Details about this collaborative project between the Broad Institute and Novartis Institutes for biomedical research can be found at http://www.broadinstitute.org/ccle/home. The legacy CCLE portal can be accessed at https://portals.broadinstitute.org/ccle_legacy/home.

As of November 2017, data generated by the collaboration covers 1457 cell lines and includes genomic, analysis, and visualization data. This covers 84,434 genes, 136,488 unique datasets, 1,159,663 mutation entries, 118,661,636 distribution scores, and 411,948,577 methylation scores as reported by the resource as of this printing. *See* Fig. 1 for data types provided by this resource.

CCLE Access

CCLE data does not require any special access permissions. You will need to create a free account requiring your email and a password for tracking purposes related to funding.

You can access the data directly through the CCLE website, and since no specific access restrictions are in place, you can download this directly. CCLE provides a file name, data, description, and download button for each set of data provided. Figure 8 provides an example of how to download this data.

Previously the data in CCLE was fetched via a tool called cgquery through CGHub. CGHub, however, has been integrated into the GDC, and so primary data otherwise available in CCLE (such as sequence and alignment data) are now available through GDC. Access to files in GDC can be found in the TCGA section above (TCGA data is also housed in GDC). This has streamlined the process of accessing data in a more central NIH location, at least for some of these large-scale studies.

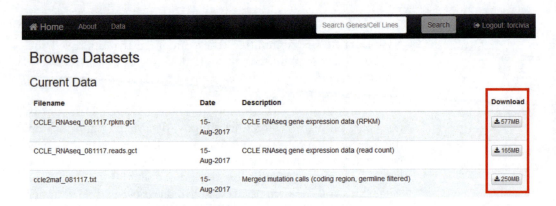

Fig. 8 Example links for downloading of the datasets from the CCLE website

ICGC

The International Cancer Genome Consortium, or ICGC [13], is a consortium that is interested in looking at 50 different tumor types or subtypes and comprehensively describing their genomic, transcriptomic, and epigenetic changes. As of November 2017, the site contained data related to: 76 cancer projects; 21 cancer primary sites; 17,570 donors with molecular data; 20,343 total donors; 63,480,214 simple somatic mutations; and 57,753 mutated genes.

Data is downloaded by project, and the type of data that is available will vary depending on the specific project. *See* Fig. 1 for data available. The data portal is explored in the following section.

ICGC Access

The data that ICGC aggregates is a mixture of publicly accessible data and protected data. Full ICGC data releases can be downloaded through the web browser starting at the URL https://dcc.icgc.org/releases (*see* Fig. 9). From here, you can navigate to your project of interest and directly download data of interest from that project through the website. Data available here are not the raw data but only include the processed and analyzed data resulting from ICGC's work.

The full ICGC repository list can be accessed at https://dcc.icgc.org/repositories. This page provides a tool that allows you to filter by various criteria and find information about your data of interest (*see* Fig. 10). You may select as many datasets as desired and can then click on the "Download manifests" button that appears at the top of the tool. This will generate an XML manifest file that can be used to directly download the actual data with an appropriate tool. Data has also been posted on several cloud services (https://dcc.icgc.org/icgc-in-the-cloud) although access through this method is beyond the scope of this chapter.

There are currently (as of this printing) 11 data repositories available in the DCC portal of ICGC. In general, raw sequencing reads and analyzed germ-line data are protected in any database, including ICGC. There are two methods of control over restricted

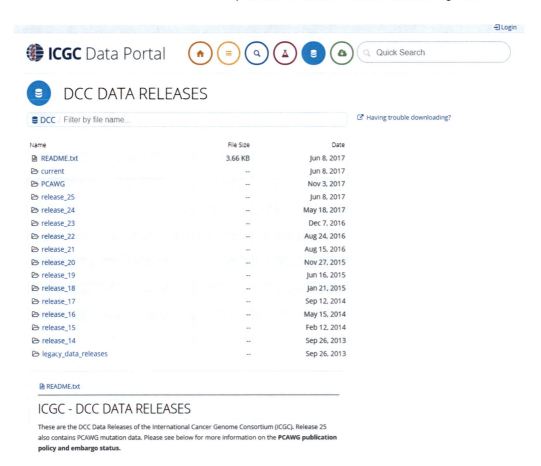

Fig. 9 List of the ICGC data releases in the ICGC Data Portal. These can be directly downloaded through the web browser

data that ICGC uses. For US-based projects, eRA Commons and dbGaP are used (similar to how they are used for TCGA access). For non-US project, the ICGC Data Access Compliance Office (DACO) is used. The form can be completed at https://icgc.org/daco where you can register, create an account, and then fill out the application. There are step-by-step videos provided by ICGC at https://icgc.org/daco/help-guide-section for creating your account, filling out your application, and submitting it to the DACO. The DACO will then generate and grant you user credentials to enable download of the controlled data (once you are approved).

Due to the nature of there being multiple data repositories, downloading the data is more difficult than would be expected. Even though all of the data is under the ICGC umbrella, each repository has its own data access guidelines (explained above) and method of actually accessing the data. The specific method of access to each repository can be found on this page http://docs.

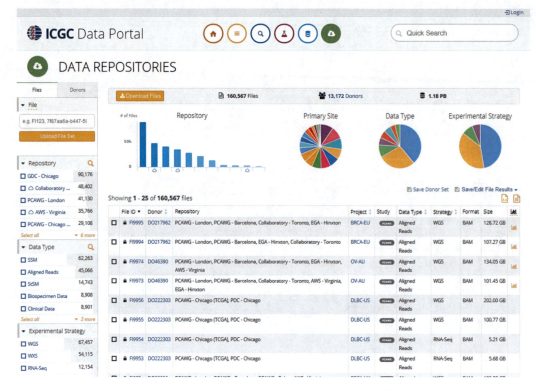

Fig. 10 ICCG Data Portal data repository page. In this page you can filter by criteria listed on the left side of the screen and files and graphical representations of the results appear on the right side

icgc.org/cloud/repositories/. However, ICGC has released a tool called icgc-get which is intended to alleviate the need to use different software across different repositories. While it is possible that for any given data, you would need to access the repository with its own tool directly, icgc-get should generally work to get data from the ICGC-related repositories. Only icgc-get will be explained below, but users should explore other access tools from the above link further if they run into difficulty with retrieving data of interest.

The user guide for icgc-get can be found at http://docs.icgc.org/cloud/icgc-get/. Accessing data in cloud repositories (such as AWS) requires icgc-get to be run directly from their servers (in your cloud instance). Otherwise icgc-get can be run locally on your computer in the same way as gdc-client (as explained above). The user guide outlines the steps needed to use the software as:

1. Download and install the client.
2. Run the icgc-get configure command to setup your environment.
3. Run the icgc-get check command to ensure your credentials are correct.

4. Generate a manifest ID via the Repository Browser.
5. Run the icgc-get report command to inspect your request before downloading.
6. Run icgc-get download –m <manifest-id> to download files in your manifest.

The software itself is supported on Mac OS and Linux and can be downloaded and unpackaged via the command line commands (**step 1**):

```
curl https://dcc.icgc.org/api/v1/ui/software/icgc-get/linux/latest -o icgc-get.latest.zip -Lunzip icgc-get.latest.zip
```

While the program is only available for Mac OS and Linux, if you are running Windows 10 you can run this program in the "Bash on Ubuntu on Windows" option available (Ubuntu is a specific version of the Linux operating system). This will require installing the Windows Subsystem for Linux (directions given at https://msdn.microsoft.com/en-us/commandline/wsl/install-win10) and will enable you to run in a virtual Linux environment on Windows. In addition to this method, a full Virtual Machine can be set up or Docker could be used. These tools can both be used to create a virtual Linux environment which would allow a user to run these tools there. The above commands can be executed in any of these environments.

Step 2 is the configuration of the icgc-get program. This will simply ask you several questions to get the program setup. Remember that this program is trying to be a meta-program to allow you to download data from multiple different repositories that are within the IGCG "family." When you run this program in configuration mode (by executing the command `./icgc-get configuration`), you will be prompted for an output directory and a log location—both of which you can answer wherever you would like. The third prompt is for which repositories you would like to be able to download from. This will depend in large part on which data you are interested in. Each repository should be entered with a space between each in the event you want to be able to download from multiple repositories. The next prompt will ask if you would like to use a docker container to encase your icgc-get actions. If you can set up Docker on your computer, you should enter true since this will give you an isolated environment where icgc-get can run that should be more consistent. In general, you should be able to install Docker on an Ubuntu (Linux)-based machine by entering in the terminal the following commands:

```
sudo apt-get update
sudo apt install docker.io
```

There are many factors outside of the scope of the chapter on why this may succeed or fail. Additional instructions can be found on Dockers website at www.docker.com. If you are unable to install Docker, enter false. Finally, you will be asked for keys/access credentials for each of the repositories you have selected. These are gathered as mentioned above (this could be a labor-intensive step).

For **step 3**, you will be able to check to see if your configuration was successful. At this point, if any errors are returned, you will need to rerun the configuration command and fix them as needed.

Step 4 is getting the manifest file. At this point the icgc-get software is set up and ready to run. The manifest file is retrieved as above—after you've selected the files you are interested in within the web page, you should click on the download files button (*see* Fig. 9 to see where the Download button is at). Once you've clicked on there, you will be given a floating window with further instructions (*see* Fig. 11).

In the floating window, you can either generate the icgc-get manifest ID or download the manifest (in Fig. 11 the icgc-get manifest ID button has already been pushed). If you generate the icgc-get manifest ID, the floating window is helpful and gives you the command to download the specific dataset you have selected. In the case of the example in Fig. 11, the command is:

```
./icgc-get download -m b0100005-f125-4472-81ec-fcb40d139f91
```

Before immediately executing your download command, you can first perform **step 5** and run a sanity check on the data you would like to download. This is done simply by running:

```
./icgc-get report -m <icgc-get manifest ID>
```

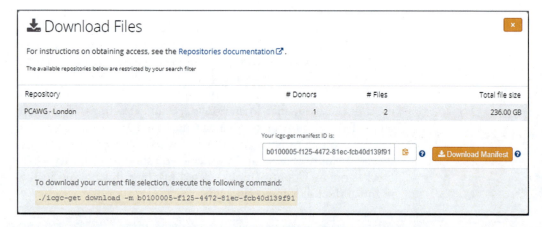

Fig. 11 The download files overlay box when trying to retrieve files through ICGC. This box will allow you to get the icgc-get manifest ID or the manifest itself in order to download the selected file(s)

Finally, you can perform **step 6** and download the data by executing the provided command in the floating window. This is the same as the above command, but with the command report replaced by the command download.

For access to data that resides on ICGC's partner clouds such as Amazon AWS or Collaboratory (OpenStack), refer to http://docs.icgc.org/cloud/guide/ for specific instructions. Accessing data in this way requires some knowledge of creating compute instances on the cloud and is outside of the scope of this chapter.

SRA

One of the most ubiquitous resources for HTS reads is NCBI's Short Read Archive (SRA). SRA contains short reads spanning many different diseases and species, but there are also large contingents of cancer-related samples that have been deposited into the repository.

See Fig. 1 for the types of data included in SRA. The web portal search is explored in depth in Subheading 2.1.1.9 below.

SRA Access

Upon navigating to SRA at http://www.ncbi.nlm.nih.gov/sra, the top of the page holds a search bar for simple keyword or accession search. A search conducted by entering a valid search term here will return a list of results, each with an SRA identifier. You can access SRA experiments, samples, or single runs and retrieve all associated data through provision of the appropriate identifiers through the SRA toolkit, which can be downloaded at the URL http://www.ncbi.nlm.nih.gov/Traces/sra/?view=software. The toolkit is available for a number of different systems including Mac OS X, Windows, and different flavors of Linux.

After installing the software, public access data can be downloaded from the terminal or command line. Most often this means retrieving FASTQ format which is easily done by entering the following command:

```
fastq-dump -split-files <SRA ID Number>
```

where <SRA ID Number> is an SRA accession number such as SRR390728. Additional applications have been bundled into the SRA toolkit, and more information on advanced uses can be found at http://www.ncbi.nlm.nih.gov/books/NBK242621/.

In order to download controlled data, you need to request access through the dbGaP system in the same way as described for TCGA above. You will be given a dbGaP repository key (".ngc" file) which is used to access the restricted data.

Using the SRA Toolkit, you will run the command `vdb-config --i` in the directory in which you installed the toolkit. This will bring you to a graphical screen where you can configure the toolkit. For this particular step, we are interested in option #4, Import

Repository Key. Press the number 4 on the keyboard and navigate to the location of the downloaded ".ngc" file retrieved from the dbGaP access request. You will also be able to change your workspace in this utility.

Now, whenever you download protected data directly into your workspace (or move it from somewhere else on your computer into your workspace), it will be de-encrypted and can be used directly at the specified location.

2.1.2 Processed Genomic Data

COSMIC

COSMIC [14, 15], or the Catalogue of Somatic Mutations in Cancer, is a data repository that contains somatic mutation information related to human cancers. The database contains data resulting from both expert curation and genome-wide screening analysis. COSMIC curators manually mine mutations (curation) from primary literature, while automated data is retained either from publications reporting large-scale genomic studies or imported from other services and databases like TCGA.

See Fig. 1 for the data types that are available in COSMIC. The web page operates as a portal allowing you to simply search for data of interest. There are additional ways to search the data, allowing you to filter based on tissue type or other criteria. Figure 12 shows the landing page, and different methods of querying the data can be

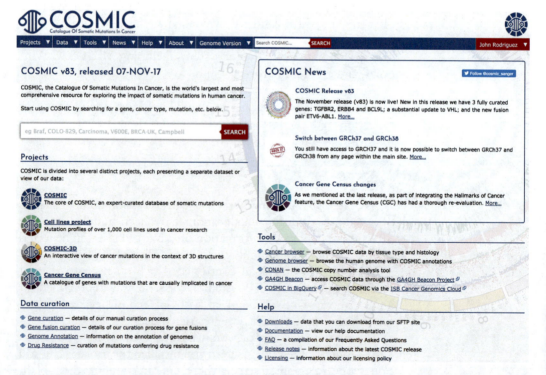

Fig. 12 COSMIC web portal and search. Under the Tools section are where the links are to further be able to filter your searches instead of using the generalized search box at the top of the page

found through the drop-down menu in the Tools, Data, and Projects sections specifically. The browser web applications provided through the Tools menu offer an easy to use and understand interface to both the cancer and the genome explorer views. These views allow you to drill down based on tissue type and see which genes are mutated.

Figure 13 shows an example use of the Cancer Browser, specifically looking at lung cancer. The selected output shows the top 20 mutated genes, an excerpt from the USCS genome browser with additional annotation information for the top gene, and a variants section which shows genes that have mutations in the tissue of interest—lung in this example.

Other tools provided such as the Genome Browser and CONAN (copy number analysis) are used in a similar manor for different results.

Coding and noncoding mutations can be downloaded as VCF files or as tab-separated files from the Data drop-down menu. The remainder of the data is available in tab-separated or comma-separated files. Files can either be downloaded directly through the website by clicking the appropriate download button near the file of interest's description or through the SFPT server provided.

COSMIC Access

No special credentials are required to use this repository: licensing for the data only permits noncommercial research. You will, however, need to create a free account on the website by providing your email address. You can access the account creation page by clicking on the log in button in the upper right corner and then clicking on the register button on the next page. As mentioned above, you can download the files in one of two ways—either directly on the website through HTTP or through the SFTP server. Direct download is available through some of the datasets available on the download page at http://cancer.sanger.ac.uk/cosmic/download (such as COSMIC Complete Mutation Data [Targeted Screens]). However, in these cases you will need to select a subset of the data, such as by gene, before downloading it through the web browser (HTTP). In order to access all of the data, you will need to access the SFTP web server. Files are kept on an SFTP server that requires an FTP client such as WinSCP or CyberDuck. Alternatively, you can directly download the files with a command line FTP program, although using one of the above graphic programs will be easier for most users. CyberDuck is available for both Windows and Mac at https://cyberduck.io, and there is a quick reference guide available at https://trac.cyberduck.io/wiki/help/en. (Note: download via the Mac App Store did have an associated charge at the time of writing.) There is also a command line version available at http://duck.sh for advanced users.

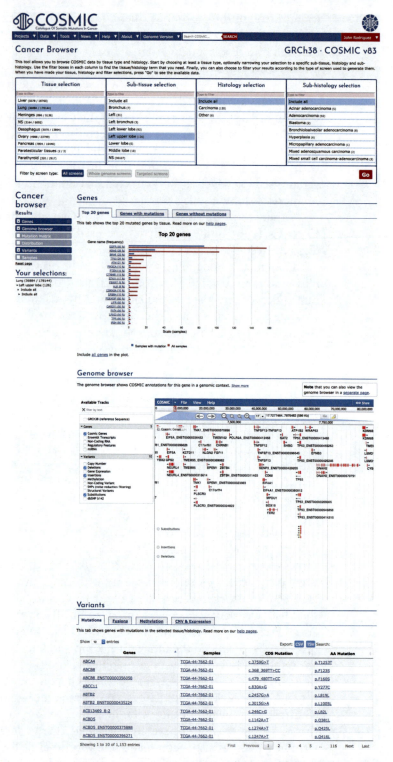

Fig. 13 COSMIC Cancer Browser tool. This is an example of using the COSMIC cancer browser tool to examine data related to lung cancer in the COSMIC repository and online tool set

BioMuta	BioMuta [16, 17] is a curated single nucleotide variation (SNV) database containing information mined from the literature along with various other cancer mutation databases. All cancer terms in the database are mapped to Disease Ontology terms [18]. Version 3.0 of BioMuta [19] contains 18,269 UniProtKB/Swiss-Prot Accessions hit, 77 Disease Ontology terms mapped, 4,684,236 non-synonymous single nucleotide variations (nsSNVs) reported in cancer, 2,304,757 predicted damaging mutations, and 980,447 mutations affecting posttranslational modification sites. BioMuta data are also now mapped to Uberon atomical structure data [20]. *See* Fig. 1 for the types of data that are available in BioMuta. In Fig. 14, the web interface is shown. Further detail on searching BioMuta is provided in Subheading 2.1.2.4 below.
BioMuta Access	To access BioMuta data, no special credentials are required. Navigate to http://hive.biochemistry.gwu.edu/biomuta on your web browser. The default search is a gene-centric search where a gene name serves as a query to retrieve relevant nsSNVs in cancer. Downloads are available in tabular format for all search results, or full version downloads are available from the Archive/Downloads page, accessible from the top right menu. In addition, BioMuta can be accessed through a robust API, which can be found documented at https://hive.biochemistry.gwu.edu/biomuta/apidoc.
BioXpress	BioXpress [19, 21] is a database of human gene and miRNA expression in cancer samples. This database includes data from TCGA, ICGC data, and manual and semiautomated literature mining evidence. This resource provides information on the fold change of expression between matched normal and adjacent tumor

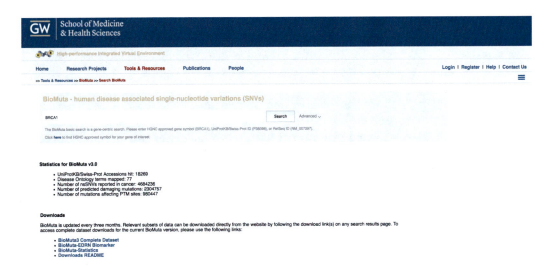

Fig. 14 BioMuta access page. This is where the database can be searched via Gene Name, UniProt Accession, or RefSeq Accession number

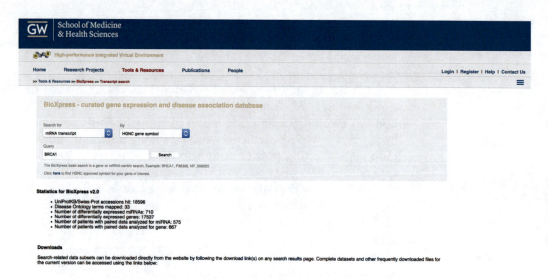

Fig. 15 BioXpress access page. This is where the database can be searched via HGNC Gene Symbol, UniProt Accession, or RefSeq Accession number

tissue as well as the significance and direction of such changes and also enables pan-sample analysis. Information available includes 18,596 UniProtKB/Swiss-Prot accessions hit, 33 Disease Ontology (DO) terms mapped, 710 differentially expressed miRNAs, 17,537 differentially expressed genes, 575 patients with paired data analyzed for miRNA, and 667 patients with paired data analyzed for genes. In addition, the data are now mapped to Uberon anatomical structures.

The types of data available in BioXpress are included in Fig. 1. *See* Fig. 15 for the web interface to BioXpress (which is explained further in Subheading 2.1.2.6).

BioXpress Access

As with BioMuta, BioXpress is a publicly available tool hosted at http://hive.biochemistry.gwu.edu/bioxpress and therefore requires no special access credentials. The home page of BioXpress allows for the querying of individual genes for discovery of significant differential expression in cancer. The database can also be searched by cancer type to return all genes known to be expressed at different levels (as interpreted from TCGA read counts and curated literature) for a cancer of interest. Search results may be downloaded for further analysis by clicking the Download table in CSV format link above the results page table. Current and previous versions of the full BioXpress dataset can be downloaded from the Archive/Downloads page in the top right menu. Like BioMuta above, BioXpress can also be accessed through API which is documented at https://hive.biochemistry.gwu.edu/bioxpress/apidoc.

ClinVar	ClinVar [22, 23] is a SNV database that links variation and phenotypes in humans. While the database allows a broader scope of exploration than phenotypes exclusively related to disease, SNV relationships with cancers and cancer-related phenotypes are included in this dataset.
ClinVar Access	There are no special requirements needed to access ClinVar data. The database is updated every Monday on the web but monthly in the full extractions. The ClinVar files are available to download directly from a web browser and include the following:

1. Complete public dataset in XML format: ftp://ftp.ncbi.nlm.nih.gov/pub/clinvar/xml/
2. Short variants in ClinVar and dbSNP in VCF format: ftp://ftp.ncbi.nlm.nih.gov/pub/clinvar/vcf_GRCh37/
   ftp://ftp.ncbi.nlm.nih.gov/pub/clinvar/vcf_GRCh38/
3. Summary data about variants or genes in TSV format: ftp://ftp.ncbi.nlm.nih.gov/pub/clinvar/tab_delimited/
4. Disease names and gene-disease relationships in TSV format: ftp://ftp.ncbi.nlm.nih.gov/pub/clinvar/

These files can also be downloaded via any FTP client or accessed by advanced users through NCBI's E-utilities API programmatically.

LNCipedia	LNCipedia [13, 24] is a data repository containing human annotated long noncoding RNAs (lncRNAs) out of Ghent University. This source is an integrated database that pulls information from many sources including Noncode, Human Body Map lincRNAs, and others. Searching on the site yields important information on particular lncRNAs including whether a particular lncRNA has been associated with cancer in the literature and its secondary structure. The web interface is shown in Fig. 16. Searches can include any combination of name, source, chromosomal location, keyword, or sequence information.
LNCipedia Access	Data in the LNCipedia database is available for public noncommercial use at the website http://lncipedia.org/download. The full database or the subset of high confidence data can be downloaded through the web browser in a variety of formats. In addition to direct downloading of data, LNCipedia provides a REST API interface for software developers. This allows developers to include in their web- and Internet-connected applications the ability to query the LNCipedia database for data in a known structure through HTTPS requests. While the use of this is beyond the scope of this chapter, the instructions on basic usage can be found at https://lncipedia.org/api.

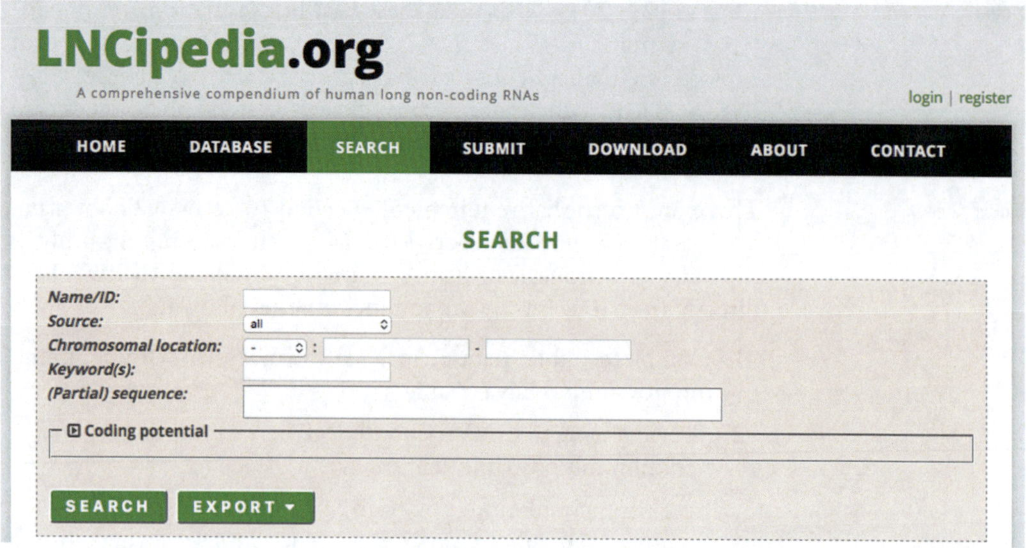

Fig. 16 LNCipedia search portal. Any combination of the input boxes can be used to search for specific information

IntOGen

Integrative Onco Genomics (IntOGen) [25, 26] is a resource developed by the BG Group out of the University Pompeu Fabra. The database created by this group contains information about genes that have been identified as driver mutations [25]. Additionally, they have a second database which characterizes interacting therapeutic agents in the context of clinical phase, cancer prescription, and other features.

When you first navigate to the site, you are able to enter any search terms of interest within the search box presented. There are a number of example searches provided to familiarize you with the search methodology employed by the site. IntOGen uses a straightforward, natural language approach, so you will likely be successful by searching for your exact topics of interest without having to compose any complex search queries.

The types of data available in IntOGen are shown in Fig. 1.

IntOGen Access

The data can be accessed directly at the URL https://www.intogen.org/downloads. An account can be created with an email address by clicking any of the "Sign in to download" buttons that are present on the screen. After prompting for an email address and password, you are then able to download either of the databases or previous releases.

EGA

EGA [27], the European Genome-phenome Archive, provides access to data from a large number of genetic studies and acts as a clearinghouse for data from many different sources such as the Wellcome Trust Case Control Consortium (https://www.wtccc.

org.uk) and the Nordic Centre of Excellence Programme in Molecular Medicine Data Access Committee (http://www.ncoedg.org). Data included varies by study and the different data types available can be found in Fig. 1.

EGA Access

EGA can be found at https://ega-archive.org. Accessing EGA [25–27] datasets requires first identifying your datasets of interest. This can be done either browsing the datasets by clicking on the "Datasets" tab on any page or by searching the site in the upper right corner of the home page. You will be given results that match your search criteria. You can select either a study or a dataset and you will see the Dataset Accession number(s) associated with your selection. On the right-hand side, there will be contact information for the DAC that controls the dataset. Simply email this address and request access to the data. They will provide you with the particular details for requesting data from that specific DAC. Once this process is completed, you will receive a onetime email request to create an EGA account (for your first time requesting access to a dataset).

In order to actually download the data, EGA provides a download client called EgaDemoClient. The most recent version of the client as of this writing is available at https://www.ebi.ac.uk/ega/sites/ebi.ac.uk.ega/files/documents/EGA_download_streamer_1.1.5.zip. The client is Java-based and requires Java 7 or higher in order to execute.

Once you have downloaded and extracted the client, the program can be run by executing the following command in either the terminal or command line:

```
java -jar EgaDemoClient.jar
```

This must be executed in the same directory to which you extracted the jar file during the download. You will then be presented with a secure data shell allowing you to log in to the system by using the following command:

```
EGA> login my@email.com mypassword
```

Replace my@email.com with your email and mypassword with your password for EGA. Once you have received the message "Login Success!," it means you have successfully logged in to the system and can proceed to download data.

The command to download data is made up of four parts: first is the type of request, in this case, "dataset"; the second part is the dataset ID; the third part is the encryption key for received data; the final part is the label that you designate for future download of the data. An example command using an encryption key called mykey.key would look like this:

```
EGA> request dataset EGAD00010000650 mykey.key request_E-
GAD00010000650
```

This command sets up a request for a dataset. To download the dataset, use the download command.

```
EGA> download request_EGAD00010000650
```

This will download the dataset that was set up in the request. Once the dataset is downloaded, you will need to decrypt it. This can be done with the following command using the name of the file downloaded and the encryption key:

```
EGA> decrypt <filename> <encryption key>
```

At this point the file is ready for use.

UniProt

UniProt [28] data contains a wealth of protein-centric information which is extremely helpful in cancer research, even though the database itself is not cancer-specific. Cancer-related information, such as mutations linked to cancer, can be found in the Feature Table (FT) for a given accession, with additional descriptive information available in the comment sections. Protein-related information, such as domain, protein family, and structural data, are also contained in the entries and can be valuable to cancer research. Additional information about the entire entry format is found throughout the manual at http://www.uniprot.org/help/?fil=section:manual.

The web interface is described under the Subheading 2.1.2.16. The interface provides simple and advanced search capabilities and also intuitive filtering of search results in order to dig down to the information of interest.

UniProt Access

UniProt data is freely accessible from the http://www.uniprot.org/ website. There are several different databases available including:

1. UniProtKB/SwissProt—manually annotated and reviewed protein sequence database
2. UniProtKB/TrEMBL—computationally annotated protein sequence database
3. UniRef—reference sets of protein clusters which hide redundant sequences and are often used as reference datasets
4. UniParc—nonredundant archive dataset that contains almost all known protein sequences without any changes or modifications once a sequence is integrated

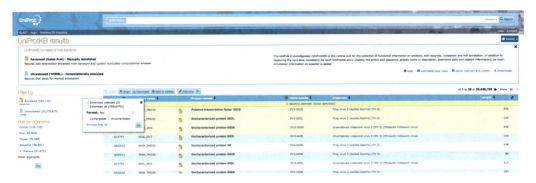

Fig. 17 UniProtKB data explorer. This is the interface where data can be filtered via option on the left side of the page, and data of interest can be placed in the "basket" for bulk access later

When you click on either UniProtKB/SwissProt or UniProtKB/TrEMBL, you are presented with a search view for sequences of interest. You can search using the tools and select whichever sequences you would like to download by checkmarking them and adding them to the basket (*see* Fig. 17). Additionally, when you select download, you are presented with different options. In order to access the FT (Feature Table) lines for the selected proteins, choose "Text" from the drop-down box of options. This will give you information similar to that in Fig. 18.

You can then process this information depending on the needs of your particular pipeline.

cBioPortal

cBioPortal [29, 30] is a website that is designed to aid in visualizing, analyzing, and downloading cancer genomics datasets primarily from TCGA and independently published datasets. The portal currently contains over 167 cancer genomics studies that are listed at http://www.cbioportal.org/data_sets.jsp. Each dataset may contain different types of information dependent on the goals of individual studies. For example, comparison of two datasets regarding liver hepatocellular carcinoma ((RIKEN, Nat Genet 2012) and (TCGA, Provisional)) demonstrates that the first dataset offers solely mutation information but the second provides mutation, copy number, and expression.

The portal itself is focused around visualizing data in the studies or performing further analytics. Instructions for accessing the data can be found in Subheading 2.1.2.18 below. Example visualizations for the acute myeloid leukemia dataset can be found in Fig. 19. For each dataset, both clinical data and mutated genes can be retrieved. Specific details on how to run analytics or create visualizations are outside of the scope of this chapter but can be found at http://www.cbioportal.org/tutorial.jsp.

Available data varies depending on the study, but possible types of data are shown in Fig. 1.

```
ID   001R_FRG3G              Reviewed;        256 AA.
AC   Q6GZX4;
DT   28-JUN-2011, integrated into UniProtKB/Swiss-Prot.
DT   19-JUL-2004, sequence version 1.
DT   01-APR-2015, entry version 30.
DE   RecName: Full=Putative transcription factor 001R;
GN   ORFNames=FV3-001R;
OS   Frog virus 3 (isolate Goorha) (FV-3).
OC   Viruses; dsDNA viruses, no RNA stage; Iridoviridae; Ranavirus.
OX   NCBI_TaxID=654924;
OH   NCBI_TaxID=8295; Ambystoma (mole salamanders).
OH   NCBI_TaxID=30343; Hyla versicolor (chameleon treefrog).
OH   NCBI_TaxID=8404; Lithobates pipiens (Northern leopard frog) (Rana pipiens).
OH   NCBI_TaxID=8316; Notophthalmus viridescens (Eastern newt) (Triturus viridescens).
OH   NCBI_TaxID=45338; Rana sylvatica (Wood frog).
RN   [1]
RP   NUCLEOTIDE SEQUENCE [LARGE SCALE GENOMIC DNA].
RX   PubMed=15165820; DOI=10.1016/j.virol.2004.02.019;
RA   Tan W.G., Barkman T.J., Gregory Chinchar V., Essani K.;
RT   "Comparative genomic analyses of frog virus 3, type species of the
RT   genus Ranavirus (family Iridoviridae).";
RL   Virology 323:70-84(2004).
CC   -!- FUNCTION: Transcription activation. {ECO:0000305}.
CC   ---------------------------------------------------------------------------
CC   Copyrighted by the UniProt Consortium, see http://www.uniprot.org/terms
CC   Distributed under the Creative Commons Attribution-NoDerivs License
CC   ---------------------------------------------------------------------------
DR   EMBL; AY548484; AAT09660.1; -; Genomic_DNA.
DR   RefSeq; YP_031579.1; NC_005946.1.
DR   ProteinModelPortal; Q6GZX4; -.
DR   GeneID; 2947773; -.
DR   KEGG; vg:2947773; -.
DR   Proteomes; UP000008770; Genome.
DR   GO; GO:0006355; P:regulation of transcription, DNA-templated; IEA:UniProtKB-KW.
DR   GO; GO:0046782; P:regulation of viral transcription; IEA:InterPro.
DR   GO; GO:0006351; P:transcription, DNA-templated; IEA:UniProtKB-KW.
DR   InterPro; IPR007031; Poxvirus_VLTF3.
DR   Pfam; PF04947; Pox_VLTF3; 1.
PE   4: Predicted;
KW   Activator; Complete proteome; Reference proteome; Transcription;
KW   Transcription regulation.
FT   CHAIN         1    256       Putative transcription factor 001R.
FT                                /FTId=PRO_0000410512.
FT   COMPBIAS     14     17       Poly-Arg.
SQ   SEQUENCE   256 AA;  29735 MW;  B4840739BF7D4121 CRC64;
     MAFSAEDVLK EYDRRRRMEA LLLSLYYPND RKLLDYKEWS PPRVQVECPK APVEWNNPPS
     EKGLIVGHFS GIKYKGEKAQ ASEVDVNKMC CWVSKFKDAM RRYQGIQTCK IPGKVLSDLD
     AKIKAYNLTV EGVEGFVRYS RVTKQHVAAF LKELRHSKQY ENVNLIHYIL TDKRVDIQHL
     EKDLVKDFKA LVESAHRMRQ GHMINVKYIL YQLLKKHGHG PDGPDILTVK TGSKGVLYDD
     SFRKIYTDLG WKFTPL
//
ID   002L_FRG3G              Reviewed;        320 AA.
AC   Q6GZX3;
DT   28-JUN-2011, integrated into UniProtKB/Swiss-Prot.
DT   19-JUL-2004, sequence version 1.
```

Fig. 18 Example data in UniProtKB. The FT lines are the functional annotations that are of interest

cBioPortal Access

From the main page, a tab is accessible that allows you to download post-processed data from these studies. First you select your cancer study, and, based on the cancer study selected, you can then select your genomic profile of interest. Only genomic profiles that exist for the cancer study selected will be included in the list.

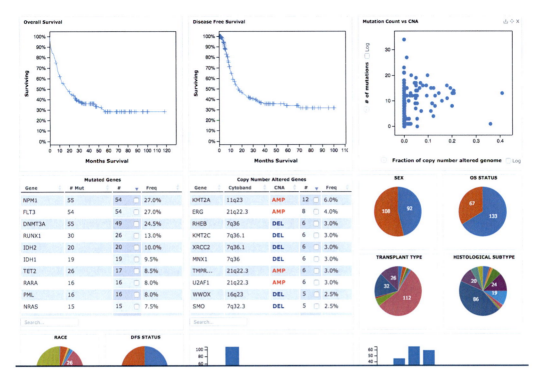

Fig. 19 Example visualizations for acute myeloid leukemia as found in cBioPortal

After selecting the genomic profile, you can limit the included data by the patient or case set. Applicable sets are listed in a drop-down menu. Finally, you can specify the gene set in which you are interested. Gene sets can be specified by typing into the text box with spaces between gene names or by selecting common groupings from the drop-down menu.

Finally, click on the submit button and your data will be displayed in the browser in a tab-separated format. You can then click on the File -> Save Page As menu (or something similar in any modern browser) to save the data as a ".tsv" formatted file. (Note: change from the save format from the default .html if you want to use the information as anything other than a web page.)

2.2 Cancer Terms

Because cancer is a complex disease that often defies easy classification, researchers have developed several approaches in standardizing cancer terms and definitions. The use of terms that are agreed upon within the research community greatly enhances the ability of scientists to communicate with each other and the general public about the significance of their research.

2.2.1 NCIt

The NCI Thesaurus (NCIt) [31] is a set of reference terminology used widely by scientists to label their work in a way that makes it easy to communicate with others.

The database itself provides information on more than 10,000 cancers subtypes. There is also a set of over 17,000 agents and related substances as well as therapies and other relevant information. Editors update the database monthly [32].

2.2.2 NCIt Access

The NCI Thesaurus can be accessed in several different ways. The first method is to directly download the entire dataset from the website https://ncit.nci.nih.gov/ncitbrowser/ at the download link (as of this publication, the direct download link is http://evs.nci.nih.gov/ftp1/NCI_Thesaurus). This method is preferred if you are planning to do any type of large-scale analysis of the terms in the dataset.

If, on the other hand, you are looking for a single term or a small group of terms, you can search directly from the website. In the upper left corner of the page is a search box in which you can enter your search term and find matches or relationships with terms in the database. In this way, you can verify you are using the same nomenclature as the broader research community.

2.2.3 OMIM

Online Mendelian Inheritance in Man, or OMIM [33], is a database that is updated daily and maintained by the McKusick-Nathans Institute of Genetic Medicine at the Johns Hopkins University School of Medicine. This resource contains a comprehensive list of human genes and disease phenotypes. These diseases include many human cancers, providing information relating to their first citation in the literature and important features such as inheritance type.

2.2.4 OMIM Access

The database can be accessed via NCBI or directly through the site's web page at http://omim.org. A direct search for terms of interest can be performed on the website via the search box. Alternatively, for larger-scale use of data, there is a drop-down downloads link at the top of the site (on the navigation ribbon) that allows you to register to download the information. Once you register, FTP access instructions are emailed to you. The database itself is composed of several files that are defined at http://omim.org/downloads.

Finally, you can register for access to OMIM's REST API if you would prefer to fetch data of interest dynamically. A REST API system allows users with some programming experience to fetch information over the http protocol (the same protocol that your web browser uses to retrieve web pages). This enables information to be retrieved through scripts and integrated with other websites created by developers. There are many resources on how to access REST APIs on the Internet, and specifics are available elsewhere.

2.2.5 Disease Ontology

The Disease Ontology (DO) [34] database provides standardized disease term (including cancer), phenotype characteristic, and related disease vocabulary for use by biomedical researchers. DO adds value to the ontology system by cross-mapping DO terms to several other databases including: MeSH, ICD, NCI's thesaurus, SNOMED, and OMIM. During the development of such terminology, many terms are often found to be overlapping and ambiguous, filled with inconsistencies when examined across publications. A specific cancer DO slim has been generated, mapping many of the terms used in databases presented in this chapter [18]: such an effort is essential for pan-cancer analysis across many datasets, including the ones presented in this chapter.

2.2.6 Disease Ontology Access

The Disease Ontology database can be accessed through GitHub at https://github.com/DiseaseOntology/HumanDiseaseOntology. GitHub files can be retrieved in several different ways. One way is to click on the "Download ZIP" button found in the upper right corner of the screen to download the entire package in .ZIP format.

A second way is to "clone" the repository in your computer. When the repository is cloned, you can easily retrieve updates to the files by the use of the Git software. This also enables you to revert to earlier versions if necessary. There are tutorials on GitHub about how to use the Git software as the usage of this versioning software is outside of the scope of this chapter.

2.3 Other Resources: Proprietary Databases/Software, Clinical Trials, and Initiatives

All of the resources discussed up to this point may require credentials for access, but do not pose any financial barriers to access. It is noteworthy to mention that there are several proprietary resources of both primary tumor data and processed data that are heavily relied upon by the cancer genomics community. An informal survey of five cancer genomics principal investigators indicated Thermo Fisher's Oncomine® https://www.oncomine.org/resource/login.html as a database critical to cancer research. Oncomine® is both a gene browser and data analysis toolbox, offering thousands of patient tumor genomes for search and study. While a research edition may be accessed by filling out the form available at https://www.oncomine.org/resource/registration.html?ACTION=SHOW_REGISTRATION, premium versions of the software must be ordered from the website or over the phone directly from a Thermo Fisher representative.

Clinical trials provide a nearly constant influx of data, but the focus is frequently narrow and accompanied by, at least temporary, access restrictions.

One example, the Adjuvant Lung Cancer Enrichment Marker Identification and Sequencing Trials (ALCHEMIST) [35, 36] is an integrated effort of three precision medicine trials designed to identify early-stage lung cancer patients with uncommon genetic factors and determine responses to targeted treatments. Although this single trial may be advantageous to a small pocket of the cancer genomics research community, an openly accessible compendium of several such trials' primary data would prove an invaluable resource to the entire field. Furthermore, the establishment of initiatives above and around clinical trials, like the exceptional responders initiative (ERI) [37] and the NCI Clinical Trial Sequencing Project (CTSP) [38], identifies important gaps or anomalies of the data, increases the generation of such data, and improves characterization and overall understanding of such events.

3 Future Outlook of Cancer Genomics

As critical to the field as each of the resources discussed above may be today, it is important to realize that the landscape of bioinformatics tools is dynamic and in constant flux at all times. While TCGA data is not in any danger of permanent deletion, the project formally concluded in 2015, marking the end of 10 years of production of cancer-related data. This will create a need for new efforts to carry on the important role that TCGA has held over the last decade, not only in ensuring the continuous generation of new cancer data but also in maintaining and disseminating that information to the cancer genomics research community in an efficient and impactful way. To this end, the NCI's Center for Cancer Genomics (CCG) has established the Genomic Data Commons with the goal of advancing molecular diagnosis of cancer and improving targeted therapeutics [39]. In conjunction with the Cancer Genomics Cloud Pilots Program, NCI is hoping to build a comprehensive infrastructure with superior capabilities for searching, navigating, analyzing, and visualizing HTS data [40]. Similarly, CCG is in the pilot phase for the Cancer Driver Discovery Program (CDDP) [41] to sequence larger numbers of samples and therefore has a greater statistical power for the determination of recurrent driver mutations, than the TCGA project.

Of equal importance, however, is the meaningful interpretation of this data: some experts are hoping that the next decade will show a paradigm shift from rapid advances in sequencing technology to rapid advances in functional validation of genetic alterations identified in sequencing experiments and subsequent alignments [42]. COSMIC, a well-used mutation database, has recently changed its licensing for a fee to commercial users. While it is hoped that the corresponding financial gains to the project would spur greater innovation in developments, it remains to be seen whether this may prove a deterrent to certain companies [43]. Small ripples created by seemingly innocuous changes can result in huge waves in the broader field, especially for a field with very little guidance and virtually no standardizations to assess the confidence or quality of this massive amount of information.

Projects like NCI's dream challenges [44] seek to identify the most effective methods from the community toward the goal of promoting a standard practice, but despite some global efforts [45], it still remains for relevant members of the academic, regulatory, and industry genomics communities to come together to agree on such standards.

4 Notes

1. There are several available cancer databases, many of which are freely accessible with little restriction. Databases that have patient-centric information, as outlined in this chapter, do require registration and present some small barriers to access for qualified researchers in order to protect patient data.

   Due to the dynamic nature of the field, it would be both impossible and presumptuous to claim to exhaustively outline all cancer databases in this chapter. In addition to the databases addressed in detail, popular initiatives like the Environment and Genetics in Lung Cancer Etiology (EAGLE) [46] project continue to add depth to the available pool of cancer-related information.

2. The specific databases discussed in this chapter represent a frequently used subset of databases and, together, compose a majority of the cancer genomics data available at this time. Researchers or interest groups often use data they extract from these databases to generate a more specific database suited to their own studies: these new and interesting research projects could grow to be of novel importance, but space constraints prevent many such databases from being described. However, these databases can easily be found as published in journal articles or even through generic web searches. In fact, the NCI Scientific Library maintains a list of cancer research databases at https://ncifrederick.cancer.gov/ScientificLibrary/ElectronicResources/CancerResearch.aspx.

3. The goal of this chapter was to provide the reader with enough information such that any new databases encountered would likely have access requirements similar to one of the databases outlined above, and, with a little creative thinking, any researcher should be able to apply these lessons to gain access and successfully navigate the next generation of cancer genomics repositories.

References

1. Cochrane G, Karsch-Mizrachi I, Takagi T (2016) The international nucleotide sequence database collaboration. Nucleic Acids Res 44: D48–D50

2. Zutter M, Bloom K, Cheng L, Hagemann I, Kaufman J, Krasinskas A, Lazar A, Leonard D, Lindeman N, Moyer A (2015) The cancer

genomics resource list. Arch Pathol Lab Med 139:989–1008

3. Yang Y, Dong X, Xie B, Ding N, Chen J, Li Y, Zhang Q, Qu H, Fang X (2015) Databases and web tools for cancer genomics study. Genomics Proteomics Bioinformatics 13:46–50

4. Simonyan V, Mazumder R (2014) High-performance integrated virtual environment (HIVE) tools and applications for big data analysis. Genes 5:957–981

5. Goecks J, Nekrutenko A, Taylor J (2010) Galaxy: a comprehensive approach for supporting accessible, reproducible, and transparent computational research in the life sciences. Genome Biol 11:R86

6. Blankenberg D, Kuster GV, Coraor N, Ananda G, Lazarus R, Mangan M, Nekrutenko A, Taylor J (2010) Galaxy: a web-based genome analysis tool for experimentalists. Curr Protoc Mol Chapter 19:Biol 19.10.1–19.10.21

7. Giardine B, Riemer C, Hardison RC, Burhans R, Elnitski L, Shah P, Zhang Y, Blankenberg D, Albert I, Taylor J (2005) Galaxy: a platform for interactive large-scale genome analysis. Genome Res 15:1451–1455

8. The Cancer Genome Atlas. http://cancergenome.nih.gov

9. Wilks C, Cline MS, Weiler E, Diehkans M, Craft B, Martin C, Murphy D, Pierce H, Black J, Nelson D et al (2014) The cancer genomics hub (CGHub): overcoming cancer through the power of torrential data. Database (Oxford) 2014:bau093

10. Therapeutically applicable research to generate effective treatments. https://ocg.cancer.gov/programs/target

11. Barretina J, Caponigro G, Stransky N, Venkatesan K, Margolin AA, Kim S, Wilson CJ, Lehar J, Kryukov GV, Sonkin D et al (2012) The Cancer Cell Line Encyclopedia enables predictive modelling of anticancer drug sensitivity. Nature 483:603–607

12. ICGC Cancer Genome Projects. https://icgc.org/icgc

13. Volders PJ, Verheggen K, Menschaert G, Vandepoele K, Martens L, Vandesompele J, Mestdagh P (2015) An update on LNCipedia: a database for annotated human lncRNA sequences. Nucleic Acids Res 43:D174–D180

14. Forbes SA, Beare D, Gunasekaran P, Leung K, Bindal N, Boutselakis H, Ding M, Bamford S, Cole C, Ward S et al (2015) COSMIC: exploring the world's knowledge of somatic mutations in human cancer. Nucleic Acids Res 43:D805–D811

15. Cancer Cell Line Encyclopedia (CCLE). https://www.broadinstitute.org/software/cprg/?q=node/11

16. Wu T-J (2014) Integration of cancer-related mutations for pan-cancer analysis. The George Washington University, Washington, DC

17. Wu T-J, Shamsaddini A, Pan Y, Smith K, Crichton DJ, Simonyan V, Mazumder R (2014) A framework for organizing cancer-related variations from existing databases, publications and NGS data using a High-performance Integrated Virtual Environment (HIVE). Database 2014:bau022

18. Wu T-J, Schriml LM, Chen Q-R, Colbert M, Crichton DJ, Finney R, Hu Y, Kibbe WA, Kincaid H, Meerzaman D (2015) Generating a focused view of disease ontology cancer terms for pan-cancer data integration and analysis. Database 2015:bav032

19. Dingerdissen HM, Torcivia-Rodriguez J, Hu Y, Chang T-C, Mazumder R, Kahsay R (2018) BioMuta and BioXpress: mutation and expression knowledge bases for cancer biomarker discovery. Nucleic Acids Res 46(D1):gkx907

20. Mungall CJ, Torniai C, Gkoutos GV, Lewis SE, Haendel MA (2012) Uberon, an integrative multi-species anatomy ontology. Genome Biol 13:R5

21. Wan Q, Dingerdissen H, Fan Y, Gulzar N, Pan Y, Wu T-J, Yan C, Zhang H, Mazumder R (2015) BioXpress: an integrated RNA-seq-derived gene expression database for pan-cancer analysis. Database 2015:bav019

22. Landrum MJ, Lee JM, Benson M, Brown G, Chao C, Chitipiralla S, Gu B, Hart J, Hoffman D, Hoover J et al (2016) ClinVar: public archive of interpretations of clinically relevant variants. Nucleic Acids Res 44(D1):D862–D868

23. Landrum MJ, Lee JM, Riley GR, Jang W, Rubinstein WS, Church DM, Maglott DR (2014) ClinVar: public archive of relationships among sequence variation and human phenotype. Nucleic Acids Res 42:D980–D985

24. Volders PJ, Helsens K, Wang X, Menten B, Martens L, Gevaert K, Vandesompele J, Mestdagh P (2013) LNCipedia: a database for annotated human lncRNA transcript sequences and structures. Nucleic Acids Res 41:D246–D251

25. Rubio-Perez C, Tamborero D, Schroeder MP, Antolin AA, Deu-Pons J, Perez-Llamas C, Mestres J, Gonzalez-Perez A, Lopez-Bigas N (2015) In silico prescription of anticancer drugs to cohorts of 28 tumor types reveals targeting opportunities. Cancer Cell 27:382–396

26. Gonzalez-Perez A, Perez-Llamas C, Deu-Pons J, Tamborero D, Schroeder MP, Jene-Sanz A, Santos A, Lopez-Bigas N (2013) IntOGen-mutations identifies cancer drivers across tumor types. Nat Methods 10:1081–1082
27. Lappalainen I, Almeida-King J, Kumanduri V, Senf A, Spalding JD, Saunders G, Kandasamy J, Caccamo M, Leinonen R, Vaughan B (2015) The European genome-phenome archive of human data consented for biomedical research. Nat Genet 47:692–695
28. Consortium U (2015) UniProt: a hub for protein information. Nucleic Acids Res 43:gku989
29. Gao J, Aksoy BA, Dogrusoz U, Dresdner G, Gross B, Sumer SO, Sun Y, Jacobsen A, Sinha R, Larsson E (2013) Integrative analysis of complex cancer genomics and clinical profiles using the cBioPortal. Sci Signal 6:pl1
30. Cerami E, Gao J, Dogrusoz U, Gross BE, Sumer SO, Aksoy BA, Jacobsen A, Byrne CJ, Heuer ML, Larsson E (2012) The cBio cancer genomics portal: an open platform for exploring multidimensional cancer genomics data. Cancer Discov 2:401–404
31. NCI Thesaurus. https://ncit.nci.nih.gov/ncitbrowser/
32. Terminology Resources. http://www.cancer.gov/research/resources/terminology
33. Online Mendelian Inheritance in Man, OMIM®. http://omim.org/
34. Schriml LM, Arze C, Nadendla S, Chang Y-WW, Mazaitis M, Felix V, Feng G, Kibbe WA (2012) Disease ontology: a backbone for disease semantic integration. Nucleic Acids Res 40:D940–D946
35. The ALCHEMIST Lung Cancer Trials. http://www.cancer.gov/types/lung/research/alchemist
36. Jänne PA, Oxnard G, Watson M, Gandara D, Ramalingam S, Vokes E, Mandrekar S, Hillman S, Watt C, Participating N. Adjuvant Lung Cancer Enrichment Marker Identification and Sequencing Trial (ALCHEMIST)
37. The "Exceptional Responders" Study. http://dctd.cancer.gov/MajorInitiatives/NCI-sponsored_trials_in_precision_medicine.htm#h06
38. An Overview of NCI's National Clinical Trials Network. http://ctep.cancer.gov/initiativesPrograms/nctn.htm
39. NCI News Note. http://www.cancer.gov/news-events/press-releases/2014/GenomicDataCommonsNewsNote
40. NCI Cancer Genomics Cloud Pilots. https://cbiit.nci.nih.gov/ncip/nci-cancer-genomics-cloud-pilots
41. CCG Programs. http://www.cancer.gov/about-nci/organization/ccg/programs
42. Anonymous (2015) The future of cancer genomics. Nat Med 21:99
43. New licensing strategy with commercial partners will spur cancer database's growth. http://cancer.sanger.ac.uk/cosmic/license
44. DREAM Challenges. http://dreamchallenges.org/project/closed/dream-7-nci-dream-drug-sensitivity-prediction-challenge/
45. FDA (2014) Public workshop: next generation sequencing standards
46. Landi MT, Consonni D, Rotunno M, Bergen AW, Goldstein AM, Lubin JH, Goldin L, Alavanja M, Morgan G, Subar AF (2008) Environment And Genetics in Lung cancer Etiology (EAGLE) study: an integrative population-based case-control study of lung cancer. BMC Public Health 8:203

Chapter 2

Building Portable and Reproducible Cancer Informatics Workflows: An RNA Sequencing Case Study

Gaurav Kaushik and Brandi Davis-Dusenbery

Abstract

The Seven Bridges Cancer Genomics Cloud (CGC) is part of the National Cancer Institute Cloud Resource project, which was created to explore the paradigm of co-locating massive datasets with the computational resources to analyze them. The CGC was designed to allow researchers to easily find the data they need and analyze it with robust applications in a scalable and reproducible fashion. To enable this, individual tools are packaged within Docker containers and described by the Common Workflow Language (CWL), an emerging standard for enabling reproducible data analysis. On the CGC, researchers can deploy individual tools and customize massive workflows by chaining together tools. Here, we discuss a case study in which RNA sequencing data is analyzed with different methods and compared on the Seven Bridges CGC. We highlight best practices for designing command line tools, Docker containers, and CWL descriptions to enable massively parallelized and reproducible biomedical computation with cloud resources.

Key words Cloud, Bioinformatics, Cancer informatics, TCGA, AWS, Docker, Reproducibility, Software design

1 Introduction

Computational reproducibility remains a significant issue when replicating studies or performing large-scale, collaborative cancer genomics [1]. Variations in software versions or parameters introduce artifacts when attempting to compare analyses from various sources or when working in large collaborations or consortia. To overcome these challenges, several methods have been developed to improve the portability and reproducibility of analysis pipelines.

In order to enable computational reproducibility, the Seven Bridges Cancer Genomics Cloud (CGC) leverages open-source and community-driven technologies for supporting reproducibility with complementary software models that enable researchers to (1) replicate analyses performed previously, (2) readily analyze large volumes of data with identical workflows, and (3) track each step, input, parameter, and output of an analysis automatically [2].

One such technology is software containers, i.e., operating-system-level virtualized environments with a complete filesystem and a unique set of resources and permissions. The Cancer Genomics Cloud specifically supports Docker [3], an implementation of software containers that is operable on all major operating systems. The only external dependency for "running" a Docker container is that the Docker daemon is installed. Because containers are isolated environments, they can be used as portable vehicles for software and their dependencies. For example, a Docker container may build upon a Linux distribution and contain a bioinformatics tool, as well as its dependencies.

Docker containers are designed to be small and intended to be easily deployed to enable sharing among data analysts. Software within containers, if deterministic, will run exactly the same regardless of where the container is deployed or by whom. The use of Docker, therefore, solves a major issue in handling software dependencies in execution environments and comparing or replicating results which may differ because of software versioning.

One issue not solved by Docker is *how* to run bioinformatics tools within a Docker container. To address this, the CGC uses the Common Workflow Language (CWL) to describe how to run software within containers [4]. CWL is an emerging standard for describing the execution of analytical tools and workflows with serialized data objects, which can use JSON or YAML documents to describe a particular set of command line executions.

For an individual tool, the CWL description contains the URL or pointer to a Docker container residing in an online registry and a set of commands which are executable within the container. In addition, CWL defines "ports" or the input objects which can be used to run analysis (e.g., files, parameters, or simple objects that the user can provide to support execution) and the output objects expected from the analysis.

Finally, Seven Bridges extends Docker and CWL to further reproducibility. Firstly, the CWL specification is extended with plug-ins to enable advanced features such as application revision history. Secondly, the platform records the explicit parameters and files used in an execution, thus allowing researchers to clone prior analyses for replication or application to new data.

2 Materials

Researchers wishing to access the Seven Bridges CGC need only a personal computer with reliable access to the Internet. For the use of Docker containers on your personal computer, we recommend that researchers follow the minimal requirement guidelines from Docker (https://docs.docker.com). Public containers for bioinformatics are also available in online repositories, such as Docker Hub

(hub.docker.com), Quay.io (quay.io), and Dockstore (dockstore.org). All containers for this study were developed using Docker for Mac version 1.12 on a 2015 MacBook Pro with four cores and 16 GB RAM (two cores and 2 GB allocated for Docker). Some familiarity with the Linux operating system, shell/bash, and bioinformatics is also assumed.

3 Methods

A frequently used analysis method for gene abundance quantification is RNA sequencing by expectation maximization (RSEM) [5], which maps reads to individual genes or isoforms. With RSEM, ambiguous reads can be mapped at the gene and isoform level based on maximum likelihood. Recently, alternative methods such as Kallisto have allowed quantifying transcript or gene abundance from reads without alignment, thereby speeding up the analysis time by orders of magnitude [6]. However, the trade-offs in accuracy for mapping- or alignment-based methods versus k-mer-based ones are still in discussion. In this protocol, we will build workflow that allows us to compare gene-level expression derived from raw RNA sequencing data (paired-end FASTQ files) from The Cancer Genome Atlas (TCGA) with RSEM and Kallisto to understand how each may affect our results and understanding of the biological data. These methods are also applicable to the Cancer Cell Line Encyclopedia [7] available on the CGC or their private RNA sequencing data. Moreover, the steps outlined here can be extended to deploy any command line tool on the CGC.

3.1 Workflow Design

For the comparison of RSEM and Kallisto, we apply the following constraints:

1. The same set of reference files are used to build indices for each tool.

2. Abundances will be compared in transcripts per million (TPM), which allows for direct comparison of relative abundance of a transcript across samples. When calculating in TPM, the total number of counts is equivalent between samples.

3. For this exercise, we will use paired-end FASTQ files from TCGA available on the CGC.

To prepare for this analysis, we must first select a set of reference files. Reference files are available from public data repositories (Ensembl, Gencode) in compressed formats [8, 9]. While Kallisto can analyze gunzipped FASTA and FASTQ files, RSEM cannot. Therefore, we will need to incorporate a decompression step (gunzip, Fig. 1) when preparing indices for RSEM (rsem-prepare reference, Fig. 1).

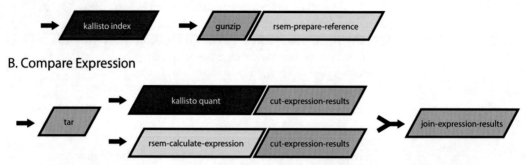

Fig. 1 Tool level description of the analysis workflow. Overall, five tools are needed for the analysis. While "kallisto quant" can accept gunzipped files, we must unzip references to pass to rsem-prepare-reference. Additionally, TCGA FASTQ files are stored as TAR.GZ files and must be decompressed before being able to be passed to kallisto quant and rsem-calculate expression. We will perform the analysis in two steps: (**a**) preparing index files which will be used as inputs and (**b**) calculating expression, along with paired-end fastq files. Colors indicate the common set of Docker containers used for each tool (blue, Kallisto; light gray, RSEM; gray, Ubuntu)

Raw sequencing data from TCGA are stored as TARGZ files, which are not interpretable by Kallisto or RSEM. Therefore, we will need to incorporate a decompression step (tar, Fig. 1) before calculating the expression (kallisto quant, rsem-calculate-expression, Fig. 1).

Finally the outputs of each tool are not directly comparable, so we will need to trim the output of RSEM and Kallisto with separate tools for direct comparison and visualization (cut-expression-results, join-rsem-kallisto, Fig. 1).

3.2 Creating Docker Containers and Testing Tools in Them

A major benefit to Docker containers is their portability; a single container running the Ubuntu Linux distribution can be smaller than 200 MB. This allows for easy and rapid sharing between researchers and platforms. In order to maintain the benefit of software containers, we recommend the following design guidelines:

- Use Dockerfiles to build your Docker containers (*see* **Note 1**).
- Package each tool in your workflow as a separate container (*see* **Note 2**).
  - Use a unique container for RSEM and its dependencies and a unique container for Kallisto.
  - For Linux tools (e.g., cut, gzip, tar, grep), we recommend using a standard Ubuntu container (`ubuntu:latest`) or a container that builds from it (*see* **Note 3**).
- In the Dockerfile, explicitly set the working directory as "/"—when we later describe how to execute commands within the

container, all arguments and file paths must be relative to "/," so it's good practice to start thinking that way early.
- In the Dockerfile, set the command option as "`/bin/bash`."

Start by building a Docker container with Kallisto, which is available on GitHub (https://pachterlab.github.io/kallisto/). First, create a folder to organize your Kallisto resources. Download the tarball for your version of choice to this folder and decompress (in this example, we use Kallisto v0.43.0 for Linux systems). Create a file called "Dockerfile" in the top directory with the following content:

```
FROM ubuntu:latest
MAINTAINER "YourFirstName YourLastName" <email@institution.io>
WORKDIR /

# Update and install necessary tools
RUN apt-get update -y
RUN apt-get install -y \
    build-essential cmake \
    python python-pip python-dev \
    hdf5-tools libhdf5-dev hdf5-helpers libhdf5-serial-dev \
    git apt-utils vim

# Add Kallisto to container and give proper permissions
RUN mkdir /opt/kallisto
COPY kallisto_linux-v0.43.0/ /opt/kallisto/
RUN chmod a+x /opt/kallisto
ENV PATH /opt/kallisto:$PATH

# Run container with bash pseudoterminal
CMD ["/bin/bash"]
```

This Dockerfile can be built with the following command:

```
$ docker build -t <repo/image:tag> </path/to/Dockerfile>
```

The first line of the Dockerfile specifies "`ubuntu:latest`" as the base image (using the `FROM` command, *see* **Note 4**). The "`MAINTAINER`" or contact information for the Dockerfile author can also be specified. The working directory is defined in the third line (`WORKDIR /`).

The second block of commands (`RUN apt-get...`) installs the dependencies for Kallisto, which are defined by the tool authors in their documentation [6]. When using "`apt-get`," include the "`-y`" or "`--yes`" option to confirm all actions ahead of time, preventing the need for intervention during install.

In the third set of actions (RUN mkdir...), we create a directory for the Kallisto executables in /opt/ and copy the local directory to this directory within the container (*see* **Note 5**). We then grant permissions to files in /opt/kallisto (chmod a+x /opt/kallisto) and add the directory to $PATH in order to invoke it from the working directory (*see* **Note 6**). Finally, we set the command to "/bin/bash" (*see* **Note 7**).

We then run the container in interactive mode to verify that the installation has occurred properly:

```
$ docker run -ti <repo/image:tag>
```

Next, verify that the software within the container (Kallisto) functions properly; examine how the files are interpreted and generated. This step will help us describe the executions more easily and reliably later on. To do this, run the commands preceded by /: #:. The expected output is shown on the indented lines.

```
/:# which kallisto
        /opt/kallisto/kallisto

/:# kallisto index -i kallisto.index opt/kallisto/transcripts.fasta.gz
        [build] loading fasta file opt/kallisto/transcripts.fasta.gz
        [build] k-mer length: 31
        [build] counting k-mers ... done.
        [build] building target de Bruijn graph ...  done
        [build] creating equivalence classes ...  done
        [build] target de Bruijn graph has 23 contigs and contains 18902 k-mers

/:# kallisto quant -i kallisto.index -o . opt/kallisto/reads_1.fastq.gz opt/kallisto/
reads_2.fastq.gz

        [quant] fragment length distribution will be estimated from the data
        [index] k-mer length: 31
        [index] number of targets: 15
        [index] number of k-mers: 18,902
        [index] number of equivalence classes: 22
        [quant] running in paired-end mode
        [quant] will process pair 1: opt/kallisto/reads_1.fastq.gz
                .................opt/kallisto/reads_2.fastq.gz
        [quant] finding pseudoalignments for the reads ... done
        [quant] processed 10,000 reads, 10,000 reads pseudoaligned
        [quant] estimated average fragment length: 178.097
        [   em] quantifying the abundances ... done
        [   em] the Expectation-Maximization algorithm ran for 52 rounds
```

This set of commands will use the example files provided by Kallisto to create an index in the working directory and then use the index file and example paired-end FASTQs (`reads_*.fastq.gz`) to quantify abundances. Because we specified the output directory ("`-o`") as "`.`" or the current directory, all outputs will appear there.

If changes need to be made to a container, we recommend recording that change in the original Dockerfile and then rebuilding the container (*see* **Note 8**).

3.3 Deploying Containers on the Seven Bridges Cancer Genomics Cloud

Once the container is tested, you can "push" it to an online registry. The Cancer Genomics Cloud can pull containers from any public registry, including Docker Hub or Quay.io. However, we recommend pushing containers to the CGC image registry for increased reliability when pulling containers for computation. To push to the CGC image registry, tag the container with the appropriate repo name:

```
docker tag <image_id> cgc-images.sbgenomics.com/<username>/<image>:<tag>
docker login cgc-images.sbgenomics.com
        <username>
        <auth_token>
docker push cgc-images.sbgenomics.com/<username>/<image>:<tag>
```

The process outlined in Subheadings 3.3 and 3.4 is then repeated for to build a Docker container for RSEM (*see* **Note 9**). We will create a Docker container for RSEM (v1.2.31) with all of its features. However, we will only use a subset of these features. Installing RSEM with all of its features increases the utility of the container by allowing reuse in multiple ways. In general, one container can spawn many tools. Often, bioinformatics tools are very comprehensive which makes it difficult to capture all of its command line arguments or utilities in a single description. Attempting to do so may require very complex wrappers, which can increase the time for debugging and testing. Wrap for your analysis, and reuse prior wrappers as your analyses change. Everything is versioned on the Seven Bridges Cancer Genomics Cloud, so it's easy to track down which applications produced which files and when and by whom by the researcher.

3.4 Describing Tools Using the Cancer Genomics Cloud

On the Cancer Genomics Cloud, tools are considered single executables or runnables, which consist of a set of command line expressions run within a Docker container. Workflows are chains of tools, in which upstream files are passed downstream until a final result is achieved.

Tools have the following major properties: Docker Container, Base Commands, Arguments, Input Ports, and Output Ports. The "Docker container" should have the `<repo/image:tag>` for the container you wish to use (e.g., "`ubuntu:latest`," "`cgc-images.sbgenomics.com/gauravcgc/rsem:1.2.31`"). Arguments are hard-coded inputs which are not user-configurable at runtime. Input Ports describe data objects that can be passed to the tool during execution. Output Ports describe data objects that will be saved from an execution, most commonly an output file or array of files (*see* **Note 10**).

3.4.1 Kallisto

Within the Kallisto suite, there are two subcommands which will enable us to calculate abundances in a format that can be compared to results from RSEM: "kallisto-index" (Fig. 2) and kallisto-quant. The "kallisto-index" tool will create an index file based on a

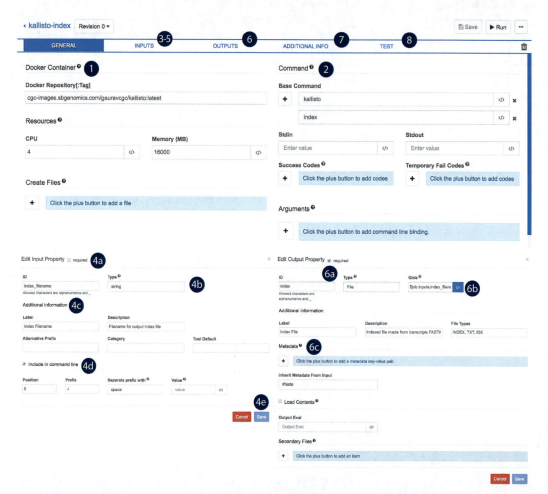

Fig. 2 Describing the "kallisto-index" tool with the CGC Tool Editor. *1* Each tool must have a Docker container, within which the command line executions are run. *2* The Base Command field is for a set of core commands for the tool, including the necessary subcommand. *3–5* The Inputs tab is where Input Ports are added and modified. *4* The Input Port menu allows the user to set the parameters and behavior for an object that can be passed to the tool (e.g., a file). *6* The Outputs menu allows the user to specify Output Ports, which describe objects produced by the tool which the user wishes to capture when the execution is completed. *7* The Additional Information field enables annotation of tool metadata, such as tool description, authors, license, and tags. *8* The Test tab allows the user to set "dummy" variables for each input field, in order to examine the behavior of the resulting command line of their tool and to determine whether the tool description is functional

reference file and a desired k-mer length. The "kallisto-quant" tool will use that index to calculate abundances for a set of paired-end FASTQ files. For each tool, we describe only the command line arguments which pertain to our use case of analyzing TCGA paired-end FASTQs (Fig. 1).

3.4.2 Kallisto Index

1. Set the Docker image URL, which can be used with a "`docker pull`" command to pull an image to your local machine.
2. Set the Base Command as "kallisto index."
3. Select the "Input" tab and then select the "+" symbol to add an Input Port for "-k," the k-mer length, which is used by "kallisto index" to construct a transcriptome de Bruijn graph, to which reads will be "pseudoaligned" during gene expression quantification [6].
4. In the Input Port menu:
   (a) Check the "required" box. A task using this tool cannot run unless this input is provided.
   (b) Set the required fields: ID as "kmer," Type as "int."
   (c) Fill out the "Additional Information" section as desired. These fields alter the UI of the Tasks page when executing this task.
   - "Label" will be how this specific port is labeled.
   - "Description" will appear in a help box. Add useful information here, such as recommended values, ranges of acceptable values, or more detail about how this port affects execution.
   - "Alternative Prefix" is where you can put the long form of a command line prefix used in this port (e.g., "`--verbose`" is the Alternative Prefix for "`-v`" in some tools).
   - "Category" lets you bin inputs in the Tasks page. This is very useful for tools with many options.
   - "Tool Default" is where you can record what the tool's own default value is if nothing is specified. For example, we can write "31" here since this is the default value used by kallisto index when "`-k`" is unspecified. Note that this field is a description and does not pass an actual value to the command line (*see* **Note 11**).
   (d) Check the "Include in Command Line" option.
   - Position: 1.
   - Prefix: -k.
   - Separate prefix with space.
   (e) Save the Input Port to return to the "Input" menu.

5. Repeat the **steps 3** and **4** for two additional Input Ports:
   (a) ID: index_filename, Type: string
      - Required: True.
      - Include in command line.
        – Position: 0.
        – Prefix: -i.
        – Separate prefix with: space.
   (b) ID: fasta, Type: File.
      - Required: True.
      - Include in command line.
        – Position: 2.
        – Separate prefix with empty string.
6. Output Ports allow you to specify which products of the execution you wish to "save." In this way, a tool may produce many files, but only those you wish to retrieve are stored. Create an Output Port for the index file created in the "Output" menu.
   (a) ID: index, Type: File.
   (b) For the glob, create a dynamic expression. Since we set the index filename as a mandatory input using a dynamic expression, we should glob the file using the same expression (*see* **Note 12**): `$job.inputs.index_filename`
   (c) Metadata:
      - Inherit Metadata From Input: #fasta.
7. Set the desired "Additional Information."
8. Verify that our dynamic expressions evaluate properly with the Test tab. Changes in "index_filename" should affect the command line printed in the "Resulting command line" pop-up field.

3.4.3 kallisto-quant

Our "kallisto-quant" tool will use the features of Kallisto which enables quantification of abundances with paired-end FASTQs, including the following arguments: index (`-i`), bias (`--bias`), bootstrap (`-b`), seed (`--seed=`), plaintext output (`--plaintext`), number of threads (`-t`), and output directory (`-o`). All but the output directory are set as Input Ports, as a user may wish to modify these values when executing a task. The output directory can be hard-coded as an Argument with a "Value" of ".". Constraining the output directory to the current working directory ("/") will remove the need to create a directory for outputs if the tool doesn't do so automatically. Finally, also include an input port for an array of FASTQ files.

In addition to describing the tool itself, we can introduce features which improve the usability of "kallisto-quant" (*see* **Note 13**). Each run of kallisto produces at least three files, "abundance.tsv," "abundance.h5," and "run_info.json," the first of which contains our desired data (transcript id and TPM). However, the user has no control over how to name each of these output files under the default Kallisto configuration. When running a large number of task with "kallisto-quant" on the CGC, this will result in each file having the same basic filename, which will encumber file management when running "kallisto-quant" at scale. However, we can provide the ability to rename the output files based on a specified input value or by modifying the filename using the input file properties (such as input filename or metadata properties). Our recommended design choice is to use the "Sample ID" of the input FASTQ files. This guarantees that, when working with TCGA data, each output file has a unique name.

In order to enable the sample-specific naming of the output files, create an additional Argument with the following expression as the "Value":

```
var sample_id = $job.inputs.fastqs[0].metadata.sample_id
"&& rename 's/^/" + sample_id + "_/' abundance*"
```

The first line creates a variable "sample_id" that evaluated to the sample_id" field for the metadata of the first element in the "fastqs" array (which should have a length of 2, for each paired-end file). The second line uses the "rename" command to rename each file that begins with "abundance" with the "sample_id" variable as a prefix. This will ensure that as we analyze a multitude of TCGA files, each output file has a unique filename.

3.4.4 RSEM

In the case of RSEM, before calculating transcript abundance, it is necessary to produce an index file. However, there are several index files generated for rsem-calculate-expression. Instead of globbing each index file individually or even as an array of files, it is more practical to create a tarball containing the index files as the final step of our "rsem-prepare-reference" tool. Decompressing the tarball will then serve as the first step of our "rsem-calculate-expression" tool. In this way, all required index files are available in a single manageable object.

3.4.5 rsem-prepare-reference

In order to prepare index files in a format which is compatible or usable with "rsem-calculate-expression," we will use an approach similar to that used in renaming files for "kallisto-quant": setting arguments that use standard bash tools (e.g., mv, tar, rename) to make asynchronous operations before and after the execution of "rsem-prepare-reference." In the case of "rsem-prepare-reference," we set the following constraints:

1. "rsem-prepare-reference" requires a GTF file and a FASTA file. Create an Input Port for each (ID: gtf, Type: File; ID: fasta, Type: File). Set Include in command line as set position as "1" and "2," respectively.

2. For this tool, we select a single aligner for our analysis (bowtie). Future versions of this tool can add Input and Output ports for commands used with other aligners (bowtie2, STAR).

   Create an "Argument" ("Value": "`--bowtie`", "Position": 0).

3. Indices will be output to a hard-coded directory "ref." This directory will be compressed as a tar.gz file which will become an output of the tool. In doing so, only the index files will be in the tarball, and when it is decompressed in the "rsem-calculate-expression" tool, they will appear in the path "/ref/".

   Set the first component(s) of the Base Command as "`mkdir ref &&,`" followed by "`rsem-prepare-reference.`" This will ensure that the "ref" directory exists before execution of the indices is produced.

   Create an Input Port (ID: output_filename, Type: string), which will be used to name the tarball containing the "ref" directory. Do not select "Include in command line."

   Create an Argument with a "Position" of "99," ensuring that it is the last operation performed, with the following dynamic expression as its value:

   "`&& tar zvcf`" + `$job.inputs.output_filename` + "`ref`"

   This operation will compress the "ref" directory and name the file with the "output_filename" given (e.g., "rsem_index.tar.gz").

   Create an Output Port (ID: output_targz, Type: File) with the glob set as the dynamic expression: `$job.inputs.output_filename`. Set "Inherit Metadata From Input" as "#fasta."

4. Create an Input Port for the type of reference used to create the indices (ID: ref, Type: enum). The "enum" type creates a dropdown list with a defined set of options. For this port, create the following options:

   (a) `ref/human_ensembl`
   (b) `ref/human_gencode`
   (c) `ref/human_refseq`

   Include in command line with "Position" as "3" to ensure that it is following the "fasta" Input Port value in the command line.

3.4.6 rsem-calculate-expression

To provide the index files to "rsem-calculate-expression" for execution, do the following:

1. Create an Input Port for the tarball created in "rsem-prepare reference" (ID: index, Type: File). This next step is vitally

important: under the "Stage Input" section, select "Link" (*see* **Note 14**). Do not include in the command line. Instead, we will use the object from this Input Port in the following step.

2. Set the Base Command as a dynamic expression: `"tar xzf "  + $job.inputs.index.path + " && rsem-calculate-expression."` This will untar the tarball. `"$job.inputs.index.path"` returns the path to the index file. The end result of this expression is that a directory "ref" containing the index files is now a subdirectory of our current working directory.

To allow batching tasks without creating output files with redundant names:

1. Create an Input Port for the "Sample Name." This is a required input for "rsem-calculate-expression" which needs to be included in the command line in the last position (set to "99").

2. Set the "Value" for this port as the following dynamic expression:

   `($job.inputs.sample_name || $job.inputs.input_fastqs[0].metadata.sample_id)`

   This will allow the user to specify a "Sample Name" when submitting a task. If none is given, the "Sample ID" for the FASTQ files is used instead.

To set the name of the reference type being used, replicate the "ref" port from "rsem-prepare-reference." Be sure to use the *exact* type (e.g., ref./human_ensembl) used in "rsem-prepare-reference" to avoid reference type mismatch.

The tool will produce two "result" files with the following names: `<sample_name>.genes.results` and `<sample_name>.isoforms.results`. You can create an Output Port for each; however, we will compare reads at the isoform level.

In addition to our Kallisto and RSEM tools, we will need to prepare a small set of tools based on Linux command line tools that will enable us to compare the outputs of RSEM and Kallisto (*see* **Note 15**).

3.5 Chaining Tools into Workflows

Workflows on the Cancer Genomics Cloud are chains of tools where input data is passed downstream. In addition, workflows expand upon tools in specific ways:

1. Explicit values can be set for Input Ports (e.g., "kmer" in "kallisto-index").

2. Workflows can be configured to "scatter" an array of parameters of values over an Input Port, creating a task for each index in the array.

3. Workflows can be "batched" based on metadata properties.

For this exercise, we're going to combine our tools into two workflows in order to process the data, one for each index file needed.

3.5.1 rsem-prepare-reference-workflow

Standard reference files are available in compressed formats. However, RSEM can only be used with uncompressed data. Therefore, when producing an index, we can create a workflow which decompresses the reference files before execution "rsem-prepare-reference." In our case, the GTF and FASTA files used to create the RSEM indices are gzipped. Therefore, we can use "gunzip" tool to decompress them.

Create a new workflow (ID: rsem-prepare-reference-workflow). In the App drawer, scroll to the project with the applications created for this workflow. Drag and drop one copy of "rsem-prepare-reference" and two copies of "gunzip." Assemble the workflow as in Fig. 2. Note that to create Input Port Nodes, click on the circular port symbol on each Tool, click and drag to the left side of the screen, and release. To connect Tools, click on a circular port you wish to connect, drag to the port which you wish to connect, and release. To create Output Port Nodes, click on the circular port and drag to the right (*see* **Note 16**).

3.5.2 compare-rsem-kallisto

The second workflow, "compare-rsem-kallisto" (Fig. 3), requires the following tools:

TCGA-untar

kallisto-quant

rsem-calculate-expression

cut-expression-results (×2)

join-rsem-kallisto

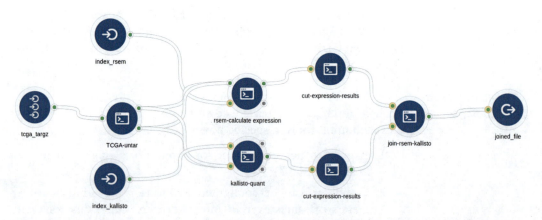

Fig. 3 Assembly of the "compare-rsem-kallisto" workflow. Workflows are described as chains of tools, in which data objects are passed downstream. Data objects (inputs/outputs) can be passed between tools by connecting the appropriate ports or can be redirected to Output Ports so they are captured and saved once execution is completed

Assemble the workflow. In addition, we will also set the parameters for each tool. To set parameters, click on an individual tool and the "Params" drawer will appear. First select the copy of "cut-expression-results" downstream of "kallisto-quant". Here, we input "1,5" as the value of "columns." For the copy of "cut-expression-results" downstream of "rsem-calculate-expression," input "1,6." Note the "lock" icon. If unlocked, this parameter field will appear in the Tasks page when executing a task. If locked, this parameter will not appear and therefore cannot be changed during task execution. Leave the parameters for "cut-expression-results" locked, as modifying them will only result in errors when comparing our results.

Additionally, we can set "default" values for parameters (Fig. 4). For example, set the following parameters for "rsem-calculate-expression":

Threads: 4 (lock)

Reference: ref/human_ensembl (unlock)

sample_name: [leave blank] (lock)

In the Tasks page, a field will appear for "Threads" and "Reference" with these values already inserted. In this way, you can use the "Params" draw to suggest values for the workflow while allowing for the user to modify them before submitting a task.

Set the following parameters for "kallisto-quant":

Threads: 4 (lock)

seed: [leave blank] (lock)

plaintext: True (lock)

bootstrap: 30 (unlock)

bias: True (lock)

Enable batching of inputs to "TCGA-untar." This will allow an array of files to be input to the workflow, and a task will be created for each TCGA TARGZ file. Select the Input Node for "TCGA-untar," and in the "Params" drawer, under "Create batch group by metadata criteria," select "Sample ID."

To perform the analysis, create an index file for RSEM and Kallisto:

Run the "rsem-prepare-reference-workflow" with the following inputs:

GTF: Homo_sapiens.GRCh38.85.gtf.gz

FASTA: Homo_sapiens.GRCh38.dna.primary_assembly.fa.gz

Reference: ref./human_ensembl

RSEM Archive Filename: rsem_GRCh38.85.tar.gz

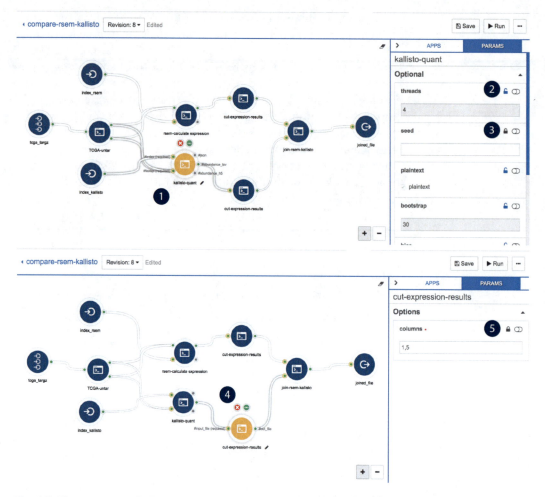

Fig. 4 Setting parameters in the "compare-rsem-kallisto" workflow. Workflows are designed such that certain ports can be "locked" with or without values (if not required), thereby preventing a user of the workflow from modifying this parameter. *1* To modify the parameters for a tool in the workflow, select the tool. It will become highlighted and the Params drawer will open on the right-hand side of the screen. *2* A parameter can have a default value set (e.g., threads = 4) and be "unlocked" such that it can be modified by a user before a task is executed with the workflow. *3* Alternatively, fields that are not "required" can be given empty values and locked such that the workflow will never use such parameters. *4* The "cut-expression-results" tool is a general-purpose tool for use with tab-delimited files, which are placed downstream from "kallisto-quant tool". *5* The columns parameter for this instance of the tool is constrained to "1,5" and locked, as this is the only setting with which the workflow will execute properly

Run the "kallisto-index" tool with the following inputs:

Transcripts: Homo_sapiens.GRCh38.rel85.cdna.all.fa.gz

kmer: 31

Run the "compare-rsem-kallisto" workflow with the following inputs:

rsem_index: rsem_index_GRCh38.85.tar.gz

kalisto_index: Homo_sapiens.GRCh38.rel85.cdna.all.fa.index

reference: ref./human_ensembl

bootstrap: 30

tcga_targz: [select array of TCGA TARGZ files containing paired-end FASTQ files]

3.6 Results

With the "compare-rsem-kallisto" workflow, we can explore how results compare between each method, as well as the computing time required. To perform this comparison, this workflow was run on every raw RNA sequencing file from the adrenocortical carcinoma cohort from TCGA (TCGA-ACC, $n = 79$). The total analysis time was 7 h, 38 min, and 26 s. We observe comparable results in transcript abundance from each method per sample (Fig. 5).

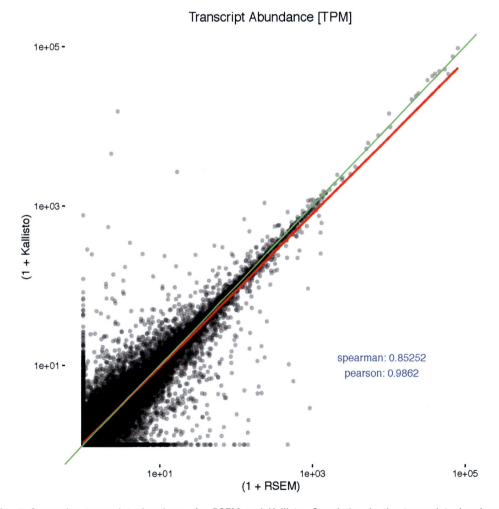

Fig. 5 Comparing transcript abundance for RSEM and Kallisto. Correlation in the transcript abundance determined from each method for an individual TCGA-ACC sample (Sample ID: TCGA-OR-A5L6-01A). Correlations were determined using a linear regression method (red line; Spearman = 0.85, Pearson = 0.98). Plot is shown as TPM + 1 for each axis in order to plot zero values. Green line indicates 1:1 correlation

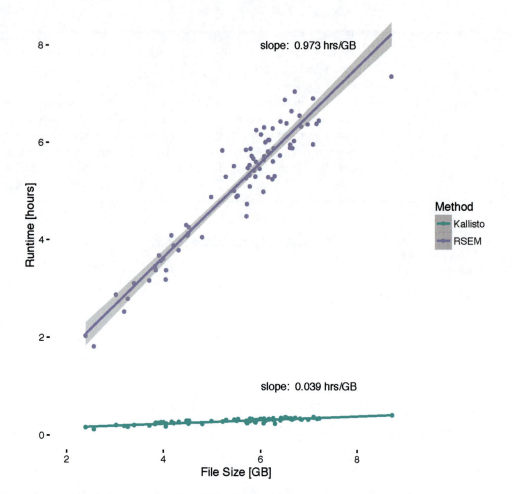

Fig. 6 Computational time as a function of file size for RSEM and Kallisto. Computational runtime (hours) versus input file size (gigabytes, GB) for the "compare-rsem-kallisto" workflow. Computation time scales linearly with input file size (TCGA TARGZ) with RSEM (Spearman = 0.91, Pearson = 0.95) and Kallisto (Spearman = 0.84, Pearson = 0.87). Solid lines indicate linear regression fit with slope (hours/GB) indicated

We can also examine differences in performance between each method. Computation time scales linearly with input file size (TAR.GZ) for both the "rsem-calculate-expression" (Fig. 6, RSEM; Spearman = 0.91, Pearson = 0.95) and "kallisto-quant" (Kallisto; Spearman = 0.84, Pearson = 0.87) components of the "compare-rsem-kallisto" workflow. From a linear regression fit, the rate of increase in computational time for RSEM is 0.973 h (58.3 min) per GB of input data, whereas Kallisto carries an additional 0.038 h (2.31 min) of computational time per additional GB of input data.

4 Notes

1. Dockerfiles should be used as a precise description of how to rebuild the container used for an analysis. Since Dockerfiles are simple text descriptions of a container using a domain-specific language, they are extremely portable and can serve as a lightweight way to enable others to reproduce your execution environments. You may want to interactively build the container and then record the steps you take in a Dockerfile—but to ensure reproducibility, the final container you use should actually be built from the Dockerfile.

2. An important aspect of Docker containers is that a group of containers in the same volume (e.g., registry, hard drive) can share layers. For example, a container that is built from another container but adds additional tools doesn't duplicate the data from the previous container. This behavior alleviates any data burden of having many function-specific containers. For this reason, we encourage that researchers optimize having many lightweight containers for easy sharing and deployment, as opposed to a few containers with all of their tools inside.

3. For simple command line tools, we recommend using standard Linux distribution containers. For example, let us examine a simple tool which saves the first 1000 lines of a FASTQ file as a new file. We can use the "head" tool to trim the top "n" lines of any file. Since head is a Linux command line tool, we can use an Ubuntu container as a bigger one is not needed. To save the first 1000 lines of a FASTQ in a new file, use head to print the first 1000 lines of the input FASTQ file then redirect stdout to a new file:

   ```
   head -1000 [input_file] > [output_file]
   ```

   This tool can then be reused on any FASTQ file to generate a plethora of outputs. Note that this tool is particularly useful for sampling FASTQs, which can then be used for rapidly testing tools or workflows which are computationally intensive. When the goal is to see if your tool runs properly, we recommend that you use sampled FASTQs to iterate more rapidly.

4. Dockerfiles use the "FROM" command to use another image as the "base" for the new image being built. We recommend that you build from trusted, standard containers (e.g., ubuntu:latest) instead of a third-party container. If you choose to rebuild your container from this Dockerfile in the future and the base image has been modified, the rebuilt container will inherit any changes within it. This may lead to errors or dependency issues if the base image has changed dramatically.

5. If you don't intend to use the software outside the container, you can use commands such as wget, curl, or other downloading software to directly download software into a container during the build.
6. Some software will automatically add itself to $PATH, and thus these steps may not be required.
7. Docker containers can be run to execute a command directly (using the CMD field). However, containers intended for use on the CGC should be built such that they can be run in "interactive mode" (e.g., docker run -it <repo/image:tag>) and a set of specified commands can be executed within them. On the Cancer Genomics Cloud, all commands are executed from the working directory ("/") by default.
8. The "docker build" command will begin to build the container layers starting from the beginning of the Dockerfile (FROM) until the end (CMD). The layers pertaining to each code block are cached during the build. If a change is made somewhere in the Dockerfile, all the layers pertaining to code blocks *above* the change will be loaded, and all layers built from the command *below* the change will be overwritten. It is recommended that any software-based changes that need to be made to container are done by modifying the original Dockerfile and then rebuilding. However, there may be cases where you wish to save an analysis or analysis output in a container for your own use (not for production). In such cases, you can commit changes made in a container back to the image with the following command: docker commit <container_id> <repo/image:tag>.
9. Here is an example Dockerfile for RSEM 1.23.1.

```
FROM ubuntu:latest
MAINTAINER "YourFirstName YourLastName" email@institution.io
WORKDIR /
# Update and install necessary tools
RUN apt-get update -y
RUN apt-get install -y \
    gcc \
    g++ \
    libdb5.1 \
    libdb5.1-dev \
    make \
    cmake \
    libboost-dev \
    libboost-thread-dev \
    libboost-system-dev \
```

```
           zlib1g-dev \
           ncurses-dev \
           libxml2-dev \
           libxslt-dev \
           build-essential \
           python \
           python-pip \
           python-dev \
           git \
           apt-utils \
           vim \
           wget \
           perl \
           perl-base \
           r-base \
           r-base-core \
           r-base-dev
    # Get RSEM-1.2.31 and install RSEM and EBSeq
    RUN wget -P opt --verbose --tries=5
    https://github.com/deweylab/RSEM/archive/v1.2.31.tar.gz
    RUN tar xzf opt/v1.2.31.tar.gz
    RUN cd RSEM-1.2.31/ && make && make install && make ebseq
    # Install bowtie
    RUN apt-get install bowtie -y
    # Open container with bash terminal
    CMD ["/bin/bash"]
```

10. There are a few important considerations when designing tools. On the CGC, you can create a "batch" of tasks based on the metadata properties of a set of input files. For example, let's say you have a tool which sorts a single bam file and outputs the sorted BAM. You can create a workflow from this tool which can instead take an array of BAM files and will create a single task for each set of files based on "Sample ID." Since each BAM file presumably has its own unique Sample ID, a single task will be created per BAM with far less user interaction (if done through the GUI) or code required (if done through the API). A major constraint for this feature is that you can only batch on a *single* Input port. This is obvious for BAM files, but when performing a batch of tasks for a set of paired-end FASTQ files, you must pass the FASTQ files as an array of files. If you create an individual port for each paired-end FASTQ (e.g., 1, 2), then you cannot currently set up a batch-able workflow.

11. We can set a default value for an Input Port by taking two steps: (1) do not make the port "required" and (2) create a dynamic expression for the "Value" of this port such that the port has a

value if unspecified. For example, if the Input Port type is an integer and we wish to specify "31" as a default value, the dynamic expression can be written as: (`$self || 31`) or (`$job.inputs.<input_id> || 31`). This expression means that if the user specifies a value for this port ($self), then that is used as the "Value" or, if unspecified, 31 is given as the value. In addition, the default value in the CWL description can be different from the tool's default.

12. Explicit values for each Input Port and Allocated Resources (CPU, Memory) are provided to the application for execution. This is referred to as the "job" object (or "job.json"). From this object, we can incorporate the properties of Input Ports into the dynamic expressions of the tool. For example, suppose that a user can specify the number of threads for a tool with an integer value (ID: threads). In order to pass this to the CPU requirements field, we can set the value for CPU as the following dynamic expression: `$job.inputs.threads`.

13. Consider how a tool will operate when it runs at scale and how you will manage the output data. Tools such as Kallisto index and rsem-calculate-expression take an input which generates the output filename or its prefix. When batching tasks, as we will do for rsem-calculate-expression, you cannot then specify an individual name per file. Only an individual value can be given. On the CGC, this will produce a number of files with the same name, with the addition of a prefix ("_#_," where # is the nth copy of a file). This will make file management difficult, as the original of a file is not readily apparent from its name. Instead, we will solve this issue by automatically passing a unique identifier, such as the input file's "Sample ID," which will scale over dozens, hundreds, or thousands of tasks.

14. This will link the index file to the working directory. When the index file is decompressed, this will place its contents into the working directory. Thus, the "ref" directory containing the index files will be a subdirectory of the working directory. Whenever decompressing input files or working with directories, we recommend setting "Stage Input" to "Link."

15. Below we describe a set of tools based on common Linux command line tools. All these can be used with the "ubuntu:latest" Docker container.

    TCGA-untar

    Paired-end reads in TCGA are stored in TARGZ files. Decompressing the file will produce the reads in the current working directory. This tool will capture paired-end FASTQ files based on the filename. It will also:

1. Create an Input Port (ID: tcga_targz, Type: File). Stage the input ("Link") and include in the command line (Position: 0).

2. Set the Base Command as "`tar xzf`".

3. Create two Output Ports, one for each FASTQ file (ID: fastq1, glob: `*_1.fastq`; ID: fastq2, glob: `*_2.fastq`).

4. For each port, add a custom metadata field "paired-end" with a value of "1" (integer) and "2," for fastq1 and fastq2, respectively.

cut-expression-results

To easily compare the transcripts per million for each sample from Kallisto and RSEM, we will use "cut" to grab the appropriate columns and "awk" to trim the headers:

```
$ cut -f 1,6 input_file.tsv | tail -n+1 | awk '{col=$1;
split(col, colArr,"."); $1=colArr[1]} 1' | sort -k1 >
input_file_cut.tsv
```

While it is possible to create a general wrapper for "cut" which can handle multiple use cases, here we create a tool that only works with tab-delimited files.

1. Set the Base Command as "`cut.`"

2. Create an Input Port for the tab-delimited input file (ID: input_file).

   (a) Include in command line (Position: 1).

3. Create an Input Port for the columns to cut (ID: columns, Type: string).

   (a) Include in command line (Position: 0).

   (b) Prefix: -f.

4. Create an Argument for trimming the header with `tail`, trim the Ensembl version from the Transcript ID (to enable joining with RSEM results later) with `awk`, and sort by the first column with `sort`:

   (a) Position: 2

   (b) Value: `| tail -n+1 | awk '{col=$1; split (col, colArr,"."); $1=colArr[1]} 1' | sort -k1`

5. Redirect to standard out (stdout) with the following set of dynamic expressions:

```
var basename = $job.inputs.input_file.path.split
('/').pop().split('.').slice(0,-1).join('_')
var ext = $job.inputs.input_file.path.split('/').
pop().split('.').pop()
basename + '_cut.' + ext
```

This will insert "_cut." between the basename of the input file and the extension. For example, "sample_abundance.tsv" becomes "sample_adundance_cut.tsv."

6. Create an output port (ID: cut_file; Type: File; glob: *_cut.*), which will capture any file with "_cut." in its name.

join-rsem-kallisto

In order to compare the results from RSEM and Kallisto, we will create a tool that joins the outputs. This can be achieved purely through command line expressions:

```
$ join -1 1 -2 1 sample_isoforms_cut.results sample_abundance_cut.tsv > joined.tsv
```

1. Set the Docker container as "ubuntu:latest."
2. Set the base command to "join -1 1 -2 1."
3. Create an Input Port for each results file and include in the command line with the RSEM results file in Position 0 and Kallisto in Position 1. The order here matters greatly since the fourth column of our output file is relative expression between the two.
4. Set the following dynamic expression for stdout:

   ```
   var rsem = $job.inputs.input_rsem.path.split('/
       ').pop().split('.').slice(0,-1)
   var kallisto = $job.inputs.input_kallisto.path.
       split('/').pop().split('.').slice(0,-1)
   var rsem_sample_id = $job.inputs.input_rsem.
       metadata.sample_id
   var kallisto_sample_id = $job.inputs.input_kallisto.metadata.sample_id
   if (rsem_sample_id == kallisto_sample_id) {
   "joined_" + rsem_sample_id + ".tsv"
   } else {
   "joined_" + rsem + "-" + kallisto + ".tsv"
   }
   ```

   This expression will check if the input files have identical Sample IDs, and then name the output file as "joined_<sample_id>.tsv." Note that the Sample IDs should be identical in order for the comparison of methods to make sense.

5. Create an Output Port for the joined file (ID: , Type: File, glob: `joined*`).

gunzip

This tool takes an input file that is gunzipped; decompress it, and return the decompressed file. The decompressed file will have the same filename without the ".gz" extension.

1. Set the Base Command as "gunzip."
2. Create an Input Port (ID: input; Type: File), Stage Input as "Link," and include in the command line (Position: 0).
3. Create an Output Port (ID: output, Type: File, glob (dynamic expression):

```
$job.inputs.input.path.split(/).pop().
split(.gz)[0]
```

16. Within workflows, if an Output Node is not created from a port, the object from that port is not saved. It is possible to both pass an output from an upstream tool downstream, as well as creating an Output Port to save it. In this way, you can also save "intermediate files" or files which can be passed to downstream tools, by creating Output Nodes for them in addition to connecting them to downstream tools.

Acknowledgements

The Cancer Genomics Cloud is powered by Seven Bridges and has been funded in whole or in part with federal funds from the NCI, NIH, Department of Health and Human Services, under contract no. HHSN261201400008C and HHSN261200800001E. We thank the entire Seven Bridges team, the Cancer Genomics Cloud Pilot teams from the NCI, the Broad Institute, and the Institute of Systems Biology, the Genomic Data Commons team, countless early users, and data donors. We also wish to further acknowledge the source of two of the datasets that are available to authorized users through the CGC and that were central to its development: The Cancer Genome Atlas (TCGA, phs000178). The resources described here were developed in part based upon data generated by The Cancer Genome Atlas managed by the NCI and NHGRI. Information about TCGA can be found at https://cancergenome.nih.gov/. And Therapeutically Applicable Research to Generate

Effective Treatments (TARGET, phs000218). The resources described here were developed in part based on data generated by the Therapeutically Applicable Research to Generate Effective Treatments (TARGET) initiative managed by the NCI.

References

1. Alioto TS et al (2015) A comprehensive assessment of somatic mutation detection in cancer using whole-genome sequencing. Nat Commun 6:10001
2. Lau JW, Lehnert E, Sethi A, Malhotra R, Kaushik G, Onder Z, Groves-Kirkby N (2017) The cancer genomics cloud: Collaborative, reproducible, and democratized-a new paradigm in large-scale computational research. Cancer Research. 77(21):e3–e6
3. Merkel D (2014) Docker: lightweight linux containers for consistent development and deployment. Linux J 2014(239):2
4. Amstutz, Peter, Crusoe, Michael R, Tijanić, Nebojša, Chapman, Brad, Chilton, John, Heuer, Michael, Kartashov, Andrey, Leehr, Dan, Ménager, Hervé, Nedeljkovich, Maya, Scales, Matt, Soiland-Reyes, Stian, Stojanovic, Luka (2016) Common workflow language, v1.0. Figshare
5. Li B, Dewey CN (2011) RSEM: accurate transcript quantification from RNA-Seq data with or without a reference genome. BMC Bioinformatics 12(1):1
6. Bray NL, Pimentel H, Melsted P, Pachter L (2016) Near-optimal probabilistic RNA-seq quantification. Nat Biotechnol 34(5):525–527
7. Barretina J, Caponigro G, Stransky N, Venkatesan K, Margolin AA, Kim S, Wilson CJ et al (2012) The Cancer Cell Line Encyclopedia enables predictive modelling of anticancer drug sensitivity. Nature 483(7391):603–607
8. Hubbard T, Barker D, Birney E, Cameron G, Chen Y, Clark L, Cox T et al (2002) The Ensembl genome database project. Nucleic Acids Res 30(1):38–41
9. Derrien T, Johnson R, Bussotti G, Tanzer A, Djebali S, Tilgner H, Guernec G et al (2012) The GENCODE v7 catalog of human long noncoding RNAs: analysis of their gene structure, evolution, and expression. Genome Res 22 (9):1775–1789

Chapter 3

Computational Analysis of Structural Variation in Cancer Genomes

Matthew Hayes

Abstract

Cancer onset and progression is often triggered by the accumulation of structural abnormalities in the genome. Somatically acquired large structural variants (SV) are one class of abnormalities that can lead to cancer onset by, for example, deactivating tumor suppressor genes and by upregulating oncogenes. Detecting and classifying these variants can lead to improved therapies and diagnostics for cancer patients.

This chapter provides an overview of the problem of computational genomic SV detection using next-generation sequencing (NGS) platforms, along with a brief overview of typical approaches for addressing this problem. It also discusses the general protocol that should be followed to analyze a cancer genome for SV detection in NGS data.

Key words Cancer, Structural variation, Sequencing, Next-generation sequencing

1 Introduction

Structural variants (SV) are widespread abnormalities that affect the genomes of living organisms. Although there is no standard requirement for the length of an SV, they are generally defined as structural abnormalities that are greater than 50–1000 bases in length [1]. Such abnormalities include deletions, inversions, insertions, tandem repeats, and interchromosomal translocations [2–5]. In addition to single nucleotide polymorphisms (SNPs), it is believed that germline SVs also contribute to the genetic diversity observed across populations. However, when SVs are acquired somatically, they can make genomic changes that engender the onset of cancer, depending on the genes that are affected. For example, the Philadelphia chromosome is a genetic abnormality caused by a reciprocal translocation between chromosomes 9 and

The original version of this chapter was revised. The correction to this chapter is available at https://doi.org/10.1007/978-1-4939-8868-6_17

22, leading to a fusion of the BCR and ABL genes. This fusion is highly oncogenic, as it is found in 95% of people with chronic myelogenous leukemia (CML) [6]. Other types of SVs can lead to oncogenic products. For example, if a genomic deletion affects the region of a tumor suppressor gene, it could inactivate the gene, which may lead to tumor onset. Similarly, a tandem replication of an oncogene can cause the gene to be overly expressed, which can also lead to tumor onset. Inversions can also be oncogenic because they can create fusion genes or they can deactivate important genes such as tumor suppressors [7].

Data produced from next-generation sequencing (NGS) platforms allows for the systematic analysis of genomes to detect and classify SVs. NGS platforms provide high-throughput sequencing of genomes, leading to faster sequencing experiments than was previously performed by older technologies like Sanger sequencing. Popular NGS platforms include those produced by Illumina, PacBio, and Ion Torrent [8]. Although the sequencing technologies differ among these different platforms, they share the same basic steps (including pre-sequencing sample preparation):

1. Isolate (genomic) DNA.
2. Amplify the DNA via PCR or by another means.
3. Randomly shear the DNA into overlapping fragments.
4. Sequence the end(s) of each fragment.

Each sequencing experiment produces a large set of sequence reads that are generated from the target DNA sequence. Figures 1, 2, and 3 present a high-level graphical overview of the process of sequence read generation. For each molecule fragment produced, one or both ends of the fragment may be sequenced depending on the experiment being performed. In the case of both ends being sequenced, the sequence dataset is said to be *paired-end*; otherwise it is a *single-end* dataset.

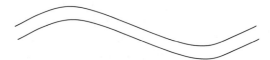

Fig. 1 The first step is to isolate the DNA that will be sequenced in the ensuing experiment. This is performed during sample preparation

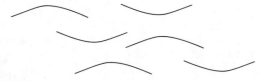

Fig. 2 The second step is to amplify and to randomly fragment the DNA into millions of fragments

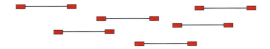

Fig. 3 For paired-end sequencing experiments (shown), both ends of each fragment are sequenced. For single-end, only one end of each fragment is sequenced

NGS platforms help researchers to answer pertinent biological and medical questions about the individual whose DNA is sequenced during the experiments. This genome is typically referred to as the test or *donor* genome. For example, it may be desirable to find regions in the genome that have been amplified, deleted, or otherwise affected by SVs. These genomic changes may result in the onset of disease, so NGS experiments are often used to determine the extent to which changes to the genome engender changes to phenotype. After sequencing, such analyses are typically performed by *aligning* the sequence reads to a *reference* genome, which is a genome that is assumed to be healthy or free from the genomic features that presumably affect the donor genome. In the context of cancer genomics, the test genome is potentially affected by oncogenic abnormalities, while the reference genome is the control. Thus, the alignment step allows researchers to compare the donor genome to the reference genome to assess their differences. Alignment is performed by short-read alignment programs such as BWA and Bowtie [9, 10]. These programs specialize in rapid alignment of short sequence reads to long reference genomes. These programs, like the vast majority of short-read aligners, produce read alignments in the Sequence Alignment/Map (SAM) format [11], which has become the standard file format for representing NGS read alignments.

Once the sequence has been aligned to the reference, structural variants like those previously mentioned can be located and classified by examining the characteristics of those aligned read pairs that span SV breakpoints. When aligned back to the reference genome, these read pairs are aligned *discordantly*, which means that their alignment features are somehow different than what is expected if there was no structural variant. Otherwise, the mapping of the read pair is said to be *concordant*. Figure 4 depicts the discordant mapping signals that are produced when a paired read is mapped back to the reference genome for each kind of basic structural variant (*see* **Note 1**). Algorithms like BreakDancer, VariationHunter, Delly, and GASV detect structural variants by locating large groups of these discordantly mapped read pairs since large groups of these pairs could indicate a structural variant [12–15]. If a single-end sequencing experiment was performed, then SV detection can be performed by using split-read programs like Pindel and SLOPE, which can detect SVs using the mapping characteristics of single reads [16, 17]. One can also implement a pipeline that uses a short-

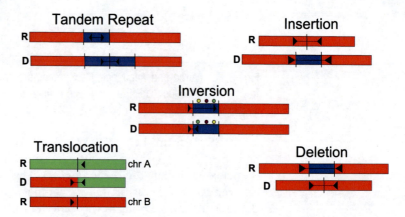

Fig. 4 Discordantly mapped paired reads and their mapping signals. Algorithms to locate SVs look for groups (or clusters) of these discordant read pairs to predict the variants shown

read aligner that produces *soft-clipped reads*, like BWA, and then by using an SV detection program like CREST or Socrates [18, 19] which can locate SVs by collecting and realigning these soft-clipped reads.

The purpose of this chapter is to describe the systematic approach typically used in the analysis of cancer genomes using NGS data, specifically on the analysis of somatic structural variants. Identifying somatic SVs has important implications in the treatment, diagnosis, and prevention of cancer, so it is important to have clearly defined steps that outline the aforementioned process.

2 Methods

2.1 Preliminaries

Analyzing cancer genomes using NGS involves several distinct steps. The major goal of these analyses is the actual prediction of SVs. There are many programs that are used to predict structural variants. These programs fall into the following categories, according to the kinds of SV signals they consider.

1. Paired-end
2. Split read
3. Depth of coverage
4. Sequence assembly

Paired-end methods identify structural variants by locating clusters of the discordant read pairs described above. If many of these read pairs align in close proximity to one another and if the pairs share the same mapping characteristics, then the region is likely predicted as an SV. The methods differ mostly by the criteria they set for determining if a group of discordant read pairs is significant enough to be an SV. Examples of paired-end methods include

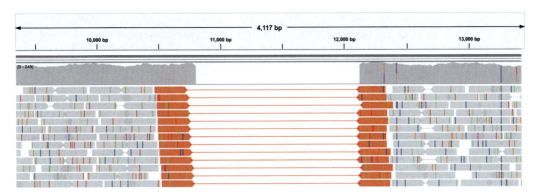

Fig. 5 A homozygous deletion that is spanned by long, discordantly mapped read pairs (red) and concordant alignments (gray) that do not span the deletion. The mapping coverage plot is shown near the top of the image. For deletion variants, the distance between flanking discordant read pairs should be larger than expected. There should be many of these read pairs for a true deletion variant. The alignment is visualized with the Integrative Genomics Viewer (IGV) [20]

BreakDancer, GASV, VariationHunter, and Delly (*see* **Note 2**). An example of a discordant read pair cluster spanning a deletion variant is shown in Fig. 5.

Split-read methods also detect structural variants by analyzing sequence reads produced by NGS platforms. However, these methods are designed to detect SVs based on the mapping characteristics of individual reads. Paired-end datasets can be used by such methods, but the programs will only consider individual reads and will ignore the mapping characteristics of discordant mate pairs like the methods described above. These methods exploit the properties of single reads or groups of reads that span SV breakpoints. These reads are often not initially mappable to the reference by short-read aligners since the reads do not form a (roughly) contiguous match to the reference. As a secondary step, however, these algorithms align the matching portions of the read to the reference, which will map at or near the variant breakpoints. Examples of such algorithms include Pindel and SPLITREAD [21]. When using a split-read method, the average read depth should be high enough to maintain sensitivity of SV predictions, as split-read methods tend to have lower sensitivity in low-coverage datasets than paired-end methods [14].

Depth-of-coverage (DOC) approaches detect variants by analyzing the number of reads that map to within a certain region on the reference. These methods are only concerned with the *abundance* of reads that align to the reference and not the mapping characteristics of read pairs or individual reads. The mapping coverage within a certain genomic region is roughly proportional to its copy number, with variations due to GC content (*see* **Note 3**), PCR amplification bias of the sequenced fragment, or natural variations in the ability of locally generated reads to map to within the same region (since many sequence reads do not align to the reference genome with high quality, which could be due to highly repetitive regions in the reference genome). DOC methods thus can only be used to detect amplified genomic segments (duplications) or genomic deletions and cannot be used to detect copy-neutral SVs like inversions and reciprocal translocations. For example, if the number of reads that align to a certain region is lower than what is expected on average, then there is a likely genomic deletion. If there are more aligned reads than what is expected on average, then the variant is a likely a genomic amplification, such as a tandem repeat. Figure 5 shows the aligned reads near a deletion event and a graph displaying the coverage depth at each position. DOC methods would likely predict this region of no read depth as a deletion. Examples of DOC approaches include SegSeq and RDXplorer [22, 23].

Methods based on sequence assembly generally search for single reads that span a structural variant breakpoint. For these reads, at least part of the read will align to the reference. These methods then take the aligned subreads of many reads that span the breakpoint and assemble them into a single contig. This contig is then mapped to the reference genome at the location of the presumed structural variant. Unlike paired-end methods, split-read and assembly-based methods excel at predicting the precise location of structural variant breakpoints [24]. CREST is an example of an SV detection program that is based on read assembly.

Before attempting to predict structural variants using the above programs, one must carefully consider the NGS dataset being used; the choice of the SV program depends on whether or not the sequencing experiments produced a paired-end dataset or a single-end dataset. If a single-end dataset was used, then algorithms that were designed for paired reads *cannot* be used. However, DOC-based algorithms and split-read algorithms can still be used. If the dataset is paired-end, then *any* kind of genomic NGS-based dataset can be used, though as stated beforehand, paired-read approaches tend to have better sensitivity for calling SVs in the presence of lower coverage, even though they are inferior at predicting precise variant breakpoints. DOC-based methods can be used on either kind of dataset, but cannot detect copy-neutral SVs.

2.2 Process

The following steps must be taken when identifying structural variants using NGS data. Without loss of generality, these steps assume that Illumina sequencing is employed. The approach can be slightly altered to accommodate other sequencing technologies.

1. Sequence patient tumor genomic DNA.
2. Sequence normal (healthy) genomic DNA belonging to the patient, preferably (but not necessarily) from the same tissue as the primary tumor.
3. Assess quality of sequence reads.
4. Align tumor reads to the reference genome.

Align normal reads to the reference genome (*see* **Note 4**).

5. Take resulting SAM alignment files for both the tumor and healthy data from **step 4** and convert them to BAM.
6. Sort the BAM files by chromosome and coordinates.
7. Remove sequence read replicates from BAM files.
8. (**Paired-end data** only) If the NGS dataset is paired-end and if no read-depth analysis is being performed, remove all concordant read alignments from the BAM files.
9. If the SV program requires it, create BAM index files (.bai) from the sorted BAM alignments.
10. Apply the structural variant detection program to the BAM files. This produces a list of predicted SVs for both the tumor dataset and the healthy dataset.
11. If the SV program does not automatically filter germline SVs, remove from the list of tumor structural variant calls all of those SVs that overlap with the healthy data SVs.

2.2.1 Sequence Patient Tumor Genomic DNA and Sequence Patient Normal (Healthy) Genomic DNA

Steps 1 and **2** are interchangeable. However, tumor cells will still share common germline structural variants with healthy cells since the tumor cells are descendent from those healthy cells. Thus, it may be desirable to remove germline SVs since somatically-acquired SVs are usually of greater clinical importance. Furthermore, normal cell contamination is a persistent problem in cancer sequencing data analysis, so even in a BAM file containing sequenced genomes from collected tumor cells, it is likely that there will be a mixture of tumor **and** healthy genome sequence data since normal cells (and their germline SVs) will invariably be collected during biopsies, for example. In the case where germline SVs are present among somatic SVs, the tumor and normal genomic DNA must both be sequenced to allow for accurate filtering of germline (inherited) structural variants, which are mostly present in the healthy (or normal) sample. After the genomes have been sequenced, the NGS machines will produce FASTQ files containing sequence reads for each sample. FASTQ format files contain the called bases of the sequence reads as well as their quality scores. A sample FASTQ record is provided in Fig. 6. Depending on the number of sequence runs performed in **step 1**, there may be more than one FASTQ file for each sample produced in **step 2**.

```
@read1
ACGGACTATATAGGACCACACAGGACCACACACAGAGTAGCAGTACCAGA
+
::??:::???AAAAFFACAFAC:FAC?A:FAC?AF:CAAFF:AC?@@AC::
```

Fig. 6 A single FASTQ record. The first line contains the read label. The second line provides the sequenced bases, while the fourth line contains the per-base quality scores reported by the sequencer in ASCII format

2.2.2 Assess Quality of Sequence Reads

After the sequence reads have been produced by the sequencer, their quality should be assessed before any further analyses take place, as per **step 3**. For example, it is possible that contaminants could have been introduced during sample preparation (e.g., adapter dimers for the Illumina HiSeq 2000), which could cause meaningless sequences to be overrepresented. It is also possible that the base quality scores are unacceptably low, which indicates that the sequencer called the bases with low confidence. There are many more potential issues that can arise during the process of sample preparation and during the sequencing experiment. These issues can indicate errors in protocol and experimental setup, so it is critical that they are discovered early. Many sequencers include built-in programs to assess the quality of the sequencing experiments, but these are primarily designed to assess the quality of only the sequence data itself and not the experiment as a whole. FastQC is a stand-alone program that is commonly used to assess the quality of sequencing experiments [25]. It takes as input FASTQ files or BAM files and produces reports that evaluate the sequencing experiment on several criteria that help the researcher determine if the experiment is of acceptable quality. Some examples of FastQC's analysis modules are (1) GC content, (2) read duplication level, (3) quality score distribution, and (4) summaries of overrepresented sequences (if they exist). For each of the evaluation analysis modules, FastQC reports the test as either "Pass," "Fail," or "Warning." The results depend on set criteria that are determined by the program. The output returned by each analysis module may help the researcher determine if any further action should be taken to improve the quality of the sequencing dataset, or in some cases, it may indicate that the sequencing experiment must be repeated due to major issues with its setup and execution (*see* **Note 5**).

2.2.3 Align Tumor Reads and Normal Reads to the Reference Genome

Once the sequencer has generated reads for both the normal and tumor samples, they can be aligned to the reference genome, as per **step 4**. During read alignment, the sequence reads (which are usually between 100 and 300 base pairs in length) are compared to the reference genome to find the location that most closely matches the sequence on the read. Of course, it is possible that a single read may closely match more than one location on the reference genome. This is especially true for highly repetitive genomic regions. These ambiguous alignments are usually assigned very low mapping quality scores by short-read aligners and are often excluded from further SV analysis.

The alignment step should produce two different SAM files, each containing the alignments for (1) the tumor cell reads and the (2) normal (healthy) cell reads. As mentioned previously, programs like BWA and Bowtie/Bowtie2 can be used to create the SAM alignments, given sequence reads in FASTQ format and a reference genome in FASTA format. The FASTQ files containing the normal and tumor reads should be aligned separately to create two different SAM files. If analyzing SVs in human cancers, the reference genome should be the current version of the human reference genome or at least a subset of the reference genome that may indicate a particular region of interest. As of the date of this publication, the current version of the Genome Reference Consortium human reference genome is GRCh38.

2.2.4 Take Resulting SAM Alignment Files for Both the Tumor and Healthy Data from *Step 4* and Convert Them to BAM

Per **step 5**, after the SAM alignment file has been created, it must be converted to a BAM file, which is the binary version of the SAM alignment file (which is a text file). BAM files are generally smaller than SAM files since they do not store text data, and many programs for SV analysis require the alignments to be stored as a BAM file. This conversion can be performed by the Samtools suite [11]. The following UNIX command is an example of how the Samtools 1.8 program can be used to convert a SAM file called "alignment.sam" into its equivalent BAM file, which is called "alignment.bam." The "-b" option tells Samtools to output binary data, and the "-h" option tells Samtools to include the SAM file header, which is required by many programs for further analysis.

```
samtools view -b -h alignment.sam > alignment.bam
```

2.2.5 Sort the BAM Files by Coordinates

Per **step 6**, we must use a BAM file that is coordinate sorted. Short-read alignment programs like BWA and Bowtie/Bowtie2 do not sort the read alignments by their position on the reference; they report the aligned position of the reads in the order by which they are encountered in the FASTQ file. Variant calling using BAM alignments requires the alignments to be sorted in increasing order by coordinate position. Samtools can be used to sort the alignments in a BAM file called "alignment.bam" as follows:

```
samtools sort -T alignment.sorted -o alignment.sorted.bam \
alignment.bam
```

The above command creates a new BAM file called "alignment.sorted.bam" that is coordinate sorted.

2.2.6 Remove Sequence Read Replicates from BAM Files

Step 7 in the aforementioned process describes sequence read replicate removal. In an ideal sequencing experiment, the target genome will be well represented at high coverage in the sequence reads in the resulting dataset. However, it is possible that during sequencing, some DNA fragment molecules may have been replicated many times over during library preparation via PCR amplification of the fragments. When sequenced, these molecules will contain reads that, when aligned, map to the same coordinates

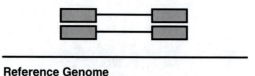

Fig. 7 The alignment of two read pairs with identical mapping coordinates for both reads. This is a likely PCR or optical artifact, so one of these read pairs should be removed before performing any analysis

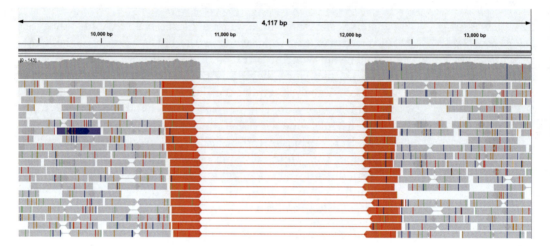

Fig. 8 The deletion event from Fig. 5, except with replicates removed. Note that the overall read depth has decreased, as shown in the coverage plot

multiple times in the SAM file. For Illumina sequencing technologies, it is also possible to have reads that are optical replicates, in which the same cluster on the flow cell is read more than once, even though it corresponds to only a single molecule. It is desirable to remove (or at least greatly reduce) the number of these replicates, because for genomic studies, they are redundant and thus add no new information that can be used in analysis. Furthermore, their inclusion increases the size of the BAM alignment file(s) which can hinder downstream analysis. Figure 7 depicts the alignment of replicated read pairs to the reference genome with identical mapping coordinates for both reads. Figure 8 presents the same deletion event shown in Fig. 5, except with duplicate read pairs removed. Furthermore, for depth-of-coverage SV analysis, replicates can confound analyses because when aligned to the reference, they can resemble copy number amplification, which is not necessarily accurate.

For paired-end data, replicates are generally identified by the following rule: if a read pair X shares (for both reads) its mapped coordinates with another read pair Y, and if the reads belonging to X and Y are of equal length, then we say that read pairs X and Y are replicates and one of them must be removed before any further

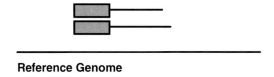

Reference Genome

Fig. 9 The two reads align the reference at identical positions in a single-end dataset. Based on the mapping of the reads, it is unknown if the molecule is a replicate since there is no second read to compare coordinates to. The reads in the figure were generated from molecules of different lengths, so these cannot be the result of a PCR or optical replicate

analyses can take place. It is possible that a replicate is not a PCR artifact or an optical replicate, however. For example, a molecule could have been generated from the sample region by chance. However, the redundancy should still be eliminated for the aforementioned reasons. For single-end sequencing data, read duplication may be determined by comparing different reads to see if they have the same mapping coordinates. However, this could be a dangerous assumption because, for example, two reads with identical mapping coordinates could belong to molecules of different lengths (*see* **Note 6**). This would suggest that the reads are in fact not replicates. Figure 9 depicts the alignment of two reads with identical coordinates in a single-end read library. Assessing the presence of read replicates is generally a much harder task for single read data, so great care must be taken before removing potential replicates in these kinds of datasets. If incorporating RNA sequencing (RNA-seq) into any analysis of DNA structural variants, caution must also be exercised before removing replicates, as a highly expressed gene will naturally produce transcripts that are repeated hundreds of times. This will create a large number of molecules that are sequenced from the same region. This level of replication is due to the gene's expression and not necessarily due to biased PCR amplification of the same molecule, for example.

Once it has been determined that the replicated sequence reads are safe to remove, they can be removed from the BAM alignments via programs such as Samtools and Picard [26]. Samtools can remove from the BAM alignment file any sequence read that is marked as a duplicate. The Picard suite contains a program called MarkDuplicates that can be used to mark duplicated reads or to remove them entirely from the BAM file(s). The following UNIX command demonstrates how Picard MarkDuplicates (version 2.18.9) can be used to remove replicates from a paired-end BAM file called "alignment.sorted.bam." In this case, a file called "alignment.sorted.nodup.bam" is created which represents the read alignments with replicates removed. In this example, we are informing Picard that the BAM file is coordinate sorted and that identified duplicates should be removed. We are also specifying "metrics.txt" as the required metrics file, which will store various statistics about the alignments in the BAM file.

```
java -jar picard.jar MarkDuplicates \
INPUT=alignment.sorted.bam \
OUTPUT=alignment.sorted.nodup.bam \
ASSUME_SORT_ORDER=coordinate REMOVE_DUPLICATES=true METRICS_-
FILE=metrics.txt
```

2.2.7 (Paired-End Data Only) If the NGS Dataset Is Paired-End and If No Read-Depth Analysis Is Being Performed, Remove All Concordant Read Alignments from the BAM Files

Per **step 8**, removing concordant read pair alignments may be necessary. Programs that find SVs by examining read pair alignments usually rely on the presence of mapped read pairs with a *discordant* alignment. As previously stated, discordantly mapped read pairs are those with mapping characteristics that are different than what is expected if there was no structural variation. For modern sequencers, the size of the sequence fragments typically ranges between 200 and 500 bases in length. For an aligned read pair that does not flank an SV breakpoint, we expect the aligned positions of the paired reads to reflect this length. We also expect reads in a pair to map to the same chromosome. For Illumina sequencing, we also expect the reads to align to different strands (forward strand and reverse strand). If **any** of these criteria are violated, however, we say that the alignment is discordant, meaning that the read pair alignment could indicate a possible nearby SV. To predict an SV, variant analysis programs require that many of these discordant read pairs to be present and in close proximity to eliminate the possibility that the ostensible variants are not there due to chance. If the paired-read alignment is "normal," then we say that the alignment is *concordant*. A concordant alignment is the opposite of a discordant alignment, and it means that all of the following criteria are true: (1) the mapped distance between reads is what is expected on average, (2) both reads map to the same chromosome, and (3) both reads align with forward-reverse orientation (for Illumina sequencing), meaning that the read alignment closest to the p-arm telomere aligns to the forward strand, while its mate aligns to the reverse strand. A concordant read alignment is a likely indicator that there is no structural variant near the read pair coordinates. Figure 5 presents discordant read pair alignments (red) that overlap a 1.2-kb deletion flanked by concordant alignments (gray) that do not overlap an SV.

Since concordant alignments are not typically indicative of an SV, programs that identify SVs using **only** discordant paired-end alignments usually ignore them. However, if performing copy number or read-depth analysis using paired-end data, concordant read pairs are useful. For example, a region with amplified copy number will have increased read depth and thus a larger number of concordant alignments. As another example, a researcher may want to determine if a variant is heterozygous, meaning that it only

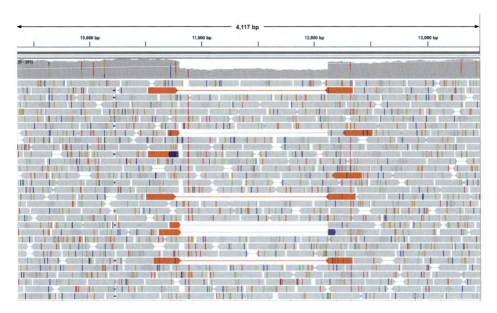

Fig. 10 A heterozygous deletion event. The deletion is spanned by long discordant read pairs (red), but concordant read pairs (gray) from the unaffected chromosome are also found within the variant's coordinates

occurs on one of the two homologous chromosomes. In this case, the SV region will contain a mixture of discordant and concordant alignments. Figure 10 depicts a region containing a heterozygous deletion that features a mixture of both discordant and concordant alignments. Without the concordant alignments, it is difficult to determine if the SV is homozygous or heterozygous (*see* **Note 7**). It is also impossible to perform accurate copy number analysis since there is no way to determine if there is a copy number amplification or deletion at that location without using concordant alignments. If any kind of read-depth analysis is being performed (e.g., using a DOC-based SV program or a program that determines if an SV is heterozygous), then concordant alignments should **not** be removed.

If no read-depth analysis is needed for paired-end data, then it is safe to remove the concordant alignments **once** we determine (or at least accurately estimate) the mean and standard deviation (or median absolute deviation) of the insert sizes for the library fragments. The average insert size is the average length of each molecule prior to sequencing. This quantity can be estimated by determining the average distance between the outer ends for each concordantly mapped read pair. Note that many SV programs estimate these values automatically **assuming that the concordant alignments have been retained.** Removing concordant paired alignments can greatly reduce the size of the BAM files. However, if concordant paired alignments must be removed, then these values must be computed and stored beforehand or else the SV program(s) will not know how to identify deletions or small insertions; it will not know how to define a read pair alignment as being longer or shorter than expected.

The following Picard 2.18.9 command will create a file called "statistics.txt" which contains the estimated mean insert length and its standard deviation, and it also creates a file called "hist.txt" which plots a histogram representing the distribution of insert sizes. Note that this command assumes the BAM file is chromosome sorted.

```
java -jar picard.jar CollectInsertSizeMetrics \ INPUT=alignment.sorted.nodup.bam \
OUTPUT=statistics.txt ASSUME_SORTED=true HISTOGRAM_FILE=hist.txt
```

Now that the statistics have been collected, we now know the mean and insert size of the mapped read pairs. To remove the concordant read pairs, the sequence reads can be realigned to the reference genome using read alignment software such as BWA. If there are enough read pairs, BWA will automatically mark alignments as not mapped in a proper pair if they are larger than what is expected, based on the distribution of insert sizes. The maximum insert length can also be set manually as a parameter to BWA; that value should be based on the insert size statistics computed in the previous step.

After marking the long insert lengths as abnormal, we can remove all concordant alignments via the following Samtools 1.8 command (which writes the alignments to a file called "alignment.sorted.nodup.nocon.bam").

```
samtools view -b -F 14 alignment.sorted.nodup.bam \
> alignment.sorted.nodup.nocon.bam
```

The "-F 14" argument tells Samtools to exclude records for reads (1) that are unmapped, (2) that are mapped in a proper pair (thus excluding abnormally long-read alignments and read pairs that do not map with forward-reverse standard Illumina orientation), and (3) where only one mate maps to the reference. Thus, the new BAM file will only contain discordant read pair alignments. However, as mentioned previously, many SV detection programs can estimate insert size mean and standard deviation given the BAM file containing concordant pairs. Thus, the step of removing concordant alignments can be skipped if disk space is not an issue. Also, if the SV program uses only signals based on the alignment of single reads and **not** discordant read pairs, this step should be skipped entirely. Such programs include CREST and Pindel.

2.2.8 Create BAM Index Files (.bai) from the Sorted BAM Alignments

Even when stored in a binary .bam file, read alignments may require a large amount of space when stored to disk. This can make the task of retrieving specific alignment records daunting. For example, for a BAM file sorted by chromosome and coordinates, if a researcher wanted to retrieve only chromosome 20 alignments, then a program that does this would have to search through all chromosome 1 through chromosome 19 alignments before finding the ones it needs. This would otherwise be an arduous process. However, per **step 9**, for any sorted BAM file, we can create an accompanying bam index file (.bai). When the index file is created, we can specify the reference genome coordinates of a read alignment anywhere in the BAM file. Index files can be created with the following Samtools command.

```
samtools index alignment.sorted.nodup.bam \
 alignment.sorted.nodup.bam.bai
```

The above command creates a BAM index file called "alignment.sorted.nodup.bam.bai." Since the index file is now created for the BAM file, we can now perform random-access retrieval of alignments. For example, the following UNIX Samtools command will print to the console all chromosome 5 read alignments that map to any coordinate position between 1 and 100,000.

```
samtools view alignment.sorted.nodup.bam chr5:1-100000
```

Retrieval of these alignments will happen immediately, and the process does not have to wait for the program to scan chromosome 1–4 alignments. Note that the above example assumes that the index file associated with the above bam file is the one with ".bai" affixed to the end of the BAM file name.

Creating index files for the BAM files is not only useful for quickly retrieving alignments, but it is usually required for many programs that analyze BAM alignments, including structural variant analysis programs. These programs will usually notify the user if an associated index file is missing (remember that for the above example, the associated index file is the one with ".bai" affixed to the end of the BAM file name).

2.2.9 Apply the Structural Variant Detection Program to the BAM Files

For **step 10**, we apply the chosen structural variant discovery program(s) to the BAM file that has been cleaned of replicates. The program can also be applied to BAM files that have been cleaned of concordant read pairs if those pairs will not be used in analysis. In the remainder of this chapter, we will assume that paired-end data has been used and that concordant read pairs have not been removed, since many SV programs ignore them anyway. For single read data, there are several programs that can be used, such as CREST and Pindel for general SV detection. For copy number variant detection, programs like SegSeq [22], CNVnator [27], and RDXplorer [23] can be used.

For **step 10**, there are several programs that exist for locating SVs using paired-end NGS data. As stated beforehand, examples of such programs include BreakDancer, VariationHunter, GASV, and SVDetect [28]. Once the BAM files have been created for both the normal dataset and the tumor dataset, and once they have undergone the treatment previously described, we can apply any of these programs to the BAM file(s) so that they can find the structural variants in each genome. As stated previously, these programs find structural variants by locating the anomalously mapped (i.e., discordant) read pairs, like those that span the deletion event in Fig. 5. Once these programs have been applied to both the normal and tumor BAM files, a list of structural variant predictions for each BAM file will be produced by the program, including the predicted type of the variants and their predicted genomic coordinates. Please consult the documentation of your desired SV analysis program for details on how to use them to analyze BAM alignment files.

2.2.10 If the SV Program Does Not Automatically Filter Germline SVs, Remove from the List of Tumor Structural Variant Calls All of Those SVs that Overlap with the Healthy Data SVs

In **step 11**, we remove germline SVs from the list of predicted variants. In the list of tumor SVs, we assume that the germline SVs are those that also occur in the healthy dataset. When samples are collected for sequencing, the tumor DNA will usually contain a mixture of tumor and healthy cells due to normal cell contamination. Thus, if SV analysis is *only* performed on the tumor data with no filtering, then it's possible that some of the predicted SVs are germline variants that occurred in the contaminating healthy cells (or were inherited from an ancestral healthy cell). Somatically acquired variants are of greater clinical significance, and we assume that these variants only occur in the tumor genome. Thus, at the end of our pipeline, we want a list of the SVs that occur **only** in the tumor sample. Several SV analysis programs perform germline variant filtering, such as VarScan [29]. If the SV analysis program does not perform automated filtering of germline variants, there are some SV analysis programs that are packaged with separate programs that perform this filtering. The DELLY program, which is a hybrid paired-end and split-read method, can also filter germline variants.

Once the somatic structural variants have been identified, they should be validated experimentally, since the analyses performed so far have been in silico. Once the variants have been identified and validated, they can be used in a clinical setting to devise specific therapies for the patient that target the SVs and the oncogenic products and symptoms they engender.

3 Notes

1. Algorithms for structural variant detection rely on the presence of *many* of these abnormally mapped read pairs.

2. DELLY considers the mapping characteristics of read pairs *and* single reads.

3. During sequencing, regions with very high (or very low) levels of G and C bases produce fewer molecular fragments from which the end(s) can be sequenced. This leads to fewer sequence reads being generated from these regions.

4. **Step 4** assumes that the tumor cells sequenced during the experiment are subject to normal cell contamination, in which a cell culture contains an admixture of healthy and tumorous cells. This is a common occurrence when collecting tumor cells (e.g., during biopsies). During sequencing, this causes the tumor sample library to contain reads generated from both tumor cells and healthy cells [30].

5. For example, as part of a previous unpublished research project undertaken by the author, FastQC revealed unacceptably high levels of sequence duplication in a sequence dataset, which was determined to be a result of errors in sample preparation. The sequence library was subsequently discarded and recreated.

6. Please note that FastQC measures sequence duplication by counting the number of replicate individual reads and not the number of replicate read pairs. Assessing sequence duplication by considering only single reads could be problematic for the reasons stated. Also, FastQC requires exact sequence matches in to call duplicates. However, PCR duplicate reads will not necessarily share the same sequence content since sequencer base-calling error is a possibility.

7. It may be possible to determine if a variant is heterozygous by only examining discordant read pairs, but this would require a read-depth analysis of discordant read pairs, which is difficult since read depth is affected by more factors than just the copy number at that location (such as PCR bias and GC-bias).

References

1. Baker M (2012) Structural variation: the genome's hidden architecture. Nat Methods 9(2):133–137. https://doi.org/10.1038/nmeth.1858
2. Tuzun E, Sharp AJ, Bailey JA, Kaul R, Morrison VA, Pertz LM, Haugen E, Hayden H, Albertson D, Pinkel D, Olson MV, Eichler EE (2005) Fine-scale structural variation of the human genome. Nat Genet 37(7):727–732. https://doi.org/10.1038/ng1562
3. Human Genome Structural Variation Working Group, Eichler EE, Nickerson DA, Altshuler D, Bowcock AM, Brooks LD, Carter NP, Church DM, Felsenfeld A, Guyer M, Lee C, Lupski JR, Mullikin JC, Pritchard JK, Sebat J, Sherry ST, Smith D, Valle D, Waterston RH (2007) Completing the map of

human genetic variation. Nature 447 (7141):161–165. https://doi.org/10.1038/447161a

4. Mills RE, Walter K, Stewart C, Handsaker RE, Chen K, Alkan C, Abyzov A, Yoon SC, Ye K, Cheetham RK, Chinwalla A, Conrad DF, Fu Y, Grubert F, Hajirasouliha I, Hormozdiari F, Iakoucheva LM, Iqbal Z, Kang S, Kidd JM, Konkel MK, Korn J, Khurana E, Kural D, Lam HY, Leng J, Li R, Li Y, Lin CY, Luo R, Mu XJ, Nemesh J, Peckham HE, Rausch T, Scally A, Shi X, Stromberg MP, Stutz AM, Urban AE, Walker JA, Wu J, Zhang Y, Zhang ZD, Batzer MA, Ding L, Marth GT, McVean G, Sebat J, Snyder M, Wang J, Ye K, Eichler EE, Gerstein MB, Hurles ME, Lee C, McCarroll SA, Korbel JO, Genomes P (2011) Mapping copy number variation by population-scale genome sequencing. Nature 470(7332):59–65. https://doi.org/10.1038/nature09708

5. Genomes Project Consortium, Abecasis GR, Altshuler D, Auton A, Brooks LD, Durbin RM, Gibbs RA, Hurles ME, GA MV (2010) A map of human genome variation from population-scale sequencing. Nature 467 (7319):1061–1073. https://doi.org/10.1038/nature09534

6. Nowell PC (1962) The minute chromosome (Phl) in chronic granulocytic leukemia. Blut 8:65–66

7. Soda M, Choi YL, Enomoto M, Takada S, Yamashita Y, Ishikawa S, Fujiwara S, Watanabe H, Kurashina K, Hatanaka H, Bando M, Ohno S, Ishikawa Y, Aburatani H, Niki T, Sohara Y, Sugiyama Y, Mano H (2007) Identification of the transforming EML4-ALK fusion gene in non-small-cell lung cancer. Nature 448(7153):561–566. https://doi.org/10.1038/nature05945

8. Liu L, Li Y, Li S, Hu N, He Y, Pong R, Lin D, Lu L, Law M (2012) Comparison of next-generation sequencing systems. J Biomed Biotechnol 2012:251364. https://doi.org/10.1155/2012/251364

9. Li H, Durbin R (2009) Fast and accurate short read alignment with Burrows-Wheeler transform. Bioinformatics 25(14):1754–1760. https://doi.org/10.1093/bioinformatics/btp324

10. Langmead B (2010) Aligning short sequencing reads with Bowtie. Curr Protoc Bioinformatics Chapter 11:Unit 11.7. doi:https://doi.org/10.1002/0471250953.bi1107s32

11. Li H, Handsaker B, Wysoker A, Fennell T, Ruan J, Homer N, Marth G, Abecasis G, Durbin R, Genome Project Data Processing Subgroup (2009) The sequence alignment/map format and SAMtools. Bioinformatics 25 (16):2078–2079. https://doi.org/10.1093/bioinformatics/btp352

12. Hormozdiari F, Alkan C, Eichler EE, Sahinalp SC (2009) Combinatorial algorithms for structural variation detection in high-throughput sequenced genomes. Genome Res 19 (7):1270–1278. https://doi.org/10.1101/gr.088633.108

13. Sindi S, Helman E, Bashir A, Raphael BJ (2009) A geometric approach for classification and comparison of structural variants. Bioinformatics 25(12):i222–i230. https://doi.org/10.1093/bioinformatics/btp208

14. Rausch T, Zichner T, Schlattl A, Stutz AM, Benes V, Korbel JO (2012) DELLY: structural variant discovery by integrated paired-end and split-read analysis. Bioinformatics 28(18): i333–i339. https://doi.org/10.1093/bioinformatics/bts378

15. Chen K, Wallis JW, McLellan MD, Larson DE, Kalicki JM, Pohl CS, McGrath SD, Wendl MC, Zhang Q, Locke DP, Shi X, Fulton RS, Ley TJ, Wilson RK, Ding L, Mardis ER (2009) BreakDancer: an algorithm for high-resolution mapping of genomic structural variation. Nat Methods 6(9):677–681. https://doi.org/10.1038/nmeth.1363

16. Ye K, Schulz MH, Long Q, Apweiler R, Ning Z (2009) Pindel: a pattern growth approach to detect break points of large deletions and medium sized insertions from paired-end short reads. Bioinformatics 25 (21):2865–2871. https://doi.org/10.1093/bioinformatics/btp394

17. Abel HJ, Duncavage EJ, Becker N, Armstrong JR, Magrini VJ, Pfeifer JD (2010) SLOPE: a quick and accurate method for locating non-SNP structural variation from targeted next-generation sequence data. Bioinformatics 26(21):2684–2688. https://doi.org/10.1093/bioinformatics/btq528

18. Schroder J, Hsu A, Boyle SE, Macintyre G, Cmero M, Tothill RW, Johnstone RW, Shackleton M, Papenfuss AT (2014) Socrates: identification of genomic rearrangements in tumour genomes by re-aligning soft clipped reads. Bioinformatics. https://doi.org/10.1093/bioinformatics/btt767

19. Wang J, Mullighan CG, Easton J, Roberts S, Heatley SL, Ma J, Rusch MC, Chen K, Harris CC, Ding L, Holmfeldt L, Payne-Turner D, Fan X, Wei L, Zhao D, Obenauer JC, Naeve C, Mardis ER, Wilson RK, Downing JR, Zhang J (2011) CREST maps somatic structural variation in cancer genomes with

base-pair resolution. Nat Methods 8(8):652–654. https://doi.org/10.1038/nmeth.1628

20. Robinson JT, Thorvaldsdottir H, Winckler W, Guttman M, Lander ES, Getz G, Mesirov JP (2011) Integrative genomics viewer. Nat Biotechnol 29(1):24–26. https://doi.org/10.1038/nbt.1754

21. Karakoc E, Alkan C, O'Roak BJ, Dennis MY, Vives L, Mark K, Rieder MJ, Nickerson DA, Eichler EE (2012) Detection of structural variants and indels within exome data. Nat Methods 9(2):176–178. https://doi.org/10.1038/nmeth.1810

22. Chiang DY, Getz G, Jaffe DB, O'Kelly MJ, Zhao X, Carter SL, Russ C, Nusbaum C, Meyerson M, Lander ES (2009) High-resolution mapping of copy-number alterations with massively parallel sequencing. Nat Methods 6(1):99–103. https://doi.org/10.1038/nmeth.1276

23. Yoon S, Xuan Z, Makarov V, Ye K, Sebat J (2009) Sensitive and accurate detection of copy number variants using read depth of coverage. Genome Res 19(9):1586–1592. https://doi.org/10.1101/gr.092981.109

24. Wu Y, Tian L, Pirastu M, Stambolian D, Li H (2013) MATCHCLIP: locate precise breakpoints for copy number variation using CIGAR string by matching soft clipped reads. Front Genet 4:157. https://doi.org/10.3389/fgene.2013.00157

25. FastQC. http://www.bioinformatics.babraham.ac.uk/projects/fastqc/. Accessed 14 Jan 2015

26. Picard Tools. http://picard.sourceforge.net. Accessed 15 Jan 2016

27. Abyzov A, Urban AE, Snyder M, Gerstein M (2011) CNVnator: an approach to discover, genotype, and characterize typical and atypical CNVs from family and population genome sequencing. Genome Res 21(6):974–984. https://doi.org/10.1101/gr.114876.110

28. Zeitouni B, Boeva V, Janoueix-Lerosey I, Loeillet S, Legoix-ne P, Nicolas A, Delattre O, Barillot E (2010) SVDetect: a tool to identify genomic structural variations from paired-end and mate-pair sequencing data. Bioinformatics 26(15):1895–1896. https://doi.org/10.1093/bioinformatics/btq293

29. Koboldt DC, Chen K, Wylie T, Larson DE, McLellan MD, Mardis ER, Weinstock GM, Wilson RK, Ding L (2009) VarScan: variant detection in massively parallel sequencing of individual and pooled samples. Bioinformatics 25(17):2283–2285. https://doi.org/10.1093/bioinformatics/btp373

30. Gusnanto A, Wood HM, Pawitan Y, Rabbitts P, Berri S (2012) Correcting for cancer genome size and tumour cell content enables better estimation of copy number alterations from next-generation sequence data. Bioinformatics 28(1):40–47. https://doi.org/10.1093/bioinformatics/btr593

Chapter 4

CORE: A Software Tool for Delineating Regions of Recurrent DNA Copy Number Alteration in Cancer

Guoli Sun and Alexander Krasnitz

Abstract

Collections of genomic intervals are a common data type across many areas of computational biology. In cancer genomics, in particular, the intervals often represent regions with altered DNA copy number, and their collections exhibit recurrent features, characteristic of a given cancer type. Cores of Recurrent Events (CORE) is a versatile computational tool for identification of such recurrent features. Here we provide practical guidance for the use of CORE, implemented as an eponymous R package.

Key words Somatic copy number alterations, Combinatorial optimization, R language, Parallelization

1 Introduction

Somatic DNA copy number alterations (SCNA) are ubiquitous in cancer [1]. SCNA arise in tumors as a result of genomic instability, owing to dysregulation of DNA replication and to abnormalities of cell division. While these genomic events occur at random in neoplastic cells, some of them confer selective advantage on the host cells, and, as a result, SCNA patterns tend to recur in cell populations within a tumor [2] and across tumors of the same type in multiple individuals [3]. Additionally, genomic instability may manifest itself in a regular, genomic region-specific manner, again leading to recurrence of copy-number alterations.

If copy-number event recurrence is driven by positive selection, the extent and boundaries of each recurrent event are determined by the genomic content of the affected region. In some cases, such as ERBB2 amplification in breast cancer [4], such region may enclose a single oncogene. Alternatively, selective advantage may be acquired by hemizygous deletion of several neighboring and cooperating tumor suppressor genes [5]. Finally, if the recurrence is a direct result of genomic instability, large portions of the genome, such as entire chromosome arms, may be gained or lost.

Thus, the study of recurrent copy number alterations in cancer requires a method capable of handling the full spectrum of copy number events, from focal to chromosome size.

Furthermore, genuine recurrence must be distinguished from a chance accumulation of copy-number events at a genomic location. To make this distinction, one must introduce a quantitative measure of recurrence and be able to assess the statistical significance of the observed value, i.e., to determine how likely this value is to arise in an appropriate null distribution.

In response to these requirements, we have developed a method termed Cores of Recurrent Events (CORE), an algorithm for quantification and statistical assessment of recurrence in interval data [6]. The idea and principles of CORE are explained in detail in our publication. Here we provide practical guidance to the use of CORE, implemented as an eponymous R package, in cancer genomics, and do not present the theory of the method beyond a brief qualitative outline.

Given a collection of genomic intervals, CORE derives a small set of intervals most representative of the collection. These are termed cores and determined in two steps. First, for any desired number of cores, we consider all possible candidate sets of cores. For each interval in the collection, we compute a score, ranging between 0 and 1, of how well the interval is represented by the candidate set. Summing these quantities over the entire collection, we obtain the overall representation score of the collection by the candidate set and choose the cores so as to maximize this overall score. As a result of this optimization, each core will approximately delineate an interval recurrent in the collection.

The overall score increases with each additional core. As we increase the number of cores, we will eventually account for all the recurrence in the collection. From that point on, any additional core, and an increase in the score that comes with it, will be as expected in a random collection of intervals with no recurrence. Based on this intuition, CORE estimates, for each additional core, the statistical significance of the corresponding increment in the score, by comparing the observed value to its null distribution in random collections of intervals. The result is tabulated as p-value and is used to determine the necessary and sufficient number of cores.

CORE is implemented in R language as an eponymous package [7]. The package contains a single function, also called CORE. The implementation is versatile thanks to the multiple arguments of the CORE function and the multiple values of each argument. We next provide an informal tutorial, illustrated by examples, of how the CORE package is applied to tumor-derived copy-number data. This type of presentation is termed a vignette in the R user community.

2 Methods

2.1 Package Installation

Both the source code and binary executables for CORE are available from The Comprehensive R Archive Network (CRAN). From an R terminal session, the package is installed on the host computer by executing install.packages("CORE",repos="@CRAN@"). The user is then presented with a menu of CRAN mirror sites. For most users, any mirror may be selected. However, in some cases, an access to HTTPS mirror sites may be blocked. If this occurs, the last item on the menu (HTTP mirrors) should be selected, resulting in an HTTP mirror menu. A selection of a site from the latter will trigger the installation. Once installed, the package must be attached to the current R session as follows: library(CORE). CORE may then be listed along with other objects attached to the session, by invoking the search() function with no arguments.

2.2 Input Preparation for CORE Analysis

CORE can analyze for recurrence any collection of intervals, with each interval specified by its start and end coordinates. In the special case of SCNA, these intervals correspond to copy-number altering events (CNAE). A CNAE is an amplification (gain) or deletion (loss) of a genomic fragment. These events are derived from raw data, which in most present-day studies are acquired by short-read sequencing of the tumor genomes of interest. CNAE derivation from this type of data is a multi-step process, described in detail in our publication [8], and we recommend the use of software tools presented therein. CNAE may also be derived from data acquired by use of earlier technologies, such as comparative genomic hybridization (CGH) [9] or single-nucleotide polymorphism (SNP) [10] microarrays. Extensive literature and multiple software tools exist for copy-number analysis of data acquired by these platforms.

In order to enable the use of CORE, this preprocessing should result in two objects corresponding to arguments dataIn and boundaries of the CORE function. For the initial CORE analysis, dataIn argument must be an integer matrix with at least three columns. The first two columns tabulate, in each row, the start and end coordinates of an interval. For the cancer-related genomic applications discussed here, the intervals each correspond to a CNAE. For the analysis to be meaningful, all CNAE tabulated in dataIn must be of the same kind, either amplifications or deletions. The third column, which is optional for a generic call to CORE but is necessary in genomic applications, must contain, for each interval, the number of the chromosome in which the interval is located.

All the data in dataIn must be integer-valued. For the chromosome column, this is achieved by denoting each autosome by its number and by enumerating X and Y chromosomes as 23 and 24 in the human or 20 and 21 in the mouse genome. It is possible to use integer genomic coordinates. However, in SCNA-related applications, the copy number is usually computed at discrete locations distributed and enumerated throughout the genome. For data from short-read sequencing, these are bins into which the genome is divided in order to estimate copy number from read counts in each bin. For data from microarrays, these are genomic locations to which oligonucleotide probes on the array map. With these enumerated locations used as coordinates, the input copy-number data are represented at the resolution at which they were derived.

As an option, the dataIn matrix may have an additional column, tabulating, for each CNAE, a nonnegative weight to be given to the CNAE when computing the core scores. For example, the weight may be made equal (or proportional) to the copy-number alteration by the CNAE. Thus, a CNAE corresponding to a homozygous deletion would have twice the weight of the one corresponding to a loss of a single copy.

It is strongly recommended that an input object also be supplied for the boundaries argument of CORE. This object should be a matrix with three columns, corresponding to the chromosome number, and the start and end coordinates for each chromosome, using the same genomic coordinate system as for the dataIn object. While optional, this additional object is required to obtain more accurate estimates for the statistical significance of cores.

2.3 A Survey of CORE Arguments

The CORE function has multiple arguments, most of which are optional and/or have default values. For many of the arguments, the meaning is self-evident, and we need not go beyond the CORE manual page to explain them. Here we focus on the few arguments for which this is not the case.

CORE computes, for each core and each CNAE in the dataIn matrix, a measure of association, i.e., a score of how closely the CNAE is approximated by the core. The measure of association is specified by assoc argument of CORE. The argument must have one of three possible values, "I," "J," or "P." For "I," the score is zero unless the core is contained in CNAE, and then the score is the ratio of the core length to that of the CNAE. For "J" the score is the Jaccard index for the core-CNAE pair of intervals, i.e., the length ratio between their intersection and union. In particular, the score vanishes if the two intervals do not overlap. The "P" score is 1 if the core is contained in the CNAE and 0 otherwise. These rules are illustrated in Fig. 1.

These definitions of the measures of association may be modified by setting the pow argument to a value different for 1. As a result, the desired power of the chosen measure of association will be used by CORE to compute scores.

Being an iterative procedure, CORE requires a terminating condition for the iteration. Two arguments, maxmark and minscore, can be used as termination criteria, separately or in combination.

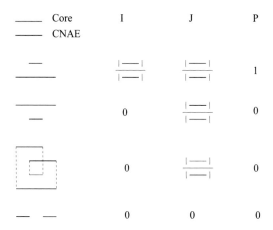

Fig. 1 The "I," "J," and "P" association rules used by the CORE. The diagrams in the leftmost column show the four possible relative positions of the CNAE and the core for which the score is computed. For each of these positions, the formulas for the score are listed in the three appropriate columns on the right. The | | symbol denotes the length of the enclosed interval

The former sets the number of cores to be computed. The latter specifies the minimal score a core is allowed to have. The iterative procedure is terminated if any one of the two conditions is met.

CORE offers the user two alternative definitions of the null distribution of scores, as set by the shufflemethod argument. These correspond each to a rule for randomizing the input collection of intervals. If the argument is set to "SIMPLE," the lengths of intervals are fixed at their original values, and each original interval is placed randomly into a new position, such that it fits entirely in one of the chromosomes. This rule is highly restrictive for long intervals; for example, a CNAE that spans most of chromosome one cannot be placed in any other chromosome. This restriction is relaxed by setting the shufflemethod argument to "RESCALE." With this choice, each original interval may be placed at random in any chromosome, and its length is changed such that it constitutes the same portion of the destination chromosome as it did of the chromosome of origin.

Multiple randomizations are required in order to assess statistical significance of the observed core scores, resulting in time-consuming computation for large input collection of intervals. The execution time may be shortened considerably by choosing one of two parallelization options offered by CORE, as determined by the distrib argument, whose default value, "vanilla," results in randomizations being performed sequentially. If the latter is set to "Rparallel," CORE will utilize the architecture of the central processing unit (CPU) on which the current R session is running to initiate a number of randomization processes in parallel.

Alternatively, if the current R session is running on a node of a computing cluster, and if the cluster uses a grid engine such as Sun Grid Engine (SGE), the distrib argument may be set to "Grid." As CORE is executed with this option, temporary files may be created in the current working directory. These files are deleted by CORE by the time the execution is completed. With either option, the number of parallel randomization processes is set to the value of the argument njobs. However, if "Rparallel" is chosen as shufflemethod, the input value of njobs may be overridden by CORE if it is inappropriately large for the host CPU. Importantly, the results of the randomization process neither depend on the value of shufflemethod nor on that of njobs.

This section has left unexplained the keep argument, which determines the policy of continuing CORE analysis from an intermediate point. This explanation is given later in the chapter, following the discussion of the CORE output object.

2.4 CORE Value and Execution from an Intermediate Point

CORE returns an R object of class "CORE," essentially a list containing as items both the results of the computation and all the data necessary to restart CORE from the point at which it exits. Among the items in the former category are coreTable and p. coreTable is a matrix with one row per core computed, with cores listed in the descending order of their scores. For each core, the start and end coordinates and the score are listed. The p object is a numeric vector of p-values for the statistical significance of cores, as estimated by randomization, and listed in the same order as the cores in coreTable.

The remaining items of the "CORE" object include the values of all the arguments with which the CORE function was called. With these data available, the CORE function may be invoked with the dataIn argument set to a "CORE" object resulting from an earlier run. This capability is useful if, for example, the earlier run has not determined all statistically significant cores, and further cores must be computed and examined for significance.

The keep argument of the CORE function allows the user some control over the CORE execution from such an intermediate point. In doing so, CORE follows the policy of making as much use as possible of the result at the intermediate point. For example, one may at first compute core positions and scores for a certain number of cores, without assessing the statistical significance of scores, then use the value from that CORE function call to set dataIn argument for a new call, in which statistical significance of scores is assessed, but no new cores are computed.

2.5 An Example

The CORE package contains two data items. One, a data frame called testInputCORE, contains a collection of CNAE (all gains) derived from a study of copy-number variation in individual cells harvested from a breast tumor [2]. The underlying copy-number profiles were obtained using next-generation sequencing, by dividing the human genome into 50009 bins and modeling the copy number from read counts in each bin. The start and end coordinates of each CNAE are the ordinal numbers of bins where, respectively, the CNAE starts and ends. The second object, called testInputBoundaries, contains, for each chromosome, the numbers of the first and the last bin in the chromosome. These objects are attached to the current session using the data function, as in data (testInputCORE). The contents and structure of each data frame can be examined, e.g., by issuing head(testInputCORE,5).

In the first example, CORE is invoked to compute the first 20 cores without statistical assessment:

> myCOREobj<-CORE(dataIn=testInputCORE,maxmark= 20,
nshuffle=0,boundaries=testInputBoundaries,seedme=123)

As a result, a "CORE" object called myCOREobj has been generated. Names of items comprising myCOREobj may be listed by issuing names(myCOREobj). One of these is coreTable, a matrix containing the locations and scores of the cores computed by the call to CORE:

> head(myCOREobj$coreTable,5)
   chrom start end score
[1,] 8 24645 26343 74.71347
[2,] 9 26674 26734 74.21248
[3,] 3 9892 10088 72.14078
[4,] 3 10530 10667 66.21470
[5,] 7 23128 23863 65.44517

Next, we compute additional cores, increasing the total number to 100. Note that, with myCOREobj as input, time will be saved, as the original 20 cores will not be recomputed. Note also that statistical assessment of all cores is performed, with eight-core parallelization to speed up the execution.

newCOREobj<-CORE(dataIn=myCOREobj,

keep=c("maxmark","seedme","boundaries"),

nshuffle=200,shufflemethod="RESCALE",njobs=8)

It is instructive to examine the results graphically. As shown in Fig. 2, the core score declines as the core number increases. The empirical core p-value, initially at the minimum of 0.00495 possible for 200 randomizations, eventually begins to grow until statistical significance is lost at the 89th core, using the customary 0.05 as the cutoff p-value.

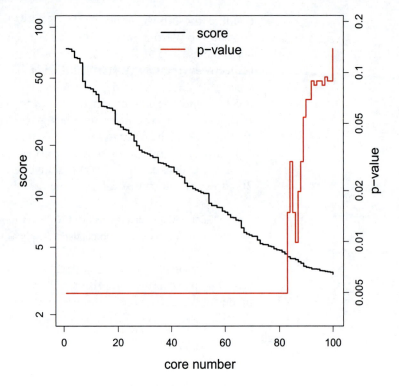

Fig. 2 Scores and empirical *p*-values for the 100 cores computed in the example (Subheading 2.5)

References

1. Beroukhim R, Mermel CH, Porter D, Wei G, Raychaudhuri S, Donovan J, Barretina J, Boehm JS, Dobson J, Urashima M, Mc Henry KT, Pinchback RM, Ligon AH, Cho YJ, Haery L, Greulich H, Reich M, Winckler W, Lawrence MS, Weir BA, Tanaka KE, Chiang DY, Bass AJ, Loo A, Hoffman C, Prensner J, Liefeld T, Gao Q, Yecies D, Signoretti S, Maher E, Kaye FJ, Sasaki H, Tepper JE, Fletcher JA, Tabernero J, Baselga J, Tsao MS, Demichelis F, Rubin MA, Janne PA, Daly MJ, Nucera C, Levine RL, Ebert BL, Gabriel S, Rustgi AK, Antonescu CR, Ladanyi M, Letai A, Garraway LA, Loda M, Beer DG, True LD, Okamoto A, Pomeroy SL, Singer S, Golub TR, Lander ES, Getz G, Sellers WR, Meyerson M (2010) The landscape of somatic copy-number alteration across human cancers. Nature 463(7283):899–905. https://doi.org/10.1038/Nature08822

2. Navin N, Kendall J, Troge J, Andrews P, Rodgers L, McIndoo J, Cook K, Stepansky A, Levy D, Esposito D, Muthuswamy L, Krasnitz A, McCombie WR, Hicks J, Wigler M (2011) Tumour evolution inferred by single-cell sequencing. Nature 472 (7341):90–94. https://doi.org/10.1038/Nature09807

3. Hicks J, Krasnitz A, Lakshmi B, Navin NE, Riggs M, Leibu E, Esposito D, Alexander J, Troge J, Grubor V, Yoon S, Wigler M, Ye K, Borresen-Dale AL, Naume B, Schlicting E, Norton L, Hagerstrom T, Skoog L, Auer G, Maner S, Lundin P, Zetterberg A (2006) Novel patterns of genome rearrangement and their association with survival in breast cancer. Genome Res 16(12):1465–1479. https://doi.org/10.1101/Gr.5460106

4. Krishnamurti U, Silverman JF (2014) HER2 in breast cancer: a review and update. Adv Anat Pathol 21(2):100–107. https://doi.org/10.1097/PAP.0000000000000015

5. Xue W, Kitzing T, Roessler S, Zuber J, Krasnitz A, Schultz N, Revill K, Weissmueller S, Rappaport AR, Simon J, Zhang J, Luo W, Hicks J, Zender L, Wang XW, Powers S, Wigler M, Lowe SW (2012) A cluster of cooperating tumor-suppressor gene candidates in chromosomal deletions. Proc

Natl Acad Sci U S A 109(21):8212–8217. https://doi.org/10.1073/pnas.1206062109
6. Krasnitz A, Sun G, Andrews P, Wigler M (2013) Target inference from collections of genomic intervals. Proc Natl Acad Sci U S A 110(25):E2271–E2278. https://doi.org/10.1073/pnas.1306909110
7. Sun G, Krasnitz A (2014) CORE: cores of recurrent events. https://cran.r-project.org/package=CORE
8. Kendall J, Krasnitz A (2014) Computational methods for DNA copy-number analysis of tumors. Methods Mol Biol 1176:243–259. https://doi.org/10.1007/978-1-4939-0992-6_20
9. Bajjani BA, Theisen AP, Ballif BC, Shaffer LG (2005) Array-based comparative genomic hybridization in clinical diagnosis. Expert Rev Mol Diagn 5(3):421–429
10. Mei R, Galipeau PC, Prass C, Berno A, Ghandour G, Patil N, Wolff RK, Chee MS, Reid BJ, Lockhart DJ (2000) Genome-wide detection of allelic imbalance using human SNPs and high-density DNA arrays. Genome Res 10(8):1126–1137. https://doi.org/10.1101/gr.10.8.1126

Chapter 5

Identification of Mutated Cancer Driver Genes in Unpaired RNA-Seq Samples

David Mosen-Ansorena

Abstract

The identification of cancer driver genes through the analysis of mutations detected with high-throughput sequencing is a useful tool and a key challenge in cancer genomics. The workflow presented here relies on unpaired RNA-seq tumoral samples, thus leveraging already available RNA-seq data and providing the intrinsical benefits of directly targeting the transcriptome. Based on well-established methods for variant detection, this workflow also involves thorough data cleaning and extensive annotation, which enable the selection for somatic mutations with functional impact and the prioritization of genes relevant to the carcinogenic processes in the input samples.

Key words High-throughput sequencing, RNA-seq, Mutations, Cancer, Driver genes

1 Introduction

High-throughput sequencing (HTS) technologies have enabled systematic genome-wide analyses that have contributed to the identification of genomic and transcriptomic signatures across cancer types. In particular, the pursuit of single nucleotide variants that underlie carcinogenic processes is a major theme in today's cancer research. Variants can be detected by sequencing the genome (whole genome sequencing, WGS), the exome (WES), or the transcriptome (RNA-seq). While either WGS or WES data are more commonly used in this kind of analysis, RNA-seq is a promising technology. For instance, the inherently available transcriptional information indicates which coding variants are expressed and, therefore, more likely to be relevant. In addition, RNA-seq data directly targets the transcriptome, providing deep coverage without target enrichment. Finally, when RNA-seq data is already available for evaluation of gene expression profiles, one can further leverage the data to define expressed mutational profiles.

It is important to understand the limitations of each sequencing approach, as there are several technical and biological factors

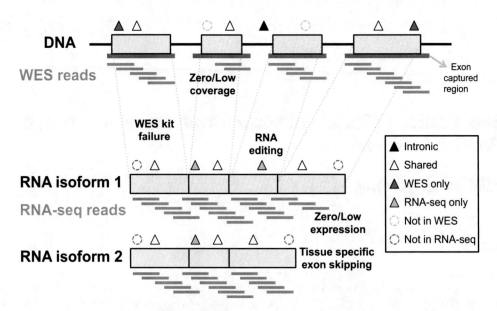

Fig. 1 Comparison between WES data and RNA-seq data. WES reads will be generated on the exome-captured regions. RNA-Seq reads will be generated based on gene expression conditions. Variants may exist in various locations of the genome, including introns adjacent to exons in the DNA and locations within the transcriptome. Variants that are in the introns, shared by WES and RNA-seq and WES only and RNA-seq only, are colored in black, white, dark gray, and light gray, respectively. Variants not included in WES due to the low coverage, WES kit failure, or RNA editing are represented with light gray dotted circles. Variants not included in RNA-seq due to the low expression or coverage are represented with dark gray dotted circles. Adapted from O'Brien et al. (2015) [22] with permission from Elsevier

that restrict which variants each technique can detect and to what extent. Figure 1 depicts some of these differences. An apparent limitation of both WES and RNA-seq is their restriction to the exome and the transcriptome, respectively. Conversely, given the same amount of reads, WES and RNA-seq provide deeper coverage of genetic regions than WGS. Coverage constraints and variability constitute yet another main source of inconsistency across technologies. For example, in the case of RNA-seq, loss-of-function mutations in tumor suppressor genes may lead to nonsense-mediated decay. In the case of WES, the exome enrichment step limits coverage to the capture regions and introduces irregularities in the coverage caused by variable GC content. In terms of purely biological factors, intra-tumoral heterogeneity and normal cell contamination are ubiquitous factors in the three technologies, while cell- and tissue-specific expression, allele- and strand-specific expression, transcriptional preference, and RNA editing are further molecular mechanisms that affect RNA-seq, given that they alter the total and relative frequency of variant alleles. While these issues specific to RNA-seq complicate variant detection, they have the potential to provide richer information on the mutational landscape.

Here, we describe a procedure to identify cancer driver genes from expressed single-nucleotide mutations, otherwise simply called mutations throughout the text. More specifically, the input to the workflow comprises two sets of RNA-seq samples, tumoral and normal, which do not need to be matched. The alignment of the RNA-seq reads is followed by a succession of extensive data cleaning that involves correction and filtering at the read level and at the variant level, once variants are called. Remaining mutations are annotated and evaluated, allowing to score and rank genes based on the mutations they harbor and their recurrence across the tumoral samples.

2 Materials

The input to this workflow is a set of FASTQ files or SAM/BAM files, depending on whether sequencing reads have already been aligned. Each file, or group of them, will correspond to either a tumoral sample or to one of the normal samples that will be used as controls. The additional required information includes an assembly of the human genome, sets of known germline variants in that genome, and a database that predicts the effects of not only such variants but of most possible genomic variants.

The human genome FASTA file should be accompanied by its corresponding index and dictionary. These files are all available at the Broad's FTP (ftp://gsapubftp-anonymous@ftp.broadinstitute.org/bundle). If you obtain the FASTA file from somewhere else, the index and the dictionary may be created with SAMtools [1] and Picard Tools [2], software packages that are described in the next section.

The workflow requires at least two sets of known variants, represented in the variant calling format (VCF), one with single-nucleotide polymorphisms (SNPs) and another one with insertions and deletions (INDELs). Generally, SNPs from the dbSNP database [3] and INDELs both detected by Mills et al. [4] and coming from the 1000 Genomes phase 1 are used. These datasets can be downloaded from the Broad's FTP as well.

Ensembl's Variant Effect Predictor (VEP) [5] consists of a set of databases and associated tools used to annotate variants, determine their consequence on the protein sequence (e.g., stop gained, missense), and provide quantitative predictions on their functional impact. The human database, together with the VEP perl script, which accesses the database, needs to be installed and is available from http://www.ensembl.org/info/docs/tools/vep/script/index.html.

3 Methods

The analysis of paired DNA-seq samples for variant detection is quite streamlined and extensive literature can be found about it [6, 7]. Recently, integrated analysis of DNA-seq and RNA-seq data has gathered some attention too, as it increases variant detection performance [8]. In turn, the focus here is on the detection of expressed mutations using RNA-seq samples in conjunction with unmatched normal samples. The rationale is that time, cost, and availability constraints can limit the analysis to tumoral RNA-seq data. We will address the limitations arising from the lack of matched normal samples and DNA-level data.

A key consideration is that an appropriate workflow should identify and control the main sources of false-positive variants derived from our unpaired RNA-seq data. False-positive mutations can be roughly classified into what are actually germline variants and technical artifacts, observed due to factors that may include PCR-related issues, sequencing errors, misalignments, and batch effects. In addition to direct containment measures on the aforementioned, it is possible to set hard thresholds on a range of indicators, such as read depth, and assess functional impact, which tends to be greater in driver mutations.

The data analysis consists of these individual steps, which are performed at the read, variant, and gene level, as shown in Fig. 2:

1. Align reads to reference.
2. Preprocess alignments.
3. Read splitting and hard clipping.

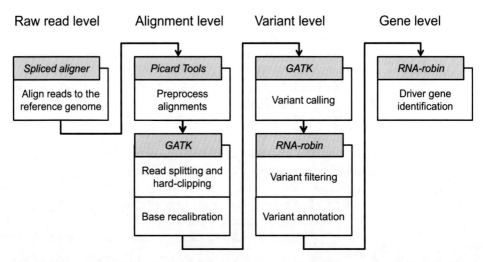

Fig. 2 Main steps in the computational workflow described in Subheading 2. After preprocessing of the alignment data, GATK bridges the gap between the alignment and variant levels, while RNA-robin takes variant information and outputs results at the gene level

4. Base recalibration.
5. Variant calling.
6. Variant filtering.
7. Variant annotation.
8. Driver gene identification.

Steps 2–4 involve data cleanup at the read level, **steps 5–7** relate variant discovery, and **step 8** is performed at the gene level. SAMtools [1] and Picard Tools [2] offer somewhat overlapping sets of tools for the manipulation, reading, writing, and indexing of raw FASTA and alignment of SAM/BAM files. Their combination is required for the preparation of non-indexed genomes prior to the workflow should it be necessary, but Picard Tools alone should suffice for **step 2** of the analysis. The Genome Analysis Toolkit or GATK [9, 10] is a software package that focuses on HTS variant discovery and genotyping. We will use GATK for further processing on the alignments and variant calling (**steps 3–5**). Finally, RNA-robin is an R package that performs variant filtering and annotation (**steps 6** and **7**), followed by driver gene identification (**step 8**), completing the set of required software. RNA-robin can be downloaded from http://scholar.harvard.edu/david/workflows/md, where indications to download the other required tools and data are provided, together with step-by-step instructions to follow the workflow.

3.1 Align Reads to the Reference

Next-generation sequencers generally produce sequences of tens to hundreds of bases that are read from the ends of DNA or RNA molecules. Typically, reads are stored in FASTQ files. Because the workflow here described involves the detection of mutations from RNA-seq, our input will be FASTQ files with RNA reads, which will already carry biases that arise in steps prior to our in silico analysis, mainly in the sample preparation and sequencing (*see* **Note 1**).

The original transcriptome represented by our short RNA reads is reconstructed by mapping, or aligning, the reads back to a reference genome. While many genome aligners can in principle be used on RNA-seq data, spliced aligners are tools specifically devised to tackle the extra tasks of detecting exon-intron boundaries and splicing reads across exons. Two interesting aligners for our purpose are the STAR 2-pass method [11], which provides high sensitivity and specificity in variant calling [12], and MapSplice [13], a conservative aligner with respect to mismatch frequency, indel and exon junction calls [14]. The output of each alignment should be a SAM file or a BAM file, its binary counterpart.

3.2 Preprocess Alignments

If you already have the alignment files, it is worthwhile to examine what the parameterization of the alignment was, as it might influence downstream results (*see* **Note 2**). In any case, before taking the subsequent steps in the analysis, each BAM file should undergo some preprocessing, in order to assign a single read group to all of its reads, sort it, mark duplicate reads, and index it. This whole preprocessing is conveniently packed into a couple of commands through Picard Tools.

Sorting and indexing BAM files allow GATK to access read information more quickly, without going through all the reads sequentially. In turn, assigning a single read group per BAM file specifies that all the reads contained in it come from the same source, regardless of whether the corresponding sample was sequenced in several lanes.

Arguably, the removal of duplicate reads also deserves further explanation, given its relevance in the analysis. Indeed, if PCR duplicates cover a putative variant, their allele will be overrepresented, skewing the allelic frequency of the variant. They can also generate false-positives if random sequencing errors occur early on during PCR and get sufficiently amplified. Duplicate reads tend to provide high read-depth support and are identifiable because their outer ends map to the same positions on the genome (*see* Fig. 3). Picard Tool's MarkDuplicates removes duplicates by first matching all reads (or read pairs) with the same 5′ coordinates and mapping orientation. It then marks as duplicates all but the best read, defined in terms of its bases' qualities. This way, the downstream GATK tool will know it should ignore the marked reads.

3.3 Read Splitting and Hard Clipping

CIGAR strings are sequences of letters that describe how reads align to the genome and, as such, they indicate if and where splicing occurs within a read, through the N operator. For instance, 20M1000N30M is indicative of a spliced read mapping 20 and

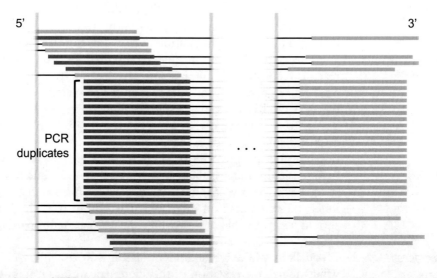

Fig. 3 Depiction of PCR duplicates for the case of paired-end reads. Once reads are aligned, duplicate fragments appear as pairs of reads with the same 5′ start position and the same length. Here, read pairs are connected by a black line, where the left read is dark and the right read is light gray

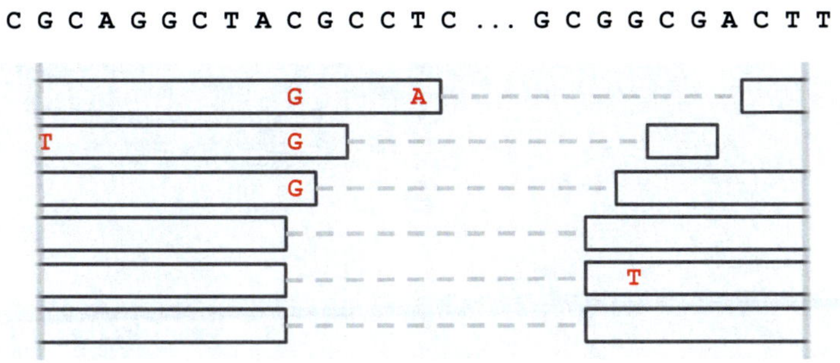

```
CGCAGGCTACGCCTC ... GCGGCGACTT
```

Fig. 4 Toy example of how reads spanning an exon-exon junction may have been aligned. The read splitting is depicted as a light-gray discontinuous line. Mismatches against the reference sequence are highlighted in the reads. The high similarity between the 5′ end of the intron and the 3′ end of the second exon is the main cause here for the overhangs, which will probably result in the call of a spurious C->G variant unless GATK's Split'N'Trim is applied

30 bases to 2 different exons, with a 1,000 bp gap between them that is likely an intron. In order to map a spliced read, spliced aligners typically require a minimum number of bases covering each of the exons involved in a junction. If there is not enough coverage in one of the exons and, especially, if there is some sequence similarity between the border of this exon and the neighboring intronic region of the other exon, a small fraction of the read will misalign into the intron (*see* Fig. 4). Therefore, without proper correction, nucleotide positions near exon junctions are prone to harboring false-positives and false-negatives due to such alignment issue. GATK's Split'N'Trim (*see* **Note 3**) gets rid of the N operators and splits each read into smaller reads corresponding to its exon segments. Then, sequences overhanging into the intronic regions are hard-clipped. This approach might be preferable to downstream filtering of variants around exon-exon junctions (*see* **Note 4**).

3.4 Base Recalibration

Base quality scores are estimates of error emitted by sequencing machines. Such scores, however, can be misestimated due to random and systematic sequencing errors at certain genomic positions, which can potentially result in false-positive variant calls. In data coming from sequencing-by-synthesis, random base mismatches with the reference are associated with sequencing technology, position in the read (machine cycle), and sequence context. For instance, the mismatches tend to occur toward the end of the reads and in AC dinucleotides, rather than in TG.

Base quality score recalibration, as performed by GATK, updates scores based on the empirically observed mismatch rate, given the aforementioned known covariates (*see* Fig. 5). This creates more accurate base qualities, which in turn improves the accuracy of variant calling. In a first step, reads are tabulated into bins using information on quality score, machine cycle, and dinucleotide

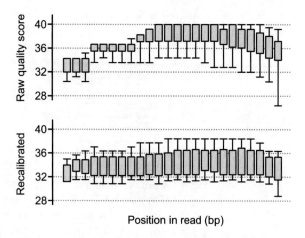

Fig. 5 Toy example showing boxplots of raw and recalibrated base quality scores by base position in the reads. Raw scores had overestimated qualities, especially in the center positions of the reads

context. Then, the new scores are calculated using the overall difference between reported and empirical scores, the effect of the covariates, and the bin-specific score shifts.

It is important to note that known SNPs, taken from dbSNP [3], are removed from the recalibration process. Otherwise, they would artificially inflate the mismatch rates, which would subsequently bring down in excess the corrected quality scores. Less common variants and somatic mutations still affect the recalibration process to a lesser extent but are not removed given that they are unknown at this point.

3.5 Variant Calling

HaplotypeCaller (HC) is GATK's recommended tool for variant calling in RNA-seq, given that it is able to incorporate into its algorithm the information that Split'N'Trim embeds in the BAM files on intron-exon split regions. In a prior step to variant calling and after some initial filtering (*see* **Note 5**), HC performs local de novo reassembly in each region around loci with evidence of containing a variant, identifying the haplotypes with highest likelihood based on the reassembly graph. This initial process has the potential to capture INDELs previously missed by the alignment software. Then, a pair hidden Markov model (pair HMM) is used to align the reads against each haplotype, resulting in a matrix of likelihoods of the haplotypes given the reads. These likelihoods are marginalized over the haplotypes to obtain the likelihoods of individual alleles given the reads. Variants are called at loci where there is sufficient evidence for an alternative allele based on the reads. Specifically, GATK's general recommendation is to use a phred-scaled confidence threshold of 20 to call variants. However, in this workflow, we want to be more stringent in order to minimize the amount of false-positives, so thresholds of 30 or even 40 are appropriate on the tumoral samples. In the case of the normal samples, it is the other way around, as our aim is to capture as many non-somatic variants as possible in order to filter them from the tumoral samples in the next step. Thus, going as low as 10 is appropriate here.

3.6 Variant Filtering

A key step to minimize the amount of false positives is the application of a range of vigorous filters. At the read level, we already removed secondary alignments and presumed PCR duplicates. Now, at the variant level, the first step taken by RNA-robin is to filter out variants that are present in the normal samples or in databases of known variants, not well supported by reads (*see* **Note 6**) or suspiciously being associated to a certain sequencing batch. The objective is to reduce the initial set of variants to a collection where most of the variants are likely to be somatic mutations, in opposition to having a germline or artifactual origin.

To elaborate, known germline variants, particularly those gathered in the dbSNP and ExAC [15] databases, are filtered out, except for variants that co-locate with well-known mutations according to the COSMIC [16] database, which are white-listed. Accompanying normal samples are used to further filter germline variants that may not be present in databases. This filtering has the additional benefit of discarding variants that were called due to, for instance, shared recurrent sequencing errors at certain loci. Any variant called in the normal samples is removed from the tumoral sample set. RNA-robin also checks whether the variants in the tumoral samples harbor significantly more alternative allele reads than the pool of normal samples, discarding those that do not.

3.7 Variant Annotation

The functional impact of a missense mutation in the coding fraction of the genome is a score that estimates its damaging effects on the protein product. This is useful here because passenger mutations tend to have lower deleterious effects and driver genes tend to accumulate mutations with greater deleterious effect. For variants with predicted functional impact, RNA-robin takes the merged predictions from several methods. In turn, it assigns the maximum functional score to mutations that result in stop codon gain or loss according to Ensembl's VEP [5]. A variant at a certain genomic locus may overlap and affect multiple transcripts. Because we do not know the relative presence of the variant in each of the transcripts, RNA-robin takes a conservative approach and computes the overall variant impact as the mean impact across transcripts.

Out of n reads aligning to a transcriptomic k-mer with uniqueness m, only n*m are expected to actually come from such region, given that 1/m k-mers exist in the transcriptome with the same sequence. Therefore, a read provides support to the corresponding allele of a variant proportionally to the uniqueness of the k-mer where it maps. More specifically, because aligners generally allow reads to map with a few mismatches, the term alignability [17] is

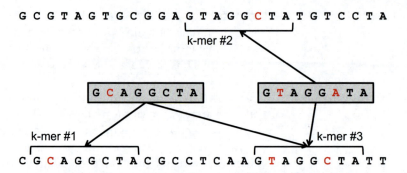

Fig. 6 Toy example depicting two 8 bp reads and how they can be aligned to a two-sequence transcriptome with up to one mismatch. K-mer #1 has a uniqueness of 1, but an alignability of 0.5, because reads with one mismatch containing its sequence can also be aligned to k-mer #3. In turn, k-mer #3 is also unique in this transcriptome, but has an alignability of 0.33, because introducing up to one mismatch in a read coming from it can result in an alignment to any of the three k-mers in the figure, depending on where the mismatch lies

more appropriate in this context, where alignability values are computed taking alignment mismatches into consideration (*see* Fig. 6). Contemplating these values provides us with information to downweigh the variants' support. Specifically, RNA-robin calculates variant alignability scores by averaging the precomputed alignabilities of k-mers to which reads supporting the alternative allele map. Such scores can be hard-filtered, which is a common approach (*see* **Note 7**), and used to weight mutational scores.

3.8 Driver Gene Identification

RNA-robin exploits a set of technical and biological indicators to score genes, predict their probability of being cancer drivers, and annotate them. Similar methods for DNA-seq exist but use other sources of information suited for their data (*see* **Note 8**). The aforementioned variant call quality, normalized by depth (*see* **Note 9**), functional impact, and alignability are used to filter and weight the individual scores of the mutations considered at this point, which are then summated gene-wise in order to get gene scores. For each gene, a p-value is assigned based on the probability of a gene randomly accumulating at least the gene's score, given the total score of all remaining mutations and the number of genes assessed in the workflow. Thus, the score and the p-value take into account the mutational frequency, as well as factors of technical origin and biological relevance.

Thanks to the extensive filtering and annotation, we were able to discard most of the germline variants in the tumoral samples. Yet, given that the workflow does not take matched normal samples as input, we have no way of knowing for sure whether our remaining variants are somatic. Importantly, this is the case of some cancer somatic mutations that co-locate with germline variants. Genes with variants in these loci are therefore flagged.

Table 1
Example of top-ranked genes in an analysis

Gene	FImpact	Alig	AFreq	AReads	#loci	#samples	#muts	Score	P-val	Flags
KRAS	0.95	0.8	0.4	10	20	50	50	700	0.001	G
TP53	0.8	0.7	0.55	500	40	35	40	500	0.002	
AHNAK	0.7	0.35	0.5	100	10	60	80	400	0.005	HNA

After the gene symbol, the first few columns displayed in this table represent the mean functional impact, alignability, alternative allele frequency, and number of reads for the mutations in the corresponding gene. The number of loci and samples contributing to the total amount of found mutations, together with the total score, corresponding p-value, and flags, as described in the main text, are also displayed

Throughout the workflow, similar processes and filtering are applied to the normal samples. Still, we might detect recurrently mutated genes in the normal samples. While this might be biologically relevant, it might also be indicative that the genes are long and highly polymorphic, making them more likely to harbor rare germline variants that are not captured in the filtering process. Therefore, while polymorphic genes have been observed to be less likely to play a central role in carcinogenesis, they tend to rank higher in this analysis. To help with such issue, RNA-robin flags genes that present mutations in the normal samples or a high amount of known germline variants. Other indicators of a given gene being a false-positive or having an inflated score include a low-average mutational functional impact and a few samples/mutations accounting for most of the gene score.

The main output from RNA-robin consists of two tables, one with detailed information on the mutations and another one with the ranked genes, including score, p-value, and the described flags. See Table 1 for an example of this latter with top-ranked genes.

4 Notes

1. The fidelity of DNA polymerases in PCR (polymerase chain reaction) amplification processes is not perfect, thus introducing errors at a small but existing rate. The earlier PCR round an error appears, the more reads will reflect it, thus being more likely to produce a false positive variant. PCR duplicates are another consequence of the amplification. Some fragments are sequenced more than once, potentially skewing the allelic frequency of the variants. Sequencing errors, especially mismatches, are yet another potential source of false positives, although they are often recognizable because they are generally random and thus unlikely to overlap.

2. If at some point of the workflow, especially at the beginning, the software complains about a BAM file not having the chromosomes properly ordered, these are likely ordered lexicographically instead of karyotypically. Running Picard's ReorderSam will solve the issue. Also, it might be worthwhile to find out whether a GTF file was used as input for the alignment. Providing a GTF file to an aligner that supports such annotation might increase the amount of exon junctions that it finds, altering the discovery of variants around these regions.

3. GATK's authors plan to integrate Split'N'Trim into the tool's engine so that it will be done automatically where appropriate, so this step might not apply here if the workflow is carried out with newer versions of the tool.

4. Some software pipelines that make use of GATK versions prior to the inclusion of Split'N'Trim filter variant sites close to exon junctions as an alternative [18, 19]. Such filtering may be used in combination with Split'N'Trim, but Split'N'Trim by itself seems to greatly alleviate the problem.

5. There are multiple filters that GATK applies automatically before running HC. Importantly, these include removing secondary alignments and marked duplicate reads.

6. Low-confidence variants present low-quality scores, provided by HC. They also tend to be supported by less reads, so it is typical to use the number of reads instead. The minimum quality or number of reads that best separates variants of biological origin from those of artifactual origin depends on factors such as sequencing depth and error rate, but variant calling algorithms typically use thresholds that range between qualities of 20 and 30, and between 4 and 10 reads supporting the alternative allele or all alleles. Importantly, a threshold in terms of alternative allele frequency is also advisable, with a sensible value standing at 0.2, that is, 20%. Much lower thresholds on the frequency begin to include many artifacts and subclonal passenger mutations, whereas higher ones would start to miss clonal heterozygous mutations with some allelic imbalance.

7. Several methods for the detection of variants in RNA-seq follow this filtering approach. There are diverse approaches for filtering low-uniqueness regions, which may involve using software to create masks (e.g., BlackOps [20]), manually using BLAT [21] or just masking repetitive sequences in the genome, among others.

8. Various methods exist for the identification of mutational driver genes through the analysis of mutations called from DNA-seq data. However, technical and biological differences

exist between workflows for unpaired RNA-seq and the more common paired DNA-seq, making the set of suitable factors for driver gene identification different. Gene expression, for instance, has been used in DNA-seq-oriented methods, but, while expression inversely correlates with true mutation rate, correlation is direct with the amount of callable mutations, therefore making it complex to correct for it in RNA-seq.

9. GATK's variant calling quality depends on the number of reads supporting the alternative allele. Quality by depth is calculated by normalizing the former over the latter, thus getting a better picture of how well supported the variant is, independently of the number of reads.

References

1. Li H, Handsaker B, Wysoker A, Fennell T, Ruan J, Homer N, Marth G, Abecasis G, Durbin R (2009) The sequence alignment/map format and SAMtools. Bioinformatics 25:2078–2079. https://doi.org/10.1093/bioinformatics/btp352
2. Picard Tools. https://broadinstitute.github.io/picard/
3. Sherry ST, Ward MH, Kholodov M, Baker J, Phan L, Smigielski EM, Sirotkin K (2001) dbSNP: the NCBI database of genetic variation. Nucleic Acids Res 29:308–311. https://doi.org/10.1093/nar/29.1.308
4. Mills RE, Pittard WS, Mullaney JM, Farooq U, Creasy TH, Mahurkar AA, Kemeza DM, Strassler DS, Ponting CP, Webber C, Devine SE (2011) Natural genetic variation caused by small insertions and deletions in the human genome. Genome Res 21:830–839. https://doi.org/10.1101/gr.115907.110
5. McLaren W, Pritchard B, Rios D, Chen Y, Flicek P, Cunningham F (2010) Deriving the consequences of genomic variants with the Ensembl API and SNP effect predictor. Bioinformatics 26:2069–2070. https://doi.org/10.1093/bioinformatics/btq330
6. Cibulskis K, Lawrence MS, Carter SL, Sivachenko A, Jaffe D, Sougnez C, Gabriel S, Meyerson M, Lander ES, Getz G (2013) Sensitive detection of somatic point mutations in impure and heterogeneous cancer samples. Nat Biotechnol 31:213–219. https://doi.org/10.1038/nbt.2514
7. Koboldt DC, Zhang Q, Larson DE, Shen D, McLellan MD, Lin L, Miller CA, Mardis ER, Ding L, Wilson RK (2012) VarScan 2: somatic mutation and copy number alteration discovery in cancer by exome sequencing. Genome Res 22:568–576. https://doi.org/10.1101/gr.129684.111
8. Radenbaugh AJ, Ma S, Ewing A, Stuart JM, Collisson EA, Zhu J, Haussler D (2014) RADIA: RNA and DNA integrated analysis for somatic mutation detection. PLoS One 9:e111516. https://doi.org/10.1371/journal.pone.0111516
9. McKenna A, Hanna M, Banks E, Sivachenko A, Cibulskis K, Kernytsky A, Garimella K, Altshuler D, Gabriel S, Daly M, DePristo MA (2010) The genome analysis toolkit: a MapReduce framework for analyzing next-generation DNA sequencing data. Genome Res 20:1297–1303. https://doi.org/10.1101/gr.107524.110
10. DePristo MA, Banks E, Poplin R, Garimella KV, Maguire JR, Hartl C, Philippakis AA, del Angel G, Rivas MA, Hanna M, McKenna A, Fennell TJ, Kernytsky AM, Sivachenko AY, Cibulskis K, Gabriel SB, Altshuler D, Daly MJ (2011) A framework for variation discovery and genotyping using next-generation DNA sequencing data. Nat Genet 43:491–498. https://doi.org/10.1038/ng.806
11. Dobin A, Davis CA, Schlesinger F, Drenkow J, Zaleski C, Jha S, Batut P, Chaisson M, Gingeras TR (2013) STAR: ultrafast universal RNA-seq aligner. Bioinformatics 29:15–21. https://doi.org/10.1093/bioinformatics/bts635
12. Van der Auwera GA, Carneiro MO, Hartl C, Poplin R, del Angel G, Levy-Moonshine A, Jordan T, Shakir K, Roazen D, Thibault J, Banks E, Garimella KV, Altshuler D, Gabriel S, DePristo MA (2013) From FastQ data to high-confidence variant calls: the Genome Analysis Toolkit best practices pipeline. Curr Protoc Bioinformatics 43:11.10.1–11.10.33

13. Wang K, Singh D, Zeng Z, Coleman SJ, Huang Y, Savich GL, He X, Mieczkowski P, Grimm SA, Perou CM, MacLeod JN, Chiang DY, Prins JF, Liu J (2010) MapSplice: accurate mapping of RNA-seq reads for splice junction discovery. Nucleic Acids Res 38:e178. https://doi.org/10.1093/nar/gkq622

14. Engström PG, Steijger T, Sipos B, Grant GR, Kahles A, Rätsch G, Goldman N, Hubbard TJ, Harrow J, Guigó R, Bertone P (2013) Systematic evaluation of spliced alignment programs for RNA-seq data. Nat Methods 10:1185–1191. https://doi.org/10.1038/nmeth.2722

15. Exome Aggregation Consortium (ExAC), Cambridge, MA. http://exac.broadinstitute.org/

16. Forbes SA, Bindal N, Bamford S, Cole C, Kok CY, Beare D, Jia M, Shepherd R, Leung K, Menzies A, Teague JW, Campbell PJ, Stratton MR, Futreal PA (2011) COSMIC: mining complete cancer genomes in the Catalogue of Somatic Mutations in Cancer. Nucleic Acids Res 39:D945–D950. https://doi.org/10.1093/nar/gkq929

17. Derrien T, Estellé J, Marco Sola S, Knowles DG, Raineri E, Guigó R, Ribeca P (2012) Fast computation and applications of genome mappability. PLoS One 7:e30377. https://doi.org/10.1371/journal.pone.0030377

18. Wang C, Davila JI, Baheti S, Bhagwate AV, Wang X, Kocher J-PA, Slager SL, Feldman AL, Novak AJ, Cerhan JR, Thompson EA, Asmann YW (2014) RVboost: RNA-seq variants prioritization using a boosting method. Bioinformatics 3:1–3. https://doi.org/10.1093/bioinformatics/btu577

19. Piskol R, Ramaswami G, Li JB (2013) Reliable identification of genomic variants from RNA-seq data. Am J Hum Genet 93:641–651. https://doi.org/10.1016/j.ajhg.2013.08.008

20. Cabanski CR, Wilkerson MD, Soloway M, Parker JS, Liu J, Prins JF, Marron JS, Perou CM, Neil Hayes D (2013) BlackOPs: increasing confidence in variant detection through mappability filtering. Nucleic Acids Res 41:1–10. https://doi.org/10.1093/nar/gkt692

21. Kent WJ (2002) BLAT—the BLAST-like alignment tool. Genome Res 12:656–664. https://doi.org/10.1101/gr.229202

22. O'Brien TD, Jia P, Xia J, Saxena U, Jin H, Vuong H, Kim P, Wang Q, Aryee MJ, Mino-Kenudson M, Engelman J, Le LP, Iafrate AJ, Heist RS, Pao W, Zhao Z (2015) Inconsistency and features of single nucleotide variants detected in whole exome sequencing versus transcriptome sequencing: a case study in lung cancer. Methods 83:118–127. https://doi.org/10.1016/j.ymeth.2015.04.016

Chapter 6

A Computational Protocol for Detecting Somatic Mutations by Integrating DNA and RNA Sequencing

Matthew D. Wilkerson

Abstract

Somatic mutation detection is a fundamental component of cancer genome research and of the molecular diagnosis of patients' tumors. Traditionally, such efforts have focused on either DNA exome or whole genome sequencing; however, we recently have demonstrated that integrating multiple sequencing technologies provides increased statistical power to detect mutations, particularly in low-purity tumors upon the addition of RNA sequencing to DNA exome sequencing. The computational protocol described here enables an investigator to detect somatic mutations through integrating DNA and RNA sequencing from patient-matched tumor DNA, tumor RNA, and germline specimens via the open source software, *UNCeqR*.

Key words Somatic, Mutation, Cancer, UNCeqR, Open source, Protocol

1 Introduction

Identifying somatic mutations is essential for cancer genome characterization, whether the focus is a cohort of tumors or a single patient's tumor. Accurate and complete identification of mutations enables identification of driver mutations that could be targeted by therapy, prediction of patient outcome based on mutation status, and other applications [1–3]. The process of somatic mutation detection operates on high-quality tumor and germline sequencing [4]. On a high level, somatic mutation detection consists of comparing the alleles at each site in the genome that are observed in tumor sequencing to those alleles observed in germline sequencing from the same patient. Different tumor alleles versus germline alleles are suggestive of a somatic mutation, with confidence in a given mutation call related to the amount and the quality of sequencing evidence supporting the non-germline allele. One of the major challenges in somatic mutation detection is the correct differentiation of true mutations that are rare within the tumor versus sequencing and alignment errors masquerading as true mutations. In recent work [5], we demonstrated that integrating RNA sequencing with DNA whole exome sequencing led to superior accuracy versus DNA sequencing alone, with a marked boost in low-purity tumors. Our published method for integrated somatic mutation detection, *UNCeqR*, was the first of its kind and is open source. In this protocol, we focus on installation and input preparation and provide an extended description of options for different mutation calling strategies.

2 Materials

This protocol requires a computer with a Linux operating system installed, such as Red Hat Enterprise Linux or Ubuntu (available at http://www.ubuntu.com/). *To analyze sequencing data, the following additional materials are required:*

1. Genome sequence in FASTA format for the organism of interest
2. Aligned, sorted, indexed germline DNA sequencing in BAM [6] format
3. Aligned, sorted, indexed tumor DNA sequencing in BAM format
4. Aligned, sorted, indexed tumor RNA sequencing in BAM format

UNCeqR has been evaluated on BWA [7] DNA alignments and MapSplice [8] RNA alignments in earlier studies [9–17]. BAM files produced by other sequence aligners can also be utilized with *UNCeqR* [18, 19]; however, investigators should confirm that the tags and flags in their BAM file are compatible with their choice of data filtering provided by *UNCeqR*, as described in Subheadings 3.5 and 3.6. All alignments are required to be based on the same assembled genome sequence, e.g., hg19 or hg38.

3 Methods

UNCeqR concurrently evaluates multiple sequence alignment files in BAM format (germline DNA sequencing, tumor DNA sequencing, tumor RNA sequencing) proceeding sitewise through the genome. This is achieved by analyzing three simultaneous streams of alignment information, thus resulting in minimal memory usage. *UNCeqR* employs several layers of data quality filtering and makes somatic mutation predictions based on tumor DNA evidence, tumor RNA evidence, and the integration of tumor DNA and tumor RNA evidence (Fig. 1). This text uses the `Courier` font to

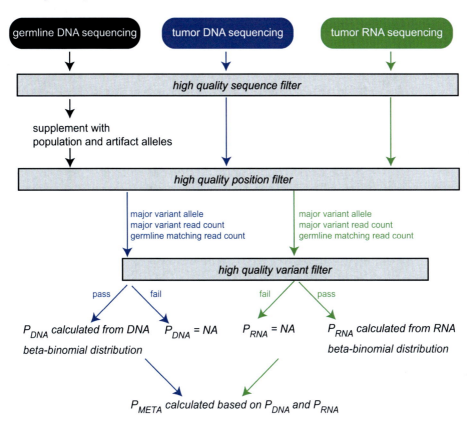

Fig. 1 Schematic of data models in integrated mutation detection

indicate the Linux command line, R commands, and options within *UNCeqR*. Bash commands are prefixed with $, and R commands are prefixed with >. The following steps are to be executed on the investigator's computer.

3.1 Install Prerequisite Software

UNCeqR requires R (available at https://www.r-project.org), one R library, and three Perl libraries. The R library VGAM [20] can be installed from within R on the investigator's computer.

The Perl libraries can be installed using cpan from the Linux command line as follows:

```
$cpan INSTALL Math::CDF
$cpan INSTALL Math::Cephes
$cpan INSTALL Getopt::Long
```

3.2 Install UNCeqR

First download *UNCeqR* from its repository by the following command:

```
$git clone https://github.com/mwilkers/unceqr.git
```

Then to install *UNCeqR*, follow the brief installation commands provided in the readme in the software. A template configuration file is included with the software, which contains computer-specific settings. To modify the template configuration file for your environment, copy this configuration file as follows:

```
$mv UNCeqR_conf.pl.template UNCeqR_conf.pl
```

Then, using a text editor, edit a few lines in the configuration file `UNCeqR_conf.pl`. Set the variable `localPath` to the full path of where you issued the git command for the *UNCeqR* installation (e.g., /home/username/unceqr/). Set the variable R to full path of the R executable on your computer. Set the variable `R_LIBS_USER` to the full path of your local R library directory (this can be verified by `>.libPaths()` from within R). Consult the example lines in `UNCeqR_conf.pl` for reference. If Perl libraries are installed in a nonstandard location, then edit `perlLib` to reflect the proper location; otherwise this string can be left "". To test your installation, enter:

```
$sh example.cmd
```

If successfully installed, the directory `test` should be created. `test/test.vcf` should be several lines representing mutations detected in the example BAM file, including a CAATT alternate allele. If `test.vcf` is not created, first examine `test/unceqr_stderror` for a potential error message, and verify that the paths above were entered correctly.

3.3 Define the Genome Regions in Which to Detect Mutations

Genome regions to be evaluated for somatic mutations are defined in the `regionsToQuery` file, which is a tab-delimited file listing the chromosome and start and stop position, with no header line. The start coordinate is 0-based and stop is 1-based. This file can be created in R, a simple text editor, or a spreadsheet program. For example:

```
1  14362  16765
1  16853  17055
```

For applications of somatic mutation calling involving DNA whole exome sequencing and RNA sequencing, an appropriate `regionsToQuery` file would contain known exons. This would restrict mutation calling to the regions expected to contain aligned sequence and would also serve as a filter against low-quality alignments. The Gene Annotation File [21] of The Cancer Genome Atlas could be used for this purpose.

For applications involving DNA whole genome sequencing, a `regionsToQuery` listing entire chromosomes would enable calling genome wide. Because particular regions of the human genome are associated with increased mutation calling errors, some investigators may opt to exclude these areas from `regionsToQuery`. For example, investigators may wish to exclude genomic regions of high repeat density, regularly low mappability, which can be obtained from sources as the UCSC genome browser [22], or by logic similar that employed by the Genome in a Bottle Consortium as callable [23]. Note that excluding regions completely prevents mutation detection in those regions by *UNCeqR*, so it is recommended to exclude only regularly problematic regions.

3.4 Compile an Allele Censor List Based on Population Polymorphisms and Sequencing Artifacts

When identifying germline alleles to be used in somatic mutation calling, *UNCeqR* takes information from three sources: germline sequencing (`normalDNA`), the reference genome (`fastaWchr` or `fastaWoChr`), and an optionable allele censor file, `snpFile`. The purpose of `snpFile` is to prevent putative false-positive alleles from being called somatic mutations; in other words, it is a hard censor list. `snpFile` contains a list of genomic sites and censor alleles at those sites, in a tab-delimited format with a header line. Multiple censor alleles at the same site are separated by a dash. For example:

```
#header line
1 100 A-T
1 101 A
1 120 ins
1 130 del
```

One type of false-positive somatic mutation is the unobserved germline polymorphism, which is a predicted tumor allele that is actually a germline variant but was not observed in germline sequencing due to shallow depth in the matched germline sequencing at a given genomic site. Common germline variants can be obtained from published sources such as the National Center for Biotechnology Information's dbSNP [24] or gnomAD [25]. Note that in addition to germline variants, these large databases can contain variants annotated as somatic, which should not be included in a `snpFile`, because they will be eliminated from somatic mutation detection. Also, these databases can contain somatic variants erroneously annotated as germline variants. The presence and extent of such possible alleles could be considered by the investigator, such as through comparing a given germline variant database version to a cancer variant database such as COSMIC [26] and determining the possible extent of such false-positive variants.

Another source of false-positive somatic mutations are "mapping-induced variants" in which highly similar short segments of related but distinct genome regions, such as from paralogous genes, are misaligned to the wrong genomic region and a true difference between the distinct paralogous gene loci is interpreted as a somatic mutation at the related, but incorrectly mapped, site. Mapping-induced variant calls can be generated for the specific read sequence lengths by the tools such as BlackOps [27] and incorporated into `snpFile`.

Another type of false-positive somatic mutations is "germline sequencing artifacts," which are variants that are commonly detected in sequencing on a given platform and sequence aligner that are not in dbSNP or other databases. This indicates that these variants are the likely consequence of common sequencing, alignment, and mutation detection errors. Germline sequencing artifacts can be generated by running *UNCeqR* on an independent cohort of germline sequencing specified (*see* **Note 4**) and selecting variants that are repeatedly called in germline samples which are not expected to contain somatic mutations. Germline sequencing artifacts are conceptually similar to the panel of normal sample filter described in [28]. For most somatic mutation calling applications, it is recommended that `snpFile` contains unobserved germline polymorphisms, mapping ambiguities, and germline sequencing artifacts.

3.5 Set Options for High-Quality Tumor Sequencing Data

Read sequences and read sequence alignments vary in their probability of being correct representations of biological truth, including base calls, aligned positions in the genome, and differences from genome sequence. Proper incorporation of sequencing data quality is important in somatic mutation detection so that low-quality data do not lead to abundant false positives [29]. *UNCeqR* applies two quality filters to sequencing data, a sequence filter and a position filter, that separate usable high-quality data from low-quality data.

The sequence filter excludes tumor sequence alignments with a mapping quality less than less than `minTMapQ`, with more than `maxNM` substitutions, insertions, or deletions derived from a read that aligns to more than `maxIH` locations in the genome or with a flag not compatible with flagFilter. Different alignment filtering is specified by value for `flagFilter` (0, no filtering; 1, only retain proper pairs; 2, remove secondary; 3, remove duplicates; 4, remove duplicates and secondary; 5, remove secondary, duplicate, and failures). The sequence filter then excludes tumor alignment bases within passed alignments that have base quality < `minTBaseQ` or are contained within the terminal `trimEnd` bases of the alignment.

The position filter excludes genomic sites with either a homopolymer exceeding `maxHomopolymer` nucleotides on either side and with a germline insertion or deletion with at least `normIndelFrac` allele fraction within `indelShadow` positions around the site and with less than `minNormCnt` germline depth. Then after this filtering, the position filter for the *UNCeqR* DNA model excludes genomic sites with less than `minDnaTumorCnt` filtered depth in tumor DNA sequencing and with greater than `maxDnaStruckProp` fraction of tumor DNA alignments filtered due to the sequence filter. For the *UNCeqR* RNA model, the position filter operates similarly but with `minRnaTumorCnt` and `maxRnaStruckProp`.

3.6 Set Options for Germline Sequencing

Germline sequencing can be filtered by the same high-quality sequence filter as for tumor sequencing; this filtering would reduce the alleles from germline sequencing that are eligible to be included in the germline allele set. Alternatively, germline sequencing does not have to be filtered which would result in all alleles from germline sequencing to be included in the germline allele set. The latter option is more aggressive in defining the germline sequencing set and thus may be more cautious in somatic calls. Readers are referred to the UNCeqR documentation to view the normal filtering options. Filtering on germline sequencing is indicated by `normal Loose`, `Y` indicates no sequence quality filtering, and `N` indicates sequence quality filtering. To restrict genome sites to those with enough germline sequencing depth in which to observe private germline variants in a given individual, sites can be restricted to those with germline sequencing depth at least `minNormCnt`.

At very high depths, a trace amount of false base calls are possible in germline sequencing. To exclude very infrequently observed alleles from being included in germline alleles, *UNCeqR* excludes alleles having a proportion less than `minInNormFrac` in germline sequencing.

3.7 Set Options for High-Quality Variant Data

With high-quality DNA or RNA tumor sequencing data for one high-quality genomic site, tumor alleles are compared to germline alleles to define a tumor allele count matching the germline alleles and variant alleles. The major variant allele is defined as the most frequent tumor allele among all variant alleles. Characteristics about the variant read evidence beyond the major variant count and reference count can affect the accuracy of the mutation prediction. To limit low-quality variants, several filters are applied to candidate variants.

The presence of multiple somatic mutations alleles in a tumor at the same site is suggestive of an artifact. An example of such a plural somatic variant site is presented in Fig. 2a. To control for such sites, the proportion of the major variant read count out of all variant read counts is required to be at least either `maxDnaTumorPluralProp` or `maxRnaTumorPluralProp`, for the respective model. Strand bias, an imbalance of variant read counts contained in forward or reverse aligning reads, is suggestive of an artifact [30]. To control for this, *UNCeqR* applies a chi-square test, on germline and variant read counts versus aligned strand, and requires the *p*-value to be greater than `maxDnaBias` or `maxRnaBias` for the respective model.

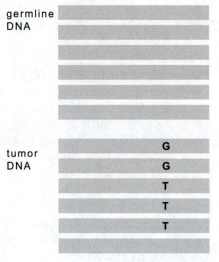
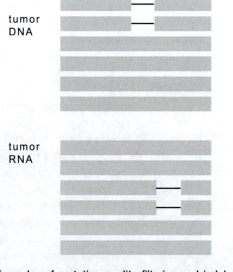

Fig. 2 Examples of mutation quality filtering and indel clustering. Gray boxes depict a sample's sequences aligned to the reference genome, which is

A lack of position variability among variants with respect to their parent alignment is suggestive of an artifact, as previously described [28, 29]. The distance of the variant's position in a read to the nearest read end is calculated. Variant sites are required to have a median absolute deviation of these distances greater than `medStart`. An example of a candidate variant with `medStart` equal to zero is presented in Fig. 2b. Candidate variants not meeting these filtering requirements are assigned a *p*-value of NA. This assignment indicates that the variant data were considered and could be considered in multiple testing correction depending on the investigator's interests.

3.8 Set Options for Insertion and Deletion Realignment

Detecting somatic insertions and deletions ("indels") in sequencing data is generally more difficult than somatic substitutions [31]. Features of neighboring genomic sequence can suggest several similar positions for an insertion or deletion mutation. These can be positioned at close but not identical sites among read alignments within the same sample. *UNCeqR* resolves indel alignment ambiguity by clustering insertions or deletions within 20 sites together. Within a cluster, the genomic site with the maximum major variant read count is selected, and all other insertion or deletion read counts in the cluster are transferred to this site. In this way, the maximum read count is considered for statistical testing. The motivation for this step relies on two principles: (1) multiple insertions or deletions are rarely expected within a short distance and (2) read aligners will often pick the true site most frequently. Investigators interested in detecting complex insertions and deletions should consider pre-processing BAM files with an indel realignment tool such as ABRA [32].

Similar to the indel placement difficulty within DNA or RNA sequencing, correspondence of indel positions between DNA and RNA is also difficult. Indels between DNA and RNA are similarly grouped together within a distance of 20 sites, for application of the meta model as described below. For example, Fig. 2c displays one case of a deletion at one position in tumor DNA (top track) and at a different position in tumor RNA (bottom track). Review of the genome sequence reveals a CTG repeating triplet, indicating the

Fig. 2 (continued) indicated in blue lettering. Different sequencing types (germline DNA, tumor DNA, tumor RNA) belonging to a sample are grouped together and labeled on the left hand side. Alleles not matching the reference sequence are depicted in black lettering or lines symbolizing missing sequence, i.e., a deletion. Two examples of putative mutations that could be filtered are displayed (**a, b**). One example of a deletion with variable position between DNA and RNA sequencing that could be clustered together by *UNCeqR* for statistical testing is displayed (**c**)

deletion of one CTG event could have been placed at either side of the repeating triplet. In practice, *UNCeqR* combines these two deletions together for statistical testing in the meta model.

3.9 Set Options for Training

UNCeqR fits beta-binomial distributions using the first `trainNum` sites in `regionsToQuery` (*see* [5] for further details). It is recommended that `trainNum` be large, e.g., 50,000, in order to observe sufficient occurrences of variant alleles. Separate beta-binomial distributions are estimated for tumor DNA and for tumor RNA, using the respective tumor germline allele count and the tumor major variant allele count. Then, *UNCeqR* calculates a DNA *p*-value (P_{DNA}) and an RNA *p*-value (P_{RNA}) based on the corresponding beta-binomial distribution. If tumor DNA and tumor RNA report the same major variant allele, then *UNCeqR* calculates a meta *p*-value (P_{META}) by combining the P_{DNA} and P_{RNA} through a combined *z*-score weighted by their respective tumor read depth (DNA or RNA), via Stouffer's method [33]. Otherwise, P_{META} is set to P_{DNA}. In summary, *UNCeqR* calculates three *p*-values per genomic site: P_{DNA}, P_{RNA}, and P_{META}.

3.10 UNCeqR Execution and Outputs

For the investigator, *UNCeqR* comes pre-configured with two modes. To discover somatic mutations in new sequencing, the de novo mode sets options that have been published on previously [5, 12, 13]. This de novo mode can be specified by running *UNCeqR* with the following Linux command line:

```
$perl UNCeqR_main_simple.pl
    -mode denovo
    -tumorDNA [insert path to tumor DNA bam]
    -tumorRNA [insert path to tumor RNA bam]
    -normalDNA [insert path to normal DNA bam]
    -resultsDir [insert sample ID for the results directory]
    -snpFile [insert path to SNP file]
    -regionsToQuery [insert path to regionsToQuery file]
    -fastaWoChr [insert path to genome FASTA file]
    -normalDNAchr N
    -tumorDNAchr N
    -tumorRNAchr N
```

Note that this example states that all BAM files are aligned to genome sequences without the chr prefix (*see* **Note 8**). In addition to de novo mutation detection, *UNCeqR* supports direct interrogation of fixed genome sites, such as for the purpose of independent mutation validation. This interrogation mode has been used to evaluate and validate somatic mutations from DNA exome sequencing in RNA sequencing [14–17]. In this context, the goal is to ascertain if there is a mutation at a given site for a particular sample because there is a prior evidence for a mutation at this site in this sample. To execute interrogation mode similar to earlier studies, set `mode` to "interrogate" and `verboseOut` to "1," which disables all sequence, position, and variant filtering and reports all variants, provide a Mutation Annotation Format file (https://docs.gdc.cancer.gov/Data/File_Formats/MAF_Format/) as `priorMutFile`, and provide the sample identifier in the context of the MAF as `sampleId` for the given sample, and dense='N' (*See* **Note 9**). *UNCeqR* will extract mutations specific to the sample from the `priorMutFile` and detect variants at those sites. To compare the *UNCeqR* mutations with the `priorMutFile`, investigators should join these files together based on genome sites and including some padding for indels. When specifying a mode, additional options can be specified to *UNCeqR*, which then override the default setting under the specified mode option set.

UNCeqR produces several output files under the directory provided by `resultsDir`. The primary output of mutation detections is comma separated value file, `unceqr_proc.all.csv`. A description of the column names can be found at https://github.com/mwilkers/unceqr. Important columns for downstream analysis are:

- *p*-values (`p.dna`, `p.rna`, `p.meta`)
- The major variant alleles: `DNA_majNonRef` and `RNA_majNonRef`
- Germline high-quality allele count: `normCnt`
- Germline high-quality alleles: `normChars`
- Major variant high-quality allele counts: `DNA_maxVal`, `RNA_maxVal`
- High-quality tumor germline allele counts: `DNA_refCnt`, `RNA_refCnt`
- Distribution of all tumor variant alleles: `DNA_str`, `RNA_str`.

The beta-binomial model parameters are listed in `unceqr_proc.all.csv.fit`. Error messages are printed to `unceqr_stderror`.

The latest instructions and complete description of options and output accompany the software.

3.11 Example Application

A hypothetical result of executing *UNCeqR* on germline DNA whole exome sequencing, tumor DNA whole exome sequencing, and tumor RNA sequencing is displayed in Fig. 3. Here, the germline DNA sequencing has sufficient depth and uniformly presents an A allele. Tumor DNA sequencing mostly presents with an A allele but also contains a trace amount of G allele. The DNA mutant allele fraction (MAF) was 29%. P_{DNA} by itself is not small enough to be considered significant given genome-wide mutation detection (typically thresholds close to 1e-9 as in [5]). In tumor RNA

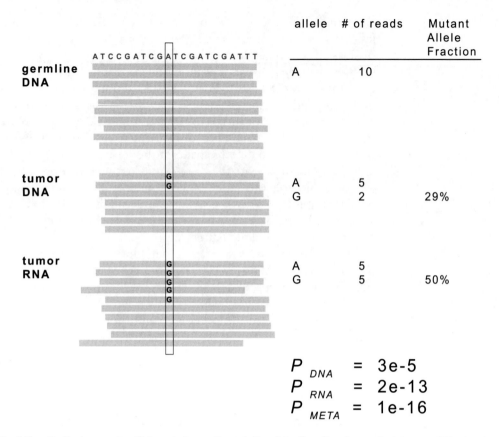

Fig. 3 Hypothetical example of integrated somatic mutation detection. Gray boxes depict a sample's sequences aligned to the reference genome, which is indicated in blue lettering. Different sequencing types (germline DNA, tumor DNA, tumor RNA) belonging to a sample are grouped together and labeled on the left hand side. Alleles not matching the reference sequence are depicted in black lettering. Allele counts and mutant allele fractions are displayed in the table. Hypothetical p-values for the different models are displayed below

sequencing, there is again the A allele; however, the RNA MAF is much greater than tumor RNA-seq, at 50%. This greater mutant allele fraction supports that mutation-specific allelic expression has occurred at this site. Correspondingly, P_{RNA} is quite small. P_{META} combines both p-values weighted by their read depth and provides a very small p-value that would be considered a significant call given genome-wide mutation detection. The advance can be summarized in three points. P_{DNA} is too large to be considered significant. P_{RNA} is small but based on RNA only, and this model tends to have many more false positives than P_{DNA} [5]. P_{META} is small and indicates that there is DNA variant support, leading to a high confident mutation detection in this gene.

3.12 Downstream Analyses

DNA and RNA integrated mutation calls from *UNCeqR* can be used for a variety of downstream analysis purposes (*see* **Note 1** for an example). Several common downstream analyses are mentioned here, and the reader is encouraged to explore the references for guidance in using these additional tools. For cohort-wide or single tumor sequencing studies, mutations detected by *UNCeqR* can be functionally annotated with gene locus and protein changes through using variant annotation programs such as ANNOVAR [34], VariantAnnotation [35], or others. For studies analyzing expressed mutations, mutation expression status can be easily queried from *UNCeqR* output by selecting those with `DNA_majNonRef` equal to `RNA_majNonRef` and a small P_{META}. For studies focused on tumor clonality or tumor purity, mutant allele fractions can be calculated from *UNCeqR* output using `DNA_maxVal`, `DNA_refCnt`, `RNA_maxVal`, and `RNA_refCnt`. For studies focused on identifying recurrent driver mutations, *UNCeqR* mutations can be analyzed by programs such as MutSig [36].

3.13 Alternate Invocations

In addition to integrated somatic mutation detection with triplet sequencing inputs (germline DNA, tumor DNA, and tumor RNA), mutation detection can also be performed with alternate varieties and combinations of sequencing input (*see* **Notes 2–6**). In some settings, reporting all possible sites rather than the default of reporting sites with a minimal amount of mutant evidence is needed (*see* **Note 7**). When detecting mutations in a large cohort for certain applications, attention to the manner in which sequence alignment files are accessed can be important to optimize the speed of mutation detection. *UNCeqR* provides several options for accelerating somatic mutation detection (*see* **Notes 9** and **10**).

4 Notes

1. In combined DNA and RNA somatic mutation detection calling mode, *UNCeqR* reports three *p*-values per site: P_{DNA}, P_{RNA}, and P_{META}. In addition to providing estimates of somatic mutation by these different models, *UNCeqR* output can be queried to investigate additional hypotheses. For instance, sites with a low P_{RNA}, large P_{DNA}, and abundant, high-quality DNA depth are suggestive of RNA editing, if RNA alignment and sequencing errors are properly controlled. Also, sites with a DNA mutant allele fraction greater than its corresponding RNA mutant allele fraction are suggestive of nonsense-mediated decay. These hypotheses are directly testable upon the UNCeqR_proc output, as it supplies all the necessary values for these calculations.

2. To detect somatic mutations without matched germline sequencing, set `normalDNA` to the string "blank" and `minNormCnt` to 0. These options enable germline-free mutation calling. False-positive somatic mutations increase without

matched germline sequencing. A large `snpFile` is recommended for this use case, as there is a large possibility of false-positive germline calls in this setting.

3. To detect somatic mutations with a single tumor sequencing (DNA or RNA) and with matched germline sequencing (DNA or RNA), the only tumor BAM should be supplied under `tumorDNA` and associated DNA filtering options. Set `dnaOnly` to 1. Set `tumorRNA` to "blank."

4. *UNCeqR* can be used to detect germline variants or possible somatic mutations in germline tissue. To detect variants in germline DNA or RNA, supply a germline BAM under `tumorDNA` and set `dnaOnly` to 1, do not provide a `snpFile`, set `normalDNA` to the string "blank," and set `minNormCnt` to 0. To detect germline variants in both DNA and RNA sequencing, add the additional BAM file but set `dnaOnly` to 0.

5. To detect somatic mutations using "quadruplets" of patient-matched germline DNA, normal RNA, tumor DNA, and tumor RNA, first merge, sort, and index the BAM files of germline DNA and normal RNA. Supply this merged BAM file as `normalDNA`. This can have the consequence of expanding the genome space with a defined germline genotype due to the inclusion of germline RNA.

6. To detect somatic mutations in nonhuman organisms (e.g., mouse), prepare the appropriate genome sequence files, alignments, `snpFile`, and `regionsToQuery`.

7. *UNCeqR* by default reports mutations with a p-value <0.25 in `unceqr_proc_all.csv`. Alternatively, all sites can be reported by setting `verboseOut` to 1, `preMinTumorCov` to 0, and `preMinNormCov` to 0.

8. *UNCeqR* can simultaneously accept alignments on "chr" prefixed genome sequences (e.g., hg19) and sequences without the prefix that represent the same genome sequence. If both forms are needed, `fastWchr` is required and is the full path to the FASTA file with the "chr" prefix, and `fastaWoChr` is also required and is the full path to the FASTA file without the "chr" prefix. `normalDNAchr`, `tumorDNAchr`, and `tumorRNAchr` are also required to be set to Y or N to indicate "chr" prefix or not for the respective sequencing.

9. *UNCeqR* accesses BAM files by two methods—a streaming fashion and a bam index lookup. These two different methods of BAM file access affect the speed of *UNCeqR*. If the investigator is analyzing 100's of regions per sample, the index lookup option (dense = "N") and supplying a brief `regionsToQuery` will be faster. If the investigator is analyzing the exome, the streaming option indicated by (dense = "Y") will be faster; in

this case, the regions specified by `regionsToQuery` are selected on the fly.

10. *UNCeqR* provides an additional two options for speed. Only genome sites with tumor depth exceeding `preMinTumorCov` in DNA or RNA and `preMinNormCov` in normal sequencing are evaluated for the detailed high-quality data and variant options. By setting these variables to `minNormCnt` and `minDnaTumorCnt`, calculation time is saved, and *UNCeqR* runs faster.

References

1. Roychowdhury S, Chinnaiyan AM (2016) Translating cancer genomes and transcriptomes for precision oncology. CA Cancer J Clin 66:75–88
2. Roychowdhury S, Iyer MK, Robinson DR, Lonigro RJ, Wu YM, Cao X, Kalyana-Sundaram S, Sam L, Balbin OA, Quist MJ et al (2011) Personalized oncology through integrative high-throughput sequencing: a pilot study. Sci Transl Med 3:111ra121
3. Clinical Lung Cancer Genome P, Network Genomic M (2013) A genomics-based classification of human lung tumors. *Sci Transl Med* 5:209ra153
4. Meyerson M, Gabriel S, Getz G (2010) Advances in understanding cancer genomes through second-generation sequencing. Nat Rev Genet 11:685–696
5. Wilkerson MD, Cabanski CR, Sun W, Hoadley KA, Walter V, Mose LE, Troester MA, Hammerman PS, Parker JS, Perou CM, Hayes DN (2014) Integrated RNA and DNA sequencing improves mutation detection in low purity tumors. Nucleic Acids Res 42:e107
6. Li H, Handsaker B, Wysoker A, Fennell T, Ruan J, Homer N, Marth G, Abecasis G, Durbin R (2009) The Sequence Alignment/Map format and SAMtools. Bioinformatics 25:2078–2079
7. Li H, Durbin R (2009) Fast and accurate short read alignment with Burrows-Wheeler transform. Bioinformatics 25:1754–1760
8. Wang K, Singh D, Zeng Z, Coleman SJ, Huang Y, Savich GL, He X, Mieczkowski P, Grimm SA, Perou CM et al (2010) MapSplice: accurate mapping of RNA-seq reads for splice junction discovery. Nucleic Acids Res 38:e178
9. Troester MA, Hoadley KA, D'Arcy M, Cherniack AD, Stewart C, Koboldt DC, Robertson AG, Mahurkar S, Shen H, Wilkerson MD et al (2016) DNA defects, epigenetics, and gene expression in cancer-adjacent breast: a study from The Cancer Genome Atlas. NPJ Breast Cancer 2:16007
10. Mertins P, Mani DR, Ruggles KV, Gillette MA, Clauser KR, Wang P, Wang X, Qiao JW, Cao S, Petralia F et al (2016) Proteogenomics connects somatic mutations to signalling in breast cancer. Nature 534:55–62
11. Liu W, Snell JM, Jeck WR, Hoadley KA, Wilkerson MD, Parker JS, Patel N, Mlombe YB, Mulima G, Liomba NG et al (2016) Subtyping sub-Saharan esophageal squamous cell carcinoma by comprehensive molecular analysis. JCI Insight 1(16):e88755
12. Fishbein L, Leshchiner I, Walter V, Danilova L, Robertson AG, Johnson AR, Lichtenberg TM, Murray BA, Ghayee HK, Else T et al (2017) Comprehensive molecular characterization of pheochromocytoma and paraganglioma. Cancer Cell 31:181–193
13. Ciriello G, Gatza ML, Beck AH, Wilkerson MD, Rhie SK, Pastore A, Zhang H, McLellan M, Yau C, Kandoth C et al (2015) Comprehensive molecular portraits of invasive lobular breast cancer. Cell 163:506–519
14. The Cancer Genome Atlas Research Network (2014) Comprehensive molecular profiling of lung adenocarcinoma. Nature 511:543–550
15. The Cancer Genome Atlas Research Network (2012) Comprehensive genomic characterization of squamous cell lung cancers. Nature 489:519–525
16. The Cancer Genome Atlas Research Network (2015) Genomic classification of cutaneous melanoma. Cell 161:1681–1696
17. The Cancer Genome Atlas Research Network (2015) Comprehensive genomic characterization of head and neck squamous cell carcinomas. Nature 517:576–582
18. Brady SW, McQuerry JA, Qiao Y, Piccolo SR, Shrestha G, Jenkins DF, Layer RM, Pedersen

BS, Miller RH, Esch A et al (2017) Combating subclonal evolution of resistant cancer phenotypes. Nat Commun 8:1231

19. Field MG, Durante MA, Anbunathan H, Cai LZ, Decatur CL, Bowcock AM, Kurtenbach S, Harbour JW (2018) Punctuated evolution of canonical genomic aberrations in uveal melanoma. Nat Commun 9:116

20. Yee T (2008) The {VGAM} package. R News 8:28–39

21. Gene Annotation File. https://api.gdc.cancer.gov/v0/data/a0bb9765-3f03-485b-839d-7dce4a9bcfeb

22. Karolchik D, Barber GP, Casper J, Clawson H, Cline MS, Diekhans M, Dreszer TR, Fujita PA, Guruvadoo L, Haeussler M et al (2014) The UCSC genome browser database: 2014 update. Nucleic Acids Res 42:D764–D770

23. Zook JM, Chapman B, Wang J, Mittelman D, Hofmann O, Hide W, Salit M (2014) Integrating human sequence data sets provides a resource of benchmark SNP and indel genotype calls. Nat Biotechnol 32(3):246–251

24. Sherry ST, Ward MH, Kholodov M, Baker J, Phan L, Smigielski EM, Sirotkin K (2001) dbSNP: the NCBI database of genetic variation. Nucleic Acids Res 29:308–311

25. Lek M, Karczewski KJ, Minikel EV, Samocha KE, Banks E, Fennell T, O'Donnell-Luria AH, Ware JS, Hill AJ, Cummings BB et al (2016) Analysis of protein-coding genetic variation in 60,706 humans. Nature 536:285–291

26. Forbes SA, Beare D, Gunasekaran P, Leung K, Bindal N, Boutselakis H, Ding M, Bamford S, Cole C, Ward S et al (2015) COSMIC: exploring the world's knowledge of somatic mutations in human cancer. Nucleic Acids Res 43: D805–D811

27. Cabanski CR, Wilkerson MD, Soloway M, Parker JS, Liu J, Prins JF, Marron JS, Perou CM, Hayes DN (2013) BlackOPs: increasing confidence in variant detection through mappability filtering. Nucleic Acids Res 41:e178

28. Cibulskis K, Lawrence MS, Carter SL, Sivachenko A, Jaffe D, Sougnez C, Gabriel S, Meyerson M, Lander ES, Getz G (2013) Sensitive detection of somatic point mutations in impure and heterogeneous cancer samples. Nat Biotechnol 31:213–219

29. Pickrell JK, Gilad Y, Pritchard JK (2012) Comment on "Widespread RNA and DNA sequence differences in the human transcriptome". Science 335:1302 author reply 1302

30. Guo Y, Li J, Li CI, Long J, Samuels DC, Shyr Y (2012) The effect of strand bias in Illumina short-read sequencing data. BMC Genomics 13:666

31. Jiang Y, Turinsky AL, Brudno M (2015) The missing indels: an estimate of indel variation in a human genome and analysis of factors that impede detection. Nucleic Acids Res 43:7217–7228

32. Mose LE, Wilkerson MD, Hayes DN, Perou CM, Parker JS (2014) ABRA: improved coding indel detection via assembly-based realignment. Bioinformatics 30:2813–2815

33. Stouffer SA, Suchman EA, DeVinney LC, Star SA, Williams RM (1949) Studies in social psychology in World War II. Princeton University Press, Princeton, NJ

34. Wang K, Li M, Hakonarson H (2010) ANNOVAR: functional annotation of genetic variants from high-throughput sequencing data. Nucleic Acids Res 38:e164

35. Obenchain V, Lawrence M, Carey V, Gogarten S, Shannon P, Morgan M (2014) VariantAnnotation: a Bioconductor package for exploration and annotation of genetic variants. Bioinformatics 30:2076–2078

36. Lawrence MS, Stojanov P, Polak P, Kryukov GV, Cibulskis K, Sivachenko A, Carter SL, Stewart C, Mermel CH, Roberts SA et al (2013) Mutational heterogeneity in cancer and the search for new cancer-associated genes. Nature 499:214–218

Chapter 7

Allele-Specific Expression Analysis in Cancer Using Next-Generation Sequencing Data

Alessandro Romanel

Abstract

Allele-specific expression arises when transcriptional activity at the different alleles of a gene differs considerably. Although extensive research has been carried out to detect and characterize this phenomenon, the landscape of allele-specific expression in cancer is still poorly understood. In this chapter, we describe a fast and reliable analysis pipeline to study allele-specific expression in cancer using next-generation sequencing data. The pipeline provides a gene-level analysis approach that exploits paired germline DNA and tumor RNA sequencing data and benefits from parallel computation resources when available.

Key words Allele-specific features, Genome analysis, Parallel computation, Transcriptome analysis, Next-generation sequencing, SNPs

1 Introduction

Allele-specific expression (ASE) is a common phenomenon observed in human cells where transcription originates predominantly from one allele [1, 2]. Imprinted genes, physiological conditions (as for chromosome X inactivation), or other ASE mechanisms affecting the human genome can contribute to the phenotypical human variability [1]. Transcript degradation by miRNA, monoallelic disruption of a regulatory region or alternative splicing patterns, and alternative polyadenylation can all initiate ASE [3–5] (*see* Fig. 1) as well as epigenetic phenomena, like inherited histone modifications or DNA methylation [2, 6]. ASE is essential for cellular programming and development as well as for the diversity of cellular phenotypes [7]. Extensive research has been carried out to detect and characterize allele-specific expression, and many different approaches have been used to study ASE, including targeted sequencing, RT-qPCR, and microarrays [8, 9].

The advent of next-generation sequencing (NGS) technology made possible an advance in the field. NGS provides unprecedented single base level information of the human genome and

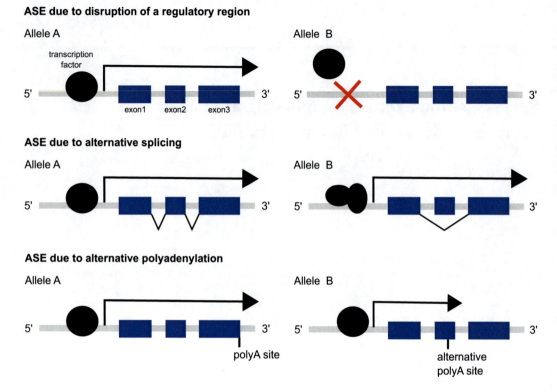

Fig. 1 Examples of biological mechanisms that can initiate allele-specific expression

transcriptome and opens up the investigation of previously unexplored biological questions. By integrating information from individuals' genetic makeup accessible in sequencing reads, it is indeed possible, among other options, to quantitatively estimate DNA somatic lesion clonality [10], to infer tumor evolution [10, 11], to describe mosaicisms [12], and to study the ASE phenomenon from an agnostic and genome-wide perspective [13, 14] . Even though ASE was demonstrated relevant to tumorigenesis, in particular with respect to tumor-suppressor genes [15], limited studies have explored the role and impact that allele-specific expression has in cancer genesis and progression [16, 17]. To this aim, large NGS datasets that are now becoming available through initiatives like The Cancer Genome Atlas (TCGA) will be fundamental in the next future, as they will provide the needed power to improve our understanding of the ASE landscape in cancer.

In this chapter we describe methodologies for allele-specific expression analysis using NGS data. Starting with a set of sequencing reads, a set of computational tools and methods are used to process and query the data with the ultimate goal to nominate ASE transcripts potentially involved in cancer.

2 Methods

Many methods to perform allele-specific studies from NGS data have been proposed in the last years. A computational pipeline called AlleleSeq was introduced in [18] to study allele-specific expression and binding. AlleleSeq requires trios (i.e., genomic information from individual's parents) and provides a built-in method to construct a diploid personal genome using genomic sequence variants. A recent tool called MBASED [19] relies instead only on RNA-seq and provides a method that combines (in a meta-analysis-based approach) evidence across single nucleotide variants within a gene to determine the extent of ASE and uses simulations to assess the statistical significance of the observed ASE events. Some other valuable approaches can be found in [20], where a hierarchical Bayesian model that combines information across loci to allow both global and locus-specific ASE inferences has been developed; in [21], where a tool called iASEq implementing a Bayesian hierarchical model to infer allele-specific binding from ChIP-seq data was presented; and in [22], where a tool called Allim that measures ASE from NGS trios data was introduced.

The analysis pipeline described in this chapter builds on the work we presented in [23] where we introduced a computational tool called ASEQ. The method consists in a complete and easy-to-use set of functionalities to optimally and rapidly perform ASE studies by exploiting single nucleotide polymorphisms (SNPs) genotype patterns. It provides a method to identify ASE transcripts/genes from paired whole exome sequencing (WES) and transcriptome sequencing (RNA-seq) data taking full advantage of a built-in fast computational engine that reduces the effort of single base level computation. To study allele-specific expression in the context of cancer, the method requires as input matched germ-line WES and tumor RNA-seq data of a set of individuals under investigation.

The complete pipeline, which includes also alignment and preprocessing of DNA and RNA reads, consists of the following steps:

- Alignment, preprocessing, and QC of WES data
- Alignment, preprocessing, and QC of RNA-seq data
- Identification of informative SNPs from WES data
- Transcript/gene-level allele-specific expression analysis
- Masking or annotation of somatic copy number alterations
- Identification of ASE specific transcript differential levels

The pipeline computational workflow is visually described in Fig. 2.

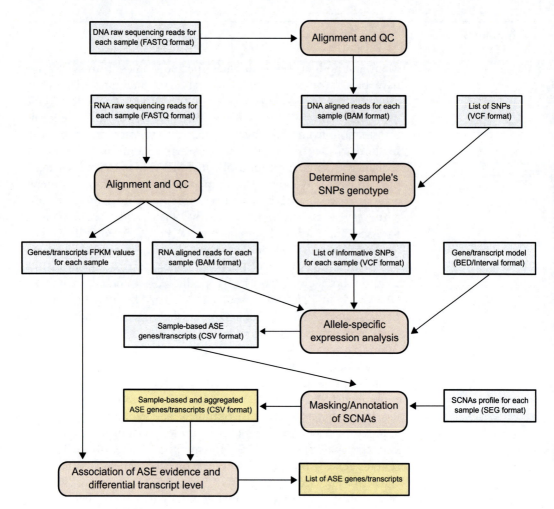

Fig. 2 Description of ASE analysis pipeline. Gray rectangles identify initial input and intermediate input/output data, while orange rectangles identify final output results. Red-rounded rectangles identify computational steps

2.1 Alignment, Preprocessing, and Quality Control of WES Reads

Reads are processed with the pipeline described in [24]. For each sequenced sample, FastQC[1] is run on the raw reads to assess their quality. Quality metrics include average base quality, sequence duplication rate, and the k-mer enrichment along the length of the reads. These measures are utilized to assess whether the sequencing and the demultiplexing of the samples was performed correctly. After initial quality control, adapter sequences are trimmed (when needed) using tools like Trimmomatic [25]. Short reads are then aligned to the reference human genome (e.g., GRC37/hg19) using BWA [26]. Picard[2] and SAMtools [27] are used to generate single-sorted BAM files for each individual's

---

[1] http://www.bioinformatics.babraham.ac.uk/projects/fastqc/.

[2] http://picard.sourceforge.net.

sample. When needed, Picard is used to remove clonal duplicates. BAM files are then realigned (to correct for possible misalignments due to indels) and recalibrated (to adjust for over- and underestimated base quality scores in the data) using GATK tools [28]. Finally SAMtools are used to adjust BAM MD tags (strings for mismatch positions). The alignment quality of the BAM files is obtained by several metrics related to the average depth of coverage and the capture rate. For any given sample, the capture rate is given by the percent of aligned reads that overlap any captured region in the considered WES kit over the total number of mapped reads. Average coverage is computed from the captured regions of the WES kit in use.

2.2 Alignment, Preprocessing, and Quality Control of RNA Reads

Also in this case, FastQC is run to assess raw read quality for each sequenced sample. Quality metrics are utilized to assess whether the sequencing and the demultiplexing of the samples was performed correctly. After initial quality control, short reads are aligned to the reference human genome (e.g., GRC37/hg19) using TopHat 2 [29]. Cufflinks [30] workflow is then applied to generate normalized expression tables both at gene and transcript levels for downstream analysis. Specifically, Cuffquant tool is used to compute genes and transcript expression profiles which are then normalized using Cuffnorm tool to generate genes and transcript FPKM tables.

2.3 SNP-Based ASE Detection Approach

Allele-specific expression analysis is performed by exploiting individual's germline heterozygous sites, also called *informative* SNPs. Sites that are inherited as heterozygous but show significant allelic imbalance in the transcriptome may be explained by ASE events. Although a powerful tool, the distribution of informative SNPs across the genome may also constitute a limitation underlying the overall power of detecting ASE through SNP-based approaches. Based on dbSNP 144 common SNP[3] data and UCSC knownGene hg19 catalog[4], we calculated that ~70% of the ~28 K genes span *coding* SNPs (i.e., SNPs lying in coding regions of the genome) and the majority (~95%) of these genes span multiple coding SNPs. The frequency of coding SNPs per gene follows the distribution reported in Fig. 3a. Based on 1000 Genome Project genotyping data and dbSNP 144 SNPs with a global minor allele frequency (MAF) greater than 1%, we computed the empirical distribution of individual's informative SNP fraction (*see* Fig. 3b) considering all available individuals and stratifying them by main ethnic groups (i.e., EUR, AFR, EAS, and SAS). Given the observed non-uniform distribution, in [23], we introduced a general approach to measure

---

[3] http://www.ncbi.nlm.nih.gov/SNP/.
[4] https://genome.ucsc.edu/.

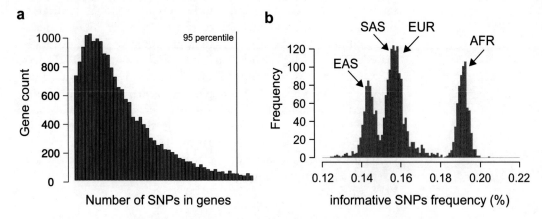

Fig. 3 (**a**) Frequency distribution of coding SNPs per gene. Frequency distribution of genes containing $N = 1, 2, \ldots$ coding SNPs based on UCSC hg19 knownGene catalog and dbSNP 144 common SNPs. (**b**) Frequency distribution of informative SNP frequencies in 1000 Genome Project genotype data

the number of genes suitable for ASE analysis; we defined a mathematical formulation (here extended) that given a value I representing the frequency of heterozygous SNPs per individual and assuming that:

- n SNPs are sufficient to perform ASE analysis on a gene
- Heterozygous SNPs are uniformly distributed across the genome of an individual
- SNPs are independent

estimates the upper bound of the number of genes available for ASE calculation. The formula

$$\sum_{i=1}^{M} D_i * (1 - P(X < n)) \quad \text{where } X = \text{Binom}(i, I)$$

calculates the estimate by combining the maximum observed number of coding SNPs overlapping a gene (M), the number of genes with I overlapping coding SNPs (D_i), and the probability that at least n of these I SNPs are heterozygous ($1 - P(X < n)$ with X to be a binomial distribution with i number of trials and I success probability).

To have a broader view of the ASE detection power, we used the formula to estimate the number of genes available for ASE calculation considering the frequency of coding SNPs per gene computed from dbSNP 144 common SNPs[5] and UCSC knownGene hg19 coding regions, and also considering captured regions from four different and commonly used WES platforms

---

[5] Only dbSNP 144 common SNPs represented in the 1000 Genome Project genotype data and with global MAF greater or equal to 1% were considered.

Table 1
Number of genes available for ASE calculation at different informative SNP fractions considering UCSC knownGene coding regions and captured regions of four commonly used WES kits

	Number of genes available for ASE calculation at different informative SNP fractions			
	10%	15%	20%	25%
1 SNP sufficient to perform ASE				
UCSC knownGene hg19 (coding)	5840 (20%)	7656 (27%)	9089 (32%)	10,249 (36%)
Agilent SureSelect v2	5127 (18%)	6760 (24%)	8060 (28%)	9123 (32%)
Agilent SureSelect v4	4976 (17%)	6601 (23%)	7909 (28%)	8987 (32%)
HaloPlex	5642 (20%)	7415 (26%)	8818 (31%)	9957 (35%)
NimbleGen SeqCapEZ_Exome_v3.0	5134 (185)	6812 (24%)	8164 (29%)	9280 (33%)
2 SNPs sufficient to perform ASE				
UCSC knownGene hg19 (coding)	1714 (6%)	2853 (10%)	3960 (14%)	4996 (18%)
Agilent SureSelect v2	1441 (5%)	2419 (9%)	3382 (12%)	4291 (15%)
Agilent SureSelect v4	1324 (5%)	2255 (8%)	3184 (11%)	4073 (14%)
HaloPlex	1622 (6%)	2718 (10%)	3789 (13%)	4796 (17%)
NimbleGen SeqCapEZ_Exome_v3.0	1368 (5%)	2322 (8%)	3273 (11%)	4183 (15%)

Estimates were computed both considering 1 SNP and 2 SNPs sufficient to perform ASE analysis

(NimbleGen SeqCapEZ_Exome_v3.0, Agilent HaloPlex, Agilent SureSelect v2, and Agilent SureSelect v4). The analysis was performed for increasing heterozygous SNP frequencies. Table 1 shows how different WES platforms may provide different powers in detecting ASE genes while highlighting the difference with respect to the ASE detection power expected considering UCSC knownGene hg19 coding regions.

2.4 Identification of Informative SNPs

Informative SNPs from germline WES data are retrieved for all individuals using the standalone *genotype* execution mode implemented in our ASEQ tool. This mode is designed to compute the genotype of an input sample at known SNP positions; an exhaustive catalog of SNPs can be obtained from dbSNP database. This method exploits a fast computational engine that, building on routines from SAMtools APIs, provides a built-in multi-threaded solution that optimizes the execution time (when multiple CPUs or cores are available) in calculating read coverage at specific genomic positions (namely, the *pileup*), which still represents one of the major bottlenecks in NGS data analysis. In [23] we show that, indicatively, our engine provides a ~11X speedup in the pileup computation of 500K SNPs on a 16-core machine with respect to the canonical SAMtools pileup implementation.

Given a list of known SNPs, the *genotype* mode first computes the pileup from each germline WES data file and then determines the genotype calls. To control the quality of the data considered for the pileup, minimum base quality score, minimum read quality score, and minimum depth of coverage can be specified. Genotype calls can be performed using two different strategies. The first method is based on alternative read count percentages. The method calls a heterozygous genotype if the proportion of coverage of the alternative base with respect to the total coverage at that position is in a specific range that by default is set to [0.2,0.8]; otherwise the method calls homozygous genotype, either for the reference or the alternative base. The second method, instead, implements a binomial test with probabilities p and q for the reference and the alternative allele, respectively. To account for the reference bias mapping [13], we apply default probabilities $p = 0.55$ and $q = 0.45$ that can be easily tuned when bias mapping deviates from default parameters. By default, no heterozygous genotypes are called for SNPs with reference or alternative allele coverage equal to zero; when too restrictive, especially in presence of low coverage, this option can be disabled hence allowing heterozygous genotypes to be called also in presence of zero reference or alternative coverage. By default, a statistical significance threshold of 5% is used. Regardless of the method chosen, read count information for reference and alternative alleles are saved and are then utilized to optimize the ASE analysis step.

In [23] we showed that these approaches, although simple, provide high precision calls. By comparing WES calls to high-quality SNP array calls (matched data available for 90 individuals), we showed that, at depth of coverage ≥ 10, the median sensitivity of both approaches with stringent significance threshold remains above 95% and median false discovery rate below 0.3%.

2.5 Allele-Specific Expression Detection

Allele-specific expression analysis is performed through the execution mode *ase* provided by ASEQ. It implements two different input options: (i) the *gene model* input that requires a list of genes start/end coordinates and a list of informative SNPs of the sample and (ii) the *transcript model* input that takes as input a list of transcripts with exonic coordinates and a list of informative SNPs of the sample. In the gene model option, SNPs are matched with gene coordinates, while in the transcript model option, SNPs are matched with transcript specific exon coordinates.

The ASE analysis method implements the following steps (sketched in Fig. 4). Given the tumor RNA-seq data file, a gene, and the list of heterozygous SNPs for a study individual, the application performs the heterozygosity test on the RNA data at each input SNP position. By default the previously described *binom*

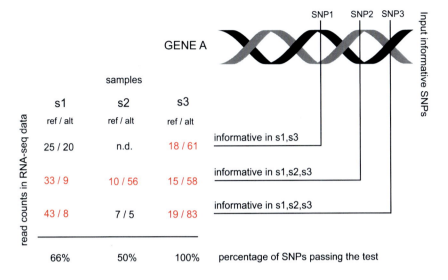

Fig. 4 Example of ASE gene computation. Gene A is overlapped by three informative SNPs in samples s1 and s3, and all three of them support ASE in sample s3, while only two of them support ASE in sample s1. Gene A is instead overlapped by two informative SNPs in samples s2, and only one of them supports ASE evidence. Overall, assuming an ASE score threshold of 66% and the requirement of at least two analyzed samples supporting ASE gene evidence, gene A is considered an ASE gene

method with $p = q = 0.5$ is applied (default a significance threshold set to 5%), but also *htperc* method can be set for the analysis. Minimum base quality score, minimum read quality score, and minimum depth of coverage can be specified to filter reads used in the pileup computations. A position is annotated as showing ASE when a non-heterozygous call in RNA-seq data is detected. False-positive ASE calls can be controlled by tuning the significance threshold or the range size when *binom* and *htperc* methods are used, respectively. Additionally, false-positive ASE calls due to different depths of coverage between the DNA- and the RNA-seq data are controlled by performing an additional statistical test (Fisher Exact test) on the reference and alternative alleles count proportions from the DNA and the RNA data.

For each sample and each gene with available heterozygous SNPs in the sample, a positive ASE result is returned only if the proportion of SNPs passing the test (denoted as *ASE score*) is greater than a predefined threshold. Different ASE score levels might be used to distinguish mechanisms involving most part of a gene (e.g., whole-gene ASE) from other ASE phenomena. For all gene-sample pair without available heterozygous SNPs or RNA-seq data coverage below the specified threshold, a flag of *not available* for ASE calculation is returned. Additionally, when multiple samples are investigated, an *ASE gene* flag is returned only if a gene shows ASE in at least N samples available for ASE calculation.

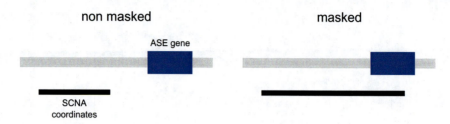

Fig. 5 Examples of SCNA masking procedure

2.6 Masking of Somatic Copy Number Alterations

The presence of somatic copy number aberrations (SCNAs) could affect the ASE analysis interpretation. A gene harboring a monoallelic deletion, for example, would appear as being an ASE gene. These ASE events may be masked, annotated, or retained in the results, depending on the final goal of the analysis. If masking (or annotation) is needed, its implementation and results depend on the availability of the SCNA profile obtained from a matching tumor tissue. Being this chapter focused on use of WES data, we refer to some tools that are commonly used to retrieve SCNA profiles from matched normal/tumor WES data [31–33]. We also remind that SCNA profiles can be computed also by matched normal/tumor WGS [31, 34, 35] and array (e.g., aCGH and SNP array) data [36]. If available, the SCNA profile makes it possible to mask (or annotate) all ASE events due to copy number aberrations. We proceed as follows. First, we identify aberrant segments in the SCNA profile. The coordinates of these regions are then matched to the coordinates of the identified ASE genes to find overlapping areas. A gene showing whole-gene ASE phenomenon is masked only if the overlapping area exceeds a specified gene size percentage. A gene showing partial ASE can be masked using the same conservative approach or, alternatively, evaluating the overlapping area by considering only the portion of the gene that shows ASE. Examples of SCNA masking are shown in Fig. 5. Overlapping areas at specific size percentage can be determined using the *intersectBed* command implemented in the BedTools [37].

2.7 Evidence of ASE and Differential Transcript Levels

When allele-specific expression analysis of multiple samples is performed, the relation between evidence of ASE and differential transcript levels is investigated using the following approach. For each transcript or gene with available ASE score and FPKM level across the investigated samples, dosage and/or allelic statistical tests are performed. A dosage test searches for an increasing or decreasing transcript level trend across a set of ASE score classes. ASE scores are usually classified as (i) *no ase* (ASE score equal to zero) and *ase* (ASE score greater than zero) and (ii) *no ase* (ASE score equal to zero), *low ase* (ASE score in [0,0.5]), and *high ase* (ASE score greater than 0.5). When the second ASE score classification is used, an allelic test is also performed to search for intra-

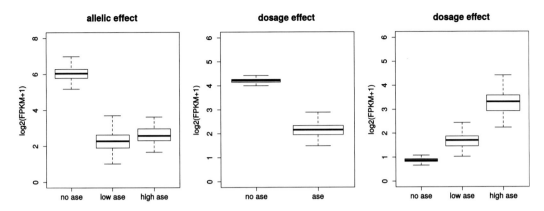

Fig. 6 Examples of differential transcript allelic and dosage effects

class transcript level differences. Both tests are implemented using a linear regression model. P-values resulting from the analysis of all available transcripts/genes might be used to select top candidates for downstream analysis; otherwise, standard methods to control for false discovery rate (e.g., Benjamini-Hochberg procedure) can be applied to select only high confident associations. Figure 6 reports some examples of genes/transcripts showing dosage and allelic effects. When regression models cannot be applied due to absence of linear regression assumptions, other methods like Mann-Whitney and Kruskal-Wallis statistics are considered.

3 Conclusion

In this chapter, we presented a computational pipeline to rapidly and reliably perform allele-specific expression studies in cancer from NGS data. The pipeline exploits parallel computation capabilities and can hence be run on computer systems with multiple CPUs and CPUs with multiple cores or across clusters of machines. The pipeline can also be applied to investigate eQTL and allele-specific binding. In the future, further improvements of the presented pipeline will be focused on dealing with tumor purity aspects. RNA data derived from tumor cells admixed with normal cells might increase the number of false-negative ASE events; informative SNP imbalance signal in the tumor transcriptome might be indeed diluted in the presence of normal admixed signal. While methods to infer tumor purity both from DNA [10, 38] and RNA [39] NGS data are already available, no ASE detection approach seems to currently provide a way to interpret ASE events in the light of tumor-normal admixture. Performances and reporting improvements will be also subjects of future work.

References

1. Lo HS, Wang Z, Hu Y, Yang HH, Gere S, Buetow KH et al (2003) Allelic variation in gene expression is common in the human genome. Genome Res 13(8):1855–1862
2. Gimelbrant A, Hutchinson JN, Thompson BR, Chess A (2007) Widespread monoallelic expression on human autosomes. Science 318 (5853):1136–1140
3. Walker EJ, Zhang C, Castelo-Branco P, Hawkins C, Wilson W, Zhukova N et al (2012) Monoallelic expression determines oncogenic progression and outcome in benign and malignant brain tumors. Cancer Res 72 (3):636–644
4. Lalonde E, Ha KCH, Wang Z, Bemmo A, Kleinman CL, Kwan T et al (2011) RNA sequencing reveals the role of splicing polymorphisms in regulating human gene expression. Genome Res 21(4):545–554
5. Meyer KB, Maia A-T, O'Reilly M, Teschendorff AE, Chin S-F, Caldas C et al (2008) Allele-specific up-regulation of FGFR2 increases susceptibility to breast cancer. PLoS Biol 6(5):e108
6. Wei Q-X, Claus R, Hielscher T, Mertens D, Raval A, Oakes CC et al (2013) Germline allele-specific expression of DAPK1 in chronic lymphocytic leukemia. PLoS One 8(1):e55261
7. Ferguson-Smith AC, Surani MA (2001) Imprinting and the epigenetic asymmetry between parental genomes. Science 293 (5532):1086–1089
8. Knight JC (2004) Allele-specific gene expression uncovered. Trends Genet 20(3):113–116
9. Pastinen T (2010) Genome-wide allele-specific analysis: insights into regulatory variation. Nat Rev Genet 11(8):533–538
10. Prandi D, Baca SC, Romanel A, Barbieri CE, Mosquera J-M, Fontugne J et al (2014) Unraveling the clonal hierarchy of somatic genomic aberrations. Genome Biol 15(8):439
11. Nik-Zainal S, Van Loo P, Wedge DC, Alexandrov LB, Greenman CD, Lau KW et al (2012) Breast Cancer Working Group of the International Cancer Genome Consortium. The life history of 21 breast cancers. Cell 149 (5):994–1007
12. Gajecka M (2016) Unrevealed mosaicism in the next-generation sequencing era. Mol Gen Genomics 291:513–530
13. Degner JF, Marioni JC, Pai AA, Pickrell JK, Nkadori E, Gilad Y et al (2009) Effect of read-mapping biases on detecting allele-specific expression from RNA-sequencing data. Bioinformatics 25(24):3207–3212
14. Pickrell JK, Marioni JC, Pai AA, Degner JF, Engelhardt BE, Nkadori E et al (2010) Understanding mechanisms underlying human gene expression variation with RNA sequencing. Nature 464(7289):768–772
15. Lee MP (2012) Allele-specific gene expression and epigenetic modifications and their application to understanding inheritance and cancer. Biochim Biophys Acta 1819(7):739–742
16. Tuch BB, Laborde RR, Xu X, Gu J, Chung CB, Monighetti CK et al (2010) Tumor transcriptome sequencing reveals allelic expression imbalances associated with copy number alterations. PLoS One 5(2):e9317
17. Ha G, Roth A, Lai D, Bashashati A, Ding J, Goya R et al (2012) Integrative analysis of genome-wide loss of heterozygosity and monoallelic expression at nucleotide resolution reveals disrupted pathways in triple-negative breast cancer. Genome Res 22(10):1995–2007
18. Rozowsky J, Abyzov A, Wang J, Alves P, Raha D, Harmanci A et al (2011) AlleleSeq: analysis of allele-specific expression and binding in a network framework. Mol Syst Biol 7:522
19. Mayba O, Gilbert HN, Liu J, Haverty PM, Jhunjhunwala S, Jiang Z et al (2014) MBASED: allele-specific expression detection in cancer tissues and cell lines. Genome Biol 15(8):405 http://genomebiology.com/2014/15/8/405
20. Skelly DA, Johansson M, Madeoy J, Wakefield J, Akey JM (2011) A powerful and flexible statistical framework for testing hypotheses of allele-specific gene expression from RNA-seq data. Genome Res 21 (10):1728–1737
21. Wei Y, Li X, Wang Q, Ji H (2012) iASeq: integrative analysis of allele-specificity of protein-DNA interactions in multiple ChIP-seq datasets. BMC Genomics 13:681
22. Pandey RV, Franssen SU, Futschik A, Schlötterer C (2013) Allelic imbalance metre (Allim), a new tool for measuring allele-specific gene expression with RNA-seq data. Mol Ecol Resour 13(4):740–745
23. Romanel A, Lago S, Prandi D, Sboner A, Demichelis F (2015) ASEQ: fast allele-specific studies from next-generation sequencing data. BMC Med Genet 8:9
24. Beltran H, Eng K, Mosquera JM, Sigaras A, Romanel A, Rennert H et al (2015) Whole-exome sequencing of metastatic cancer and biomarkers of treatment response. JAMA Oncol 1(4):466

25. Bolger AM, Lohse M, Usadel B (2014) Trimmomatic: a flexible trimmer for Illumina sequence data. Bioinformatics 30(15):2114–2120
26. Li H, Durbin R (2009) Fast and accurate short read alignment with Burrows-Wheeler transform. Bioinformatics 25(14):1754–1760
27. Li H, Handsaker B, Wysoker A, Fennell T, Ruan J, Homer N et al (2009) 1000 genome project data processing subgroup. The sequence alignment/map format and SAMtools. Bioinformatics 25(16):2078–2079
28. McKenna A, Hanna M, Banks E, Sivachenko A, Cibulskis K, Kernytsky A et al (2010) The genome analysis toolkit: a MapReduce framework for analyzing next-generation DNA sequencing data. Genome Res 20(9):1297–1303
29. Kim D, Pertea G, Trapnell C, Pimentel H, Kelley R, Salzberg SL (2013) TopHat2: accurate alignment of transcriptomes in the presence of insertions, deletions and gene fusions. Genome Biol 14(4):R36
30. Trapnell C, Williams BA, Pertea G, Mortazavi A, Kwan G, Van Baren MJ et al (2010) Transcript assembly and quantification by RNA-Seq reveals unannotated transcripts and isoform switching during cell differentiation. Nat Biotechnol 28(5):511–515
31. Boeva V, Popova T, Bleakley K, Chiche P, Cappo J, Schleiermacher G et al (2012) Control-FREEC: a tool for assessing copy number and allelic content using next-generation sequencing data. Bioinformatics 28(3):423–425
32. Amarasinghe KC, Li J, Halgamuge SK (2013) CoNVEX: copy number variation estimation in exome sequencing data using HMM. BMC Bioinformatics 14(Suppl 2):S2
33. Magi A, Tattini L, Cifola I, D'Aurizio R, Benelli M, Mangano E et al (2013) EXCAVATOR: detecting copy number variants from whole-exome sequencing data. Genome Biol 14(10):R120
34. Chiang DY, Getz G, Jaffe DB, O'Kelly MJT, Zhao X, Carter SL et al (2009) High-resolution mapping of copy-number alterations with massively parallel sequencing. Nat Methods 6(1):99–103
35. Xi R, Hadjipanayis AG, Luquette LJ, Kim T-M, Lee E, Zhang J et al (2011) Copy number variation detection in whole-genome sequencing data using the Bayesian information criterion. Proc Natl Acad Sci U S A 108(46):E1128–E1136
36. Olshen AB, Venkatraman ES, Lucito R, Wigler M (2004) Circular binary segmentation for the analysis of array-based DNA copy number data. Biostatistics 5(4):557–572
37. Quinlan AR, Hall IM (2010) BEDTools: a flexible suite of utilities for comparing genomic features. Bioinformatics 26(6):841–842
38. Su X, Zhang L, Zhang J, Meric-Bernstam F, Weinstein JN (2012) PurityEst: estimating purity of human tumor samples using next-generation sequencing data. Bioinformatics 28(17):2265–2266
39. Yoshihara K, Shahmoradgoli M, Martínez E, Vegesna R, Kim H, Torres-Garcia W et al (2013) Inferring tumour purity and stromal and immune cell admixture from expression data. Nat Commun 4:2612 http://www.nature.com/doifinder/10.1038/ncomms3612

Chapter 8

Computational Analysis of lncRNA Function in Cancer

Xu Zhang and Tsui-Ting Ho

Abstract

Long noncoding RNAs (lncRNAs) have been shown to play crucial roles in cancer biology. With the help of computational analysis illustrated here, the joint effects of lncRNAs and clinical variables can be quantified in a Cox model on cancer recurrence. Of importance, the predictive accuracy was then validated with the prognostic scores computed based on the suggested model. Further investigation of these potential lncRNAs would provide useful insights following the study of the mechanisms underlying the differential expression of these lncRNAs in association with and possibly contributing to cancer recurrence. Ultimately, the expanding knowledge of the function of lncRNAs curated by computational analysis will suggest new targets for cancer treatment.

Key words lncRNA, Cancer, Cox model, Lasso method, Model validation, Experimental validation

1 Introduction

The human genome is vigorously transcribed. Of interest, protein-coding genes only account for ~2% of the human genome, whereas the majority of transcripts are noncoding RNAs (ncRNAs) [1], which contribute to gene expression and genome maintenance without being translated to proteins [2]. A subset of these noncoding transcripts are termed long noncoding RNAs (lncRNAs), arbitrarily defined with molecular weight larger than 200 nucleotides in length [3], located nearby or within protein-coding genes (exonic, intronic, overlapping), or isolated from any protein-coding genes (intergenic) [4]. In contrast to well-studied small noncoding RNAs such as microRNAs (miRNAs), lncRNAs are poorly characterized. However, emerging evidence suggests that mutations and dysregulation of lncRNAs are often associated with diseases, including cancer [5].

Similar to protein-coding genes or miRNAs, lncRNAs can function as tumor-suppressive or oncogenic genes, thus constituting an important component of tumor biology [6]. With regard to clinical medicine, lncRNA-based diagnostics have begun to develop. For example, PCAT-1 [7] and PCA3 [8] serve as biomarkers as they exhibit tissue-specific and cancer-specific expression patterns. In addition, aberrant lncRNA function drives cancer [9]. It has been reported that while loc285194 [10] and GAS5 [11] may play a tumor-suppressive role, RoR [12, 13], UCA1 [14], and BC200 [15] may have an oncogenic role. Furthermore, PCGEM1 appears to contribute to cancer treatment resistance [16]. Together, these findings highlight the clinical significance of lncRNAs in cancer. In light of this, the systematic identification and annotation of lncRNAs is a critical need and will aid in the development of novel strategies for cancer therapy.

1.1 lncRNA Databases

Two of the most well-known lncRNA databases are lncRNAdb [17] and NONCODE [18]. lncRNAdb is a curated reference database of 287 eukaryotic lncRNAs with annotations, including gene expression data, structural information, and functional evidence supported by the literature. On the other hand, NONCODE is an interactive database about noncoding RNAs, especially lncRNAs, featured with the relationships between lncRNAs and diseases. The annotations of NONCODE were also generated based on literature mining. These two databases provide great convenience for further analysis and applications of well-characterized lncRNAs.

1.2 Function Prediction of lncRNAs

Unlike protein-coding genes whose sequence motifs are indicative of their functions or miRNAs which in general complementarity bind to 3′-untranslated region of their targets, the sequence and secondary structure of lncRNAs are usually not conserved [19]. Thus, it impedes the development of computational methods to precisely predict the functions of lncRNAs. As a result, function prediction of lncRNAs currently mainly depends on their relationships with other components [20]. Accordingly, integrative analysis of protein-coding genes (*see* **Note 1**) or miRNAs (*see* **Note 2**) and lncRNAs has emerged as an approach to understand the functions of lncRNAs.

2 Methods

There are a rich collection of computational methods to study gene expression and various diseases. Here we try to discuss the methods most relevant to lncRNAs and cancer research and how to utilize public database such as The Cancer Genome Atlas (TCGA) to search for lncRNAs predictive of cancer progression.

A large amount of genomics data are sharable among researchers through online repositories. Among them, TCGA and International Cancer Genome Consortium (ICGC) collect and publish genomic and clinical data of cancer studies. Throughout this paper, the TCGA colorectal cancer cohort is analyzed to illustrate the methodologies on predictive model building and validation, as well as considerations related to cancer studies.

2.1 Survival Data and Endpoint Consideration

When researchers started to systematically decipher gene signatures for various cancer, many studies focused on exploring differentially expressed genes between normal and cancer specimens. The primary endpoint in this context is dichotomous and the goal is to classify a subject. The classification techniques can be grouped into two categories, the statistical methods such as logistic regression and k-nearest neighbors and the computing-intensive techniques such as random forest and support vector machines.

It soon became clear that identification of genes predictive of cancer progression is practically needed. Such studies yield the survival data in which time to some endpoint is recorded. The common endpoints are death and cancer recurrence, leading to overall survival (OS) and disease-free survival (DFS), respectively. Though OS is the most important quantity in cancer epidemiological studies, cancer recurrence should be a more meaningful endpoint for discovering predictive lncRNAs. More cancer patients are diagnosed in early stages and are expected to have good survival prospect due to adoption of cancer screening and therapeutic advances. When a cancer patient expired, the cause of death may be unrelated to cancer. We would like to recommend cancer recurrence as endpoint so that a study can target at gene functions related to cancer progression. We also want to recommend to consider early-stage cancer patients as the study population because the impact of gene expression level on cancer progression is a systematic process and may take long time to have effect. Survivorship of patients with advanced-stage cancer may be greatly influenced by age and clinical conditions and only remotely related to the biological functions of genes.

We followed these two principles to define the study cohort and survival endpoint for our illustrative example. The TCGA colorectal cancer cohort consist of 631 patients diagnosed in 1998–2013. We considered 627 having primary tumor as the sample type but excluded 92 with stage IV cancer and 19 with unknown stage. Among 516 stage I–III patients, 307 had mRNA expression level measured. Four were further excluded because of unavailability of survival times. Therefore, our final study cohort consist of 303 stage I–III colorectal cancer patients. The cohort was further split into the estimation set ($N = 219$) and the validation set ($N = 84$). The demographic and clinical characteristics of these two sets are depicted in Table 1. Screening and selection of lncRNA were conducted in the estimation set, while the validation set was reserved for assessing the accuracy of the predictive models. More details about validation are provided in Subheading 2.4.

Table 1
Table of demographic and clinical characteristics

	Estimation set (N = 219)	Validation set (N = 84)	P value
Year of diagnosis	1998–2010	2011–2013	
Age, median (min, max)	68 (31, 90)	64 (31, 90)	0.327
Male	120 (55%)	46 (55%)	1.000
Race			<0.001
White	159 (73%)	58 (69%)	
Black	23 (10%)	24 (29%)	
Other	11 (5%)	2 (2%)	
Unknown	26 (12%)	0 (0%)	
Stage			0.848
I	38 (17%)	17 (20%)	
II	98 (45%)	37 (44%)	
III	83 (38%)	30 (36%)	
Vascular invasion			0.003
Yes	41 (19%)	8 (10%)	
No	142 (65%)	71 (84%)	
Unknown	36 (16%)	5 (6%)	
Lymphovascular invasion			0.002
Yes	57 (26%)	12 (14%)	
No	132 (60%)	68 (81%)	
Unknown	30 (14%)	4 (5%)	

The TCGA colorectal cancer cohort was divided into the estimation set and validation set

As we mentioned, cancer recurrence is the meaningful endpoint and was considered in this example. Among 303 patients, cancer progression/recurrence was observed in 65 patients and 29 expired without information on cancer recurrence. We considered the composite endpoint cancer recurrence or death and studied DFS. In real-life studies, it often happens that both time to disease recurrence and time to death are observed on one patient. It is always more meaningful to utilize the time to disease recurrence when exploring gene markers.

2.2 Screening of lncRNA

Several online analytical tools perform basic analysis of TCGA genomic data. One commonly used tool, cBioPortal for Cancer Genomics [21, 22], provides the z-scores of mRNA expression levels which are computed by finding the relative mRNA expression levels compared to the normal population. These z-scores offer an objective assessment of the expression levels in the cancer samples to the normal samples. It also offers easy comparisons between different cancer cohorts so that data consolidation and model validation across different studies become smooth. Because of these advantages, we chose to download the lncRNA z-scores of the TCGA colorectal cohort from cBioPortal.

At our search dated on May 16, 2016, a total of 2775 lncRNA symbols were reported at www.genenames.org. These symbols were broken down into groups of size 100 and submitted at cBioPortal to download the lncRNA z-scores. Many lncRNAs lack expression data. We got the expression data set of 272 lncRNAs. We would prefer using the upregulation or downregulation status of an lncRNA so that it is straightforward to design the potential validation experiment. For the expression levels of the normal population, we classified the top 10% as upregulated expression levels and the bottom 10% as downregulated expression levels. We applied the z-score cut points 1.28 and -1.28 on the downloaded lncRNA z-scores to find cancer cases with upregulated or downregulated lncRNAs. The next step was to screen the dichotomized lncRNAs to find those possibly associated with DFS. However we had to exclude the lncRNAs with very few upregulated or downregulated cases. We kept only the lncRNAs with at least ten upregulated or downregulated cases. Two hundred and three lncRNAs met this condition.

Screening was conducted to search for lncRNAs predictive of DFS, in order to obtain a smaller pool for further selection. In this step, the univariate analysis between each lncRNA and survival outcome was performed using the log-rank test [23]. The lncRNAs were sorted by their log-rank p values. Those with p values less than 0.1 are shown in Table 2. This set of lncRNAs was considered for building predictive models. One can see from the table that upregulation status of many lncRNAs and the downregulation status of a few lncRNAs were associated with DFS. It is necessary to examine the effect of both upregulation and downregulation of an lncRNA on cancer progression. The screening greatly reduces the dimensionality of high-throughput genomic data. One can focus on the meaningful markers on the model building step, so that the computational time can be affordable.

2.3 Predictive Model Building

Cancer progression is driven by the demographic and clinical factors as well as the interplay of genetic markers. The Cox model [24] is the most popular regression model to quantify the joint effects of predictors on a survival outcome. The instantaneous probability of experiencing the failure event given a set of characteristics, x, is specified in a Cox model,

Table 2
lncRNAs associated with DFS in univariate analysis (log-rank $P < 0.10$)

lncRNA	P	lncRNA	P	lncRNA	P
Upregulated lncRNAs associated with DFS					
LINC00634	0.001	SNHG10	0.024	LINC00115	0.058
LINC00705	0.002	DLEU1	0.025	FAM138B	0.063
LINC00936	0.007	LINC00473	0.031	PIK3CD_AS1	0.067
LINC00264	0.009	OLMALINC	0.037	ARRDC1_AS1	0.072
LINC00691	0.019	LINC00161	0.044	TLX1NB	0.077
LINC00174	0.022	LINC00158	0.045	LINC00493	0.086
DANCR	0.023	FAM138E	0.051	MIMT1	0.100
LINC00957	0.024	LINC00341	0.052		
LINC00593	0.024	HCG11	0.053		
Downregulated lncRNAs associated with DFS					
FAM201A	0.041	JPX	0.077	HCG11	0.082

$$\lambda(t;x) = \lambda_0(t)\exp(\beta^T x).$$

The instantaneous probability of experiencing the event is known as the hazard function. In the above model, $\lambda_0(t)$ is the baseline hazard function. There is no restriction on its form so that the flexible trend of the risk over time can be captured. β is the vector of regression coefficients, measuring the effects of covariates on the hazard function. For a binary covariate such as lncRNA LINC00634 which was coded as 1 for upregulation and 0 otherwise, a positive regression coefficient indicates the increased risk of cancer recurrence for upregulated LINC00634, while a negative regression coefficient shows a protective effect against cancer recurrence for upregulated LINC00634. In general clinical and epidemiological studies, the hazard ratios (HR $= e^\beta$) for covariates are routinely calculated and interpreted. In terms of genetic markers, one is less interested in interpreting the hazard ratio of a single gene. It is more important to determine the prognostic score for an individual with specific characteristics and gene expression levels. Regression coefficients are directly related to computation of prognostic scores. Therefore, we report the estimated regression coefficients for each predictive model built in this subsection.

In this subsection we discuss the routine forward selection method for building a Cox model. In forward selection either p value or Akaike Information Criterion (AIC) [25] can be used as the selection criterion. We also discuss the Lasso method, which is relatively new and better fits the context of gene selection. To illustrate these methods, we built three predictive models for colorectal cancer recurrence using the estimation set ($N = 219$) depicted in Table 1.

2.3.1 Forward Selection Using P Value as Criterion

We first examined which demographic and clinical variables were associated with DFS. Cancer stage and age (<70 and ≥70) turned out to be significant and were included in the models. The main goal was to choose the lncRNAs in the pool specified in Table 2. Variable selection can be conducted by adding significant variables one by one to the model or eliminating insignificant variables from the full model including all the variables. They are known as the forward selection and backward elimination methods, respectively. When selection is performed among a large number of genetic markers, the forward selection is easier to operate and was employed in our study.

The p value for a regression coefficient is a routine criterion for variable selection. At each round of selection, the variable associated with the smallest p value should enter the model. However, if any previously selected variable becomes insignificant, the variable with the smallest p value should be discarded, and the variable with the next smallest p value is considered. Variable addition should continue until all the remaining variables have p values above the significance threshold. We implemented this method to build the Cox model on DFS using the estimation set derived from TCGA colorectal cancer cohort. At the significance level 0.05, a total of seven lncRNAs were selected. The estimates of regression coefficients are shown in Table 3. Upregulations of LINC00634, LINC00705, LINC00691, DLEU1, LINC00473, and PIK3CD_AS1 are associated with the increased risk of colorectal cancer recurrence. Downregulation of FAM201A is protective against colorectal cancer recurrence.

2.3.2 Forward Selection Using AIC as Criterion

A regression model including all significant variables may not best describe the data. For likelihood-based model, how well a model fits the data is usually measured by the log likelihood. The partial likelihood [26] is routinely used for estimating the regression coefficients for a Cox model. Let $\log(L)$ be the log partial likelihood. The statistic evaluating goodness of fit of a model is $-2\log(L)$, for which a smaller value indicates a better fitting model. However, this statistic is not proper to evaluate two models with different number of covariates. The statistic AIC makes adjustment on $-2\log(L)$ by adding the term $2k$, where k is the number of covariates in a Cox model,

$$\text{AIC} = -2\log(L) + 2k.$$

AIC can be used as a criterion for variable selection. At each round of forward selection, AIC is evaluated for tentatively adding each variable. The variable yielding the smallest AIC value is chosen

Table 3
Clinical variables and lncRNAs selected by different methods

Variables	Effect	Selection method		
		Forward selection (P)	Forward selection (AIC)	Lasso
Stage	2 vs. 1	0.652	0.445	
Stage	3 vs. 1	0.812	0.276	
Age	≥70 vs. <70	0.583	0.602	0.306
LINC00634	Upregulation	1.624	1.843	0.137
LINC00705	Upregulation	1.256	0.953	0.152
LINC00936	Upregulation		1.407	0.433
LINC00691	Upregulation	0.834	0.971	0.298
LINC00174	Upregulation			0.416
DANCR	Upregulation			0.163
LINC00957	Upregulation			0.700
LINC00593	Upregulation		1.118	
DLEU1	Upregulation	0.609	0.562	0.100
LINC00473	Upregulation	1.181		0.140
OLMALINC	Upregulation			0.414
LINC00161	Upregulation			−0.056
LINC00158	Upregulation		1.325	0.514
FAM138E	Upregulation			1.043
LINC00341	Upregulation			0.588
HCG11	Upregulation		0.517	0.764
LINC00115	Upregulation			0.773
FAM138B	Upregulation			0.078
PIK3CD_AS1	Upregulation	0.888		0.067
ARRDC1_AS1	Upregulation			0.278
TLX1NB	Upregulation			0.400
FAM201A	Downregulation	−1.761	−2.485	−1.415

to enter the model. The AIC of the new model should be compared to the AIC of the model of the previous round. The new model is accepted, and the forward selection continues only if the AIC value decreases.

We implemented the AIC-based forward selection to build the Cox model using the colorectal cancer estimation set. The final model is depicted in Table 3. A few more lncRNAs were selected by AIC compared to the model built by the p value criterion.

2.3.3 Lasso Method

Biological functions are regulated by a large number of interacted genes. An important step in analyzing genomic data is to explore gene co-expression because highly correlated genes may work together to determine some biological function. The statistical method to measure the degree of correlation for expression data is Pearson or Spearman correlation coefficient, in conjunction with the scatter plot which provides graphical assessment of the relationship between a pair of continuous variables. The Spearman correlation coefficient should be recommended because it does not require bivariate normal distribution for the target variables. When a sample correlation coefficient is reported, many statistical software also report the accompanying p value for the null hypothesis that the correlation coefficient is zero by default. However, such a p value is not very useful since a nonzero correlation coefficient covers a wide range of correlation level. It is more informative to obtain a confidence interval of a correlation coefficient. The correlation is believed to be weak, medium, strong, and very strong when the absolute value of a correlation coefficient falls in the ranges <0.3, 0.4–0.6, 0.7–0.9, and >0.9, respectively. Association of categorical data is usually evaluated by Pearson chi-square test or Fisher's exact test. Table 4 depicts the pairs of lncRNAs strongly

Table 4
Pairs of categorized lncRNAs with high level of association (Fisher's exact test $P < 0.001$)

lncRNA 1	lncRNA 2	P
ARRDC1_AS1	LINC00115	0.0003
DANCR	SNHG10	0.0000
DLEU1	SNHG10	0.0006
DLEU2	ZFAS1	0.0005
FAM138E	LINC00634	<0.0001
LINC00115	LINC00174	<0.0001
LINC00115	TLX1NB	0.0009
LINC00264	LINC00341	0.0010
LINC00341	LINC00936	<0.0001
LINC00341	PIK3CD_AS1	<0.0001
LINC00473	LINC00936	0.0001

associated with each other as indicated by Fisher's exact test p value <0.001.

In building a regression model, the problem of highly correlated predictors is known as multicollinearity. It poses the challenges on variable selection and stability of the regression coefficient estimates. Principle component analysis (PCA) is the routine method to solve the problem of multicollinearity with continuous predictors. The large number of continuous predictors can be reduced to a few uncorrelated principle components that explain the majority of the variation and are fitted as covariates in the regression model. However, PCA may not be feasible in many real-world studies because many demographic and clinical characteristics are categorical such as gender, race, and cancer stage. The more practically feasible solution is the penalized regression models such as the ridge regression [27] and Lasso regression model [28]. A penalized regression model shrinks the regression coefficients to reduce over-fitting. The Lasso penalty can shrink the regression coefficients of the variables contributing less to the response toward zero; therefore, it is considered a useful variable selection method for correlated predictors. The Cox model with a Lasso penalty was studied by Tibshirani [29] and Zhang and Lu [30] among others. We installed the R package "glmnet" [31] and run the function "glmnet" to obtain the Lasso model with the variables age, cancer stage, and lncRNAs given in Table 2. The estimation result is shown in Table 3. Compared to the two models built by the forward selection method, a lot more lncRNAs were selected in the Lasso model, but cancer stage was excluded. Inclusion of a good number of genetic markers can better differentiate the individuals.

2.4 Predictive Model Validation

When a predictive model is built, one should validate whether the model will work fine with actual data. If multiple predictive models are built by the study design, model validation and evaluation is an inherent step to guide the decision on choosing a model. A general guideline for model validation is to use a data set different from the one on which the models are built. Here we discuss two simple ways of obtaining a validation data set.

First, one can split the whole data set of the study into the estimation set and the validation set. These two data sets are used for building the model and validating the model, respectively. This method is a good choice with a large study cohort. Allocation of the subjects into these two sets can be guided by random mechanism. Randomization usually yields two cohorts of similar characteristics given a large study. An alternative allocation method can be considered if subject enrollment lasts a fairly long period of time. We can let the early enrolled participants to be the estimation set and the participants enrolled at the late study period go to the validation set. This kind of allocation creates a pseudo setting to use the prospectively collected data to validate a predictive model. When there is concern about the size, one may explore other means of acquiring the validation set.

Second, one can try to find and use data of a similar study as the validation set. The major concern is difficult to justify the equivalence between the target study and the study used for validation purpose. Various sources can cause inequality. First, the demographic and clinical variables collected in different studies are not exactly the same. Second, spatial and temporal differences may be present and difficult to quantify. Third, it has been a challenging issue to consolidate data from different sequencing experiments. The mRNA expression z-score provided by cBioPortal is a feasible solution because the expression levels of different studies have been aligned to the distribution of the normal population. Since cBioPortal hosts data of cancer studies other than TCGA, it offers a convenient route to use a cancer cohort of other cBioPortal study as the validation set. Nowadays, some researchers employ the big data concept in bioinformatics applications. They consolidate data from all possible sources together and then split the pooled data into the estimation set and validation set. This is an innovative approach that should be employed in cancer studies though statisticians and computing scientists need to deal with many challenges such as missing data and across-study normalization.

For our illustrative study, we let the relative new cases, those diagnosed in 2011–2013, as the validation set ($N = 84$). To evaluate the predictive accuracy of the Cox model built by forward selection method using the p value criterion, the prognostic score should be calculated for everyone in the validation set by the equation,

$$\text{Score} = 0.652 \times \text{stage}\,2 + 0.812 \times \text{stage}\,3 + 0.583 \times \text{ageGE70} \\ + 1.624 \times \text{LINC00634} + 1.256 \times \text{LINC00705} + 0.834 \\ \times \text{LINC00691} + 0.609 \times \text{DLEU1} + 1.181 \\ \times \text{LINC00473} + 0.888 \times \text{PIK3CD\_AS1} - 1.761 \\ \times \text{FA201A}$$

In the above equation, LINC00634, LINC00705, LINC00691, DLEU1, LINC00473, and PIK3CD_AS1 are all binary variables indicating whether upregulation of these lncRNAs occurred. FA201A is the binary variable indicating downregulation of this lncRNA. For example, one individual in the validation set was diagnosed at 60 with stage 2 colorectal cancer, upregulation occurred on LINC00705 and DLEU1, and FA201A was downregulated. The prognostic score for this patient should be evaluated as

$$\text{Score} = 0.652 + 1.256 + 0.609 - 1.761 = 0.756$$

After all the scores were computed, the validation set was split into high- and low-score groups of nearly equal size. The Kaplan-Meier curves [32] of DFS were obtained for these two groups and depicted in Fig. 1a. There is a good separation between two curves with a log-rank test p value 0.009. The significant p value proved the predictive accuracy of the suggested model.

The other two models specified in Table 3 can be similarly evaluated. Figure 1b, c shows the DFS curves of the high- and low-score groups of the validation set where the prognostic scores were computed from the second and third model in Table 3. Both sets of curves are well separated, together with log-rank test p value 0.039 and 0.055, respectively. These two models were successfully validated for precisely predicting DFS. In this particular study, the Lasso model happened to perform not as good as the two models built by forward selection method. It should be noted that more lncRNAs were selected by the Lasso method. The prognostic scores derived from the Lasso model are more distinct between individuals; consequently, the individuals can be better differentiated in a general sense.

2.5 Experimental Validation

In addition to in silico model validation, experimental approaches are needed to understand the effects of hit lncRNAs on cellular functions. The main strategies require lncRNA manipulations. That being said, overexpress the hit if it's predicted to be downregulated (supposedly tumor-suppressive gene), whereas knock down/knock out it if it's upregulated (supposedly oncogenic gene). For example, to validate the functions of LINC00657, which is upregulated and associated with overall survival or recurrence in human breast cancer based on TCGA at cBioPortal, Liu et al. demonstrated that LINC00657 knockout with the use of CRISPR/Cas9 system [33] suppresses tumor cell growth, suggesting that LINC00657 is a potential oncogene [34]. Overall functional validation of lncRNAs is critical to understand their biological consequence: in vitro cell line experiments can be performed to assess alterations in oncogenic properties; in vivo xenograft models can be used to compare tumor growth between control and dysregulated lncRNAs. Moreover, the expression of a given lncRNA can be investigated in cancer tissue cDNA arrays for high-throughput molecular profiling of hundreds of specimens. It would offer the opportunity to conduct pilot and validation studies of potential lncRNAs using clinical samples linked to clinicopathological databases.

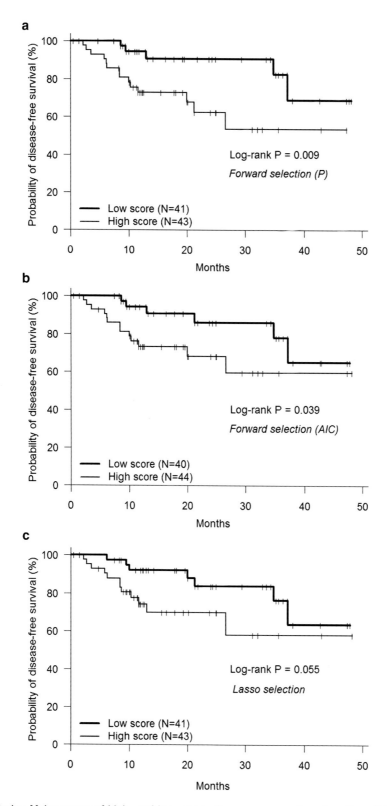

Fig. 1 The Kaplan-Meier curves of high- and low-prognostic-score groups based on the validation set. The prognostic scores were computed from three models. (**a**) The model was built using the forward selection method. The variables were selected by their *p* values. (**b**) The model was built using the forward selection method. The variables were selected by AIC values. (**c**) The model was built using the Lasso method

3 Notes

1. Co-expression of lncRNAs and protein-coding genes

    Genomic loci analysis revealed that some lncRNAs showed co-regulated expression patterns with their neighboring protein-coding genes [35], suggesting the involvement of lncRNAs in regulating the expression of neighboring coding genes. Therefore, identifying coding genes that are co-expressed with lncRNAs may help to infer lncRNA function. One of the earliest reports has utilized a Gene Set Enrichment Analysis (GSEA) to identify enriched functional terms corresponding to the lncRNAs at genome scale [36], whereas later an advanced coding-noncoding (CNC) gene co-expression network was constructed to elucidate the co-expression within lncRNAs group and protein-coding gene group in addition to the co-expression between lncRNAs and protein-coding genes [37].

2. Interaction of lncRNAs and miRNAs

    Some lncRNAs appear to share a synergism with miRNA in the regulatory network [38]; thus, lncRNAs may function by binding miRNA. Moreover, mounting evidence suggests that lncRNAs can function as miRNA sponges and compete for miRNA binding to protein-coding transcripts [39]. Therefore, identifying well-established miRNAs that interact with lncRNAs may also help to infer lncRNA function. Once a lncRNA-miRNA correlation network is constructed, gene ontology (GO) [40] and Kyoto Encyclopedia of Genes and Genomes (KEGG) [41] pathway analysis can be performed to predict specific molecular function associating lncRNAs as well as target genes enriched in signaling pathways. Several articles have reported potential targets of lncRNAs in cancer using the above methods [42–44].

References

1. Consortium EP, Birney E, Stamatoyannopoulos JA, Dutta A, Guigo R, Gingeras TR, Margulies EH, Weng Z, Snyder M, Dermitzakis ET, Thurman RE, Kuehn MS, Taylor CM, Neph S, Koch CM, Asthana S, Malhotra A, Adzhubei I, Greenbaum JA, Andrews RM, Flicek P, Boyle PJ, Cao H, Carter NP, Clelland GK, Davis S, Day N, Dhami P, Dillon SC, Dorschner MO, Fiegler H, Giresi PG, Goldy J, Hawrylycz M, Haydock A, Humbert R, James KD, Johnson BE, Johnson EM, Frum TT, Rosenzweig ER, Karnani N, Lee K, Lefebvre GC, Navas PA, Neri F, Parker SC, Sabo PJ, Sandstrom R, Shafer A, Vetrie D, Weaver M, Wilcox S, Yu M, Collins FS, Dekker J, Lieb JD, Tullius TD, Crawford GE, Sunyaev S, Noble WS, Dunham I, Denoeud F, Reymond A, Kapranov P, Rozowsky J, Zheng D, Castelo R, Frankish A, Harrow J, Ghosh S, Sandelin A, Hofacker IL, Baertsch R, Keefe D, Dike S, Cheng J, Hirsch HA, Sekinger EA, Lagarde J, Abril JF, Shahab A, Flamm C, Fried C, Hackermuller J, Hertel J, Lindemeyer M, Missal K, Tanzer A, Washietl S, Korbel J, Emanuelsson O, Pedersen JS, Holroyd N, Taylor R, Swarbreck D, Matthews N, Dickson MC, Thomas DJ, Weirauch MT, Gilbert J, Drenkow J, Bell I, Zhao X, Srinivasan KG, Sung WK, Ooi HS, Chiu KP, Foissac S, Alioto T, Brent M, Pachter L, Tress ML, Valencia A, Choo SW, Choo CY, Ucla C, Manzano C, Wyss C, Cheung E, Clark TG,

Brown JB, Ganesh M, Patel S, Tammana H, Chrast J, Henrichsen CN, Kai C, Kawai J, Nagalakshmi U, Wu J, Lian Z, Lian J, Newburger P, Zhang X, Bickel P, Mattick JS, Carninci P, Hayashizaki Y, Weissman S, Hubbard T, Myers RM, Rogers J, Stadler PF, Lowe TM, Wei CL, Ruan Y, Struhl K, Gerstein M, Antonarakis SE, Fu Y, Green ED, Karaoz U, Siepel A, Taylor J, Liefer LA, Wetterstrand KA, Good PJ, Feingold EA, Guyer MS, Cooper GM, Asimenos G, Dewey CN, Hou M, Nikolaev S, Montoya-Burgos JI, Loytynoja A, Whelan S, Pardi F, Massingham T, Huang H, Zhang NR, Holmes I, Mullikin JC, Ureta-Vidal A, Paten B, Seringhaus M, Church D, Rosenbloom K, Kent WJ, Stone EA, Program NCS, Baylor College of Medicine Human Genome Sequencing Center, Washington University Genome Sequencing Center, Broad Institute, Children's Hospital Oakland Research Institute, Batzoglou S, Goldman N, Hardison RC, Haussler D, Miller W, Sidow A, Trinklein ND, Zhang ZD, Barrera L, Stuart R, King DC, Ameur A, Enroth S, Bieda MC, Kim J, Bhinge AA, Jiang N, Liu J, Yao F, Vega VB, Lee CW, Ng P, Shahab A, Yang A, Moqtaderi Z, Zhu Z, Xu X, Squazzo S, Oberley MJ, Inman D, Singer MA, Richmond TA, Munn KJ, Rada-Iglesias A, Wallerman O, Komorowski J, Fowler JC, Couttet P, Bruce AW, Dovey OM, Ellis PD, Langford CF, Nix DA, Euskirchen G, Hartman S, Urban AE, Kraus P, Van Calcar S, Heintzman N, Kim TH, Wang K, Qu C, Hon G, Luna R, Glass CK, Rosenfeld MG, Aldred SF, Cooper SJ, Halees A, Lin JM, Shulha HP, Zhang X, Xu M, Haidar JN, Yu Y, Ruan Y, Iyer VR, Green RD, Wadelius C, Farnham PJ, Ren B, Harte RA, Hinrichs AS, Trumbower H, Clawson H, Hillman-Jackson J, Zweig AS, Smith K, Thakkapallayil A, Barber G, Kuhn RM, Karolchik D, Armengol L, Bird CP, de Bakker PI, Kern AD, Lopez-Bigas N, Martin JD, Stranger BE, Woodroffe A, Davydov E, Dimas A, Eyras E, Hallgrimsdottir IB, Huppert J, Zody MC, Abecasis GR, Estivill X, Bouffard GG, Guan X, Hansen NF, Idol JR, Maduro VV, Maskeri B, JC MD, Park M, Thomas PJ, Young AC, Blakesley RW, Muzny DM, Sodergren E, Wheeler DA, Worley KC, Jiang H, Weinstock GM, Gibbs RA, Graves T, Fulton R, Mardis ER, Wilson RK, Clamp M, Cuff J, Gnerre S, Jaffe DB, Chang JL, Lindblad-Toh K, Lander ES, Koriabine M, Nefedov M, Osoegawa K, Yoshinaga Y, Zhu B, de Jong PJ (2007) Identification and analysis of functional elements in 1% of the human genome by the ENCODE pilot project. Nature 447(7146):799–816

2. Cech TR, Steitz JA (2014) The noncoding RNA revolution-trashing old rules to forge new ones. Cell 157(1):77–94
3. Kapranov P, Cheng J, Dike S, Nix DA, Duttagupta R, Willingham AT, Stadler PF, Hertel J, Hackermuller J, Hofacker IL, Bell I, Cheung E, Drenkow J, Dumais E, Patel S, Helt G, Ganesh M, Ghosh S, Piccolboni A, Sementchenko V, Tammana H, Gingeras TR (2007) RNA maps reveal new RNA classes and a possible function for pervasive transcription. Science 316(5830):1484–1488
4. Derrien T, Johnson R, Bussotti G, Tanzer A, Djebali S, Tilgner H, Guernec G, Martin D, Merkel A, Knowles DG, Lagarde J, Veeravalli L, Ruan X, Ruan Y, Lassmann T, Carninci P, Brown JB, Lipovich L, Gonzalez JM, Thomas M, Davis CA, Shiekhattar R, Gingeras TR, Hubbard TJ, Notredame C, Harrow J, Guigo R (2012) The GENCODE v7 catalog of human long noncoding RNAs: analysis of their gene structure, evolution, and expression. Genome Res 22(9):1775–1789
5. Ulitsky I, Bartel DP (2013) lncRNAs: genomics, evolution, and mechanisms. Cell 154(1):26–46
6. Prensner JR, Chinnaiyan AM (2011) The emergence of lncRNAs in cancer biology. Cancer Discov 1(5):391–407
7. Prensner JR, Iyer MK, Balbin OA, Dhanasekaran SM, Cao Q, Brenner JC, Laxman B, Asangani IA, Grasso CS, Kominsky HD, Cao X, Jing X, Wang X, Siddiqui J, Wei JT, Robinson D, Iyer HK, Palanisamy N, Maher CA, Chinnaiyan AM (2011) Transcriptome sequencing across a prostate cancer cohort identifies PCAT-1, an unannotated lncRNA implicated in disease progression. Nat Biotechnol 29(8):742–749
8. Lee GL, Dobi A, Srivastava S (2011) Prostate cancer: diagnostic performance of the PCA3 urine test. Nat Rev Urol 8(3):123–124
9. Iyer MK, Niknafs YS, Malik R, Singhal U, Sahu A, Hosono Y, Barrette TR, Prensner JR, Evans JR, Zhao S, Poliakov A, Cao X, Dhanasekaran SM, Wu YM, Robinson DR, Beer DG, Feng FY, Iyer HK, Chinnaiyan AM (2015) The landscape of long noncoding RNAs in the human transcriptome. Nat Genet 47(3):199–208
10. Liu Q, Huang J, Zhou N, Zhang Z, Zhang A, Lu Z, Wu F, Mo YY (2013) LncRNA loc285194 is a p53-regulated tumor suppressor. Nucleic Acids Res 41(9):4976–4987

11. Zhang Z, Zhu Z, Watabe K, Zhang X, Bai C, Xu M, Wu F, Mo YY (2013) Negative regulation of lncRNA GAS5 by miR-21. Cell Death Differ 20(11):1558–1568
12. Zhang A, Zhou N, Huang J, Liu Q, Fukuda K, Ma D, Lu Z, Bai C, Watabe K, Mo YY (2013) The human long non-coding RNA-RoR is a p53 repressor in response to DNA damage. Cell Res 23(3):340–350
13. Huang J, Zhang A, Ho TT, Zhang Z, Zhou N, Ding X, Zhang X, Xu M, Mo YY (2016) Linc-RoR promotes c-Myc expression through hnRNP I and AUF1. Nucleic Acids Res 44(7):3059–3069
14. Huang J, Zhou N, Watabe K, Lu Z, Wu F, Xu M, Mo YY (2014) Long non-coding RNA UCA1 promotes breast tumor growth by suppression of p27 (Kip1). Cell Death Dis 5:e1008
15. Singh R, Gupta SC, Peng WX, Zhou N, Pochampally R, Atfi A, Watabe K, Lu Z, Mo YY (2016) Regulation of alternative splicing of Bcl-x by BC200 contributes to breast cancer pathogenesis. Cell Death Dis 7(6):e2262
16. Zhang Z, Zhou N, Huang J, Ho TT, Zhu Z, Qiu Z, Zhou X, Bai C, Wu F, Xu M, Mo YY (2016) Regulation of androgen receptor splice variant AR3 by PCGEM1. Oncotarget 7(13):15481–15491
17. Quek XC, Thomson DW, Maag JL, Bartonicek N, Signal B, Clark MB, Gloss BS, Dinger ME (2015) lncRNAdb v2.0: expanding the reference database for functional long non-coding RNAs. Nucleic Acids Res 43(Database issue):D168–D173
18. Zhao Y, Li H, Fang S, Kang Y, Wu W, Hao Y, Li Z, Bu D, Sun N, Zhang MQ, Chen R (2016) NONCODE 2016: an informative and valuable data source of long non-coding RNAs. Nucleic Acids Res 44(D1):D203–D208
19. Mercer TR, Dinger ME, Mattick JS (2009) Long non-coding RNAs: insights into functions. Nat Rev Genet 10(3):155–159
20. Ma H, Hao Y, Dong X, Gong Q, Chen J, Zhang J, Tian W (2012) Molecular mechanisms and function prediction of long noncoding RNA. Scientific World Journal 2012:541786
21. Cerami E, Gao J, Dogrusoz U, Gross BE, Sumer SO, Aksoy BA, Jacobsen A, Byrne CJ, Heuer ML, Larsson E, Antipin Y, Reva B, Goldberg AP, Sander C, Schultz N (2012) The cBio cancer genomics portal: an open platform for exploring multidimensional cancer genomics data. Cancer Discov 2(5):401–404
22. Gao J, Aksoy BA, Dogrusoz U, Dresdner G, Gross B, Sumer SO, Sun Y, Jacobsen A, Sinha R, Larsson E, Cerami E, Sander C, Schultz N (2013) Integrative analysis of complex cancer genomics and clinical profiles using the cBioPortal. Sci Signal 6(269):pl1
23. Mantel N (1966) Evaluation of survival data and two new rank order statistics arising in its consideration. Cancer Chemother Rep 50(3):163–170
24. Cox DR (1972) Regression models and life-tables. J R Stat Soc B 34:187–220
25. Akaike H (1973) Information theory and an extension of the maximum likelihood principle. 2nd International Symposium on Information Theory, Tsaghkadzor, Armenia, USSR, Budapest: Akadémiai Kiadó, pp 267–281
26. Cox DR (1975) Partial likelihood. Biometrika 62(2):269–276
27. Hoerl AE, Kennard RW (1970) Ridge regression: biased estimation for nonorthogonal problems. Technometrics 12(1):55–67
28. Tibshirani R (1996) Regression shrinkage and selection via the lasso. J R Stat Soc B 58:267–288
29. Tibshirani R (1997) The lasso method for variable selection in the Cox model. Stat Med 16(4):385–395
30. Zhang HH, Lu W (2007) Adaptive lasso for Cox's proportional hazards model. Biometrika 94(3):691–703
31. Friedman J, Hastie T, Tibshirani R (2016) glmnet: Lasso and elastic-net regularized generalized linear models. R package version 2.0-5. http://CRAN.R-project.org/package=glmnet
32. Kaplan EL, Meier P (1958) Nonparametric estimation from incomplete observations. J Am Stat Assoc 53:457–481
33. Ho TT, Zhou N, Huang J, Koirala P, Xu M, Fung R, Wu F, Mo YY (2015) Targeting non-coding RNAs with the CRISPR/Cas9 system in human cell lines. Nucleic Acids Res 43(3):e17
34. Liu H, Li J, Koirala P, Ding X, Chen B, Wang Y, Wang Z, Wang C, Zhang X, Mo YY (2016) Long non-coding RNAs as prognostic markers in human breast cancer. Oncotarget 7(15):20584–20596
35. Chen X, Liu B, Yang R, Guo Y, Li F, Wang L, Hu H (2016) Integrated analysis of long non-coding RNAs in human colorectal cancer. Oncotarget. https://doi.org/10.18632/oncotarget.8192
36. Guttman M, Amit I, Garber M, French C, Lin MF, Feldser D, Huarte M, Zuk O, Carey BW, Cassady JP, Cabili MN, Jaenisch R, Mikkelsen TS, Jacks T, Hacohen N, Bernstein BE, Kellis M, Regev A, Rinn JL, Lander ES

(2009) Chromatin signature reveals over a thousand highly conserved large non-coding RNAs in mammals. Nature 458 (7235):223–227

37. Liao Q, Liu C, Yuan X, Kang S, Miao R, Xiao H, Zhao G, Luo H, Bu D, Zhao H, Skogerbo G, Wu Z, Zhao Y (2011) Large-scale prediction of long non-coding RNA functions in a coding-non-coding gene co-expression network. Nucleic Acids Res 39(9):3864–3878

38. Salmena L, Poliseno L, Tay Y, Kats L, Pandolfi PP (2011) A ceRNA hypothesis: the Rosetta Stone of a hidden RNA language? Cell 146 (3):353–358

39. Du Z, Sun T, Hacisuleyman E, Fei T, Wang X, Brown M, Rinn JL, Lee MG, Chen Y, Kantoff PW, Liu XS (2016) Integrative analyses reveal a long noncoding RNA-mediated sponge regulatory network in prostate cancer. Nat Commun 7:10982

40. Ashburner M, Ball CA, Blake JA, Botstein D, Butler H, Cherry JM, Davis AP, Dolinski K, Dwight SS, Eppig JT, Harris MA, Hill DP, Issel-Tarver L, Kasarskis A, Lewis S, Matese JC, Richardson JE, Ringwald M, Rubin GM, Sherlock G (2000) Gene ontology: tool for the unification of biology. The Gene Ontology Consortium. Nat Genet 25(1):25–29

41. Ogata H, Goto S, Sato K, Fujibuchi W, Bono H, Kanehisa M (1999) KEGG: Kyoto encyclopedia of genes and genomes. Nucleic Acids Res 27(1):29–34

42. Lin XC, Zhu Y, Chen WB, Lin LW, Chen DH, Huang JR, Pan K, Lin Y, Wu BT, Dai Y, Tu ZG (2014) Integrated analysis of long non-coding RNAs and mRNA expression profiles reveals the potential role of lncRNAs in gastric cancer pathogenesis. Int J Oncol 45(2):619–628

43. Xu J, Gao C, Zhang F, Ma X, Peng X, Zhang R, Kong D, Simard AR, Hao J (2016) Differentially expressed lncRNAs and mRNAs identified by microarray analysis in GBS patients vs healthy controls. Sci Rep 6:21819

44. Dong R, Jia D, Xue P, Cui X, Li K, Zheng S, He X, Dong K (2014) Genome-wide analysis of long noncoding RNA (lncRNA) expression in hepatoblastoma tissues. PLoS One 9(1): e85599

Chapter 9

Computational Methods for Identification of T Cell Neoepitopes in Tumors

Vanessa Isabell Jurtz and Lars Rønn Olsen

Abstract

Cancer immunotherapy has experienced several major breakthroughs in the past decade. Most recently, technical advances in next-generation sequencing methods have enabled discovery of tumor-specific mutations leading to protective T cell neoepitopes. Many of the successes are enabled by computational methods, which facilitate processing of raw data, mapping of mutations, and prediction of neoepitopes. In this book chapter, we provide an overview of the computational tasks related to the identification of neoepitopes, propose specific tools and best practices, and discuss strengths, weaknesses, and future challenges.

Key words Cancer immunotherapy, Bioinformatics, Epitope prediction, Next-generation sequencing, Nonsynonymous mutations

1 Introduction

Effective therapeutic cancer immunotherapy has been long awaited, and emerging technologies are likely to put it within reach. Numerous advances have been made in recent years to help fulfill the massive potential of harnessing the immune system's natural ability to fight cancer. There are multiple ways with which the immune system can be utilized to target tumor cells, and T cell-based therapies have shown great promise in recent years [1–3]. This form of therapy is enabled using next-generation sequencing (NGS) methods to map somatic mutations in tumor genomes, thereby elucidating subtle changes in tumor cells' proteins, which can lead to powerful responses by cytotoxic T lymphocytes (CTLs) [4]. These tumor antigens not only hold immense therapeutic potential but also diagnostic [5] and prognostic potential [6], and common to all these applications is the need for a wide range of computational methods to interpret data and predict useful therapy targets [7]. In this book chapter, we will discuss the computational methods and the typical workflow for neoepitope identification, assuming that the reader has a basic understanding of tumor biology and immunology.

2 Methods

2.1 Next-Generation Sequencing

NGS methods provide high-throughput sequencing of DNA or RNA. The target DNA or RNA is extracted from the cells or organism of interest and randomly digested into smaller pieces, which are then sequenced individually. The result is millions of short sequence reads that can be mapped to a reference genome or de novo assembled if a reference is not available. NGS for identification of neoepitopes can be done using whole genome (WGS), whole exome (WES), transcriptome (RNA) sequencing, or targeted DNA or RNA sequencing (TDS/TRS). Disease mutations can occur in both coding and noncoding parts of the genome. Mutations causing amino acid changes (nonsynonymous nucleotide substitutions or indels in CDS regions) account for approximately 60% of all disease mutations [8] and are the primary interest of neoepitope studies. Most recent studies of neoepitopes rely on WES of paired tumor and native cognate tissue, sometimes in combination with TDS sequencing to confirm the discovered variations. However, refined computational methods for variant calling may also enable identification of neoepitopes from RNA sequencing, which is not only a more cost-effective approach but also provides transcriptomic information, such as splice variations and mRNA expression.

Whether choosing WGS, WES, or RNA sequencing, computational tools play a central role in virtually every step of the process. These tools are constantly updated, and new applications are made to address these tasks. It is beyond the scope of this chapter to review them all (for a comprehensive listing, explore https://bio.tools/), rather, I will focus on the overall workflow for computational discovery of neoepitopes (Fig. 1), providing recommendations for tools and best practices for each step.

2.2 Preprocessing: From Base Calling to Read Mapping

Countless articles and entire books have been written about the process of transforming the raw output from sequencing platforms to fully sequenced genes or genomes. The tasks and tools needed are dependent on the choice of sequencing platform, whether one is performing WGS, WES, or RNA sequencing, as well as personal preferences for tools. Here, I will sketch out the general process, focusing on Illumina's HTS technologies, and refer readers to more in-depth reviews of the various steps. The reason I focus on Illumina is that their technologies are currently the most widely used, as they offer a good balance between depth, quality, and cost. For a

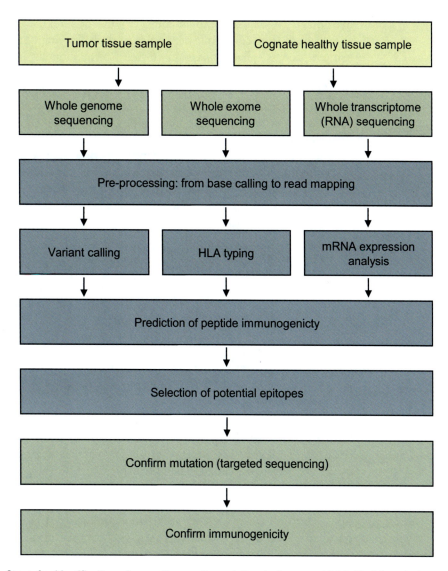

Fig. 1 Steps for identification of neoepitopes. Computational steps are highlighted in petroleum, sample collection in yellow, and experimental steps in green. Update so that computational steps match section titles

comprehensive review of other commercial systems, please see this current review by Snyder and colleagues [9].

2.2.1 Sequencing

The first step of sequencing on the Illumina MiSeq, NextSeq, and HiSeq series platforms consists of preparing the sequence library. This is done by extracting genomic DNA or RNA from the source material and fragmenting these into smaller pieces using enzymatic digestion or mechanically by sonication or nebulization. Then, an end-repair and adapter ligation step and a size filtering step are applied to select fragments of the desired size and to remove residual adapters. The resulting fragments are amplified and hybridized to oligos complementary to the adapters, which are fixated on a flow cell. Multiple copies of each fragment are made using a process called bridge amplification. The clonally amplified fragments are located in clusters of the fragment copies on the flow cell. Sequencing is done by a process called sequencing by synthesis. In this process, fluorescently labeled nucleotides are incrementally added and excited to emit a nucleotide characteristic signal with each round of addition. In the end, each cluster is sequenced in this fashion, and the process is repeated but this time synthesizing the reverse complement strand creating signals for paired-end reads. Lastly, inferring the nucleotide bases from the intensity signals recorded from each run is done in the process referred to as base calling [10].

2.2.2 Base Calling

Illumina's proprietary base caller, Bustard, performs reasonably well but is outperformed by a number of academically developed third-party base callers. Cacho et al. recently published a comprehensive review of these base callers, in which they recommend the three base callers AYB [11], Ibis [12], and freeIbis [13]. For runs without a control, or if high-quality bases are required by the downstream analyses, Cacho et al. recommend the AYB base caller [11]. On the other hand, if the speed of the base calling is important, the algorithms Ibis [12] or freeIbis [13] are recommended [14].

2.2.3 Quality Control

Before using sequencing data to draw biological conclusions, it is essential to identify and remove potential biases and errors. The quality of base calls can be assessed using FastQC (http://www.bioinformatics.babraham.ac.uk/projects/fastqc/), which provides a thorough report for each submitted sample. Among other features, FastQC scans for regions of low probability base calls or uncalled bases, overrepresented bases, GC content, and contamination from adapters, primers, or other sources. Details and instructions are provided at the FastQC website.

2.2.4 Trimming

If end-specific poor quality base calls or adapter sequences were found in the reads, one solution is to trim away low-quality portions of reads. This is not without risk, though shortening the reads will not only discard potentially valuable information but may also affect the mapping accuracy and the sequencing depth, so this step should only be done if necessary. Like every other step in the preprocessing pipeline, a large number of tools have been developed for read trimming. Although a number of popular trimmers have been reviewed, there is no clear "best trimmer" as this is highly dependent on the data and downstream analyses [15]. The quality of trimming by almost any tool is also highly dependent on the user selecting the optimal software options for the task at hand [16]. If the primary purpose of trimming is to remove adapter contamination, the cutadapt tool offers a useful relatively conservative trimming feature (https://cutadapt.readthedocs.org). After trimming the reads, one should rerun the quality control to make sure the poor quality regions have been removed.

2.2.5 Read Mapping

Once the quality of the reads is acceptable, it is time to map the reads to the reference genome. This is done by aligning the reads to the reference using a short read aligner. There are two main "flavors" of short read aligners: those that filter mapping regions by seed-extend methods and those that utilize an indexing strategy. Both strategies can lead to high-performance mapping algorithms, the main noticeable difference being that index-based aligners are much faster than seed-extend methods [17]. The most widely used methods for read mapping are BWA [18] and Bowtie 2 [19] for DNA sequence data. For RNA sequence data, it is recommended to choose a read aligner that is able to handle splice junctions, such as TopHat [20] or Kallisto [21]. An updated list of read mappers and their features is located at http://www.ebi.ac.uk/~nf/hts_mappers/.

When in doubt about which tools to use for sequence processing, a good resource is the Broad Institute's Genome Analysis Toolkit best practices (https://www.broadinstitute.org/gatk/guide/best-practices). This is a regularly updated resource, which contains recommendations for tools and workflows for most common sequencing tasks.

2.3 Variant Calling

Somatic variant calling from genomic DNA is a nontrivial task that requires specialized tools. There are a number of differences between somatic and germline variant calling. When calling germline variants from normal tissue, one expects the nucleotide variant frequencies to be either 50% or 100%, depending on whether they are heterozygous or homozygous. When calling variants in tumor tissue, the distribution of frequencies falls in a continuous range due to normal/tumor tissue admixture, subclonal variations, copy number variations, loss of heterozygosity, or ploidy changes. Standard germline variant callers are therefore not equipped to deal with somatic mutations, and a number of specialized tools have been developed for this purpose [22]. Currently, the best performing tool is VarScan 2 [23], and another commonly used tool is MuTect [24]. Both enable users to load tumor and normal samples in the same run.

Note that even the best variant callers will not be able to achieve perfect accuracy as long as sequencing technologies are imperfect. Process-related errors such as PCR artifacts, biases in library preparation, base-calling errors, and mismapped reads potentially lead to errors in variant calls. Additionally, biological challenges such as tumor heterogeneity and tissue admixture will invariably result in variant calling errors as well. False-positive variant calls can be filtered out through downstream validation analyses using TDS or TRS, whereas missed (false-negative) calls lead to undetected mutations that would otherwise be potentially valuable [25].

2.4 HLA Typing

The genes encoding the HLA are the most polymorphic in the human genome, and more than 10,000 HLA-I and 3500 HLA-II alleles have been sequenced and catalogued in the IMGT/HLA database (https://www.ebi.ac.uk/ipd/imgt/hla/) [26]. In spite of this vast allelic variety, differences between some alleles come down to single nucleotide variations, making it highly complex to uniquely identify individual alleles. To give a sense of the polymorphism of the HLA gene cluster, consider that approximately 40% of all registered HLA alleles are defined as "very rare," having only been observed in a single individual [27], and the definition of a common allele is an allele that is estimated to be prevalent in just 0.001% of the population [28]. Traditionally, typing an individual's HLA haplotype has been performed using serological or probe-based methods, but sequence-based typing is becoming more and more advanced. Although these methods are a lot more specific than antibody and probe-based methods, it is a nontrivial task to detect the subtle differences leading to an individual's HLA haplotype. Firstly, one must account for the errors invariably introduced by high-throughput sequencing methods; secondly, the high sequence homology between loci makes it difficult to unambiguously map reads to the correct allele; and lastly, the vast majority of known HLA sequences consider only the gene exons, thus making it impossible to consider intronic variance as factor. A large number of bioinformatics tools have been developed to address this problem, of which the best performing algorithm is currently OptiType [29].

2.5 Prediction of Peptide Immunogenicity

When the HLA haplotype has been established, one last step remains before HLA binders can be predicted: identifying all non-synonymous mutations located in CDS regions. Genes, transcripts, and functional annotations can be extracted from GENCODE [30], in order to filter out mutations in noncoding regions. This can be done locally using, for example, the R package GenomicFeatures along with a transcript database (TxDb) for the human genome assembly used for mapping (e.g., TxDb.Hsapiens.UCSC. hg19.knownGene for the hg19 assembly), on the command line using ANNOVAR [31], or online by submitting mutation calls to The Broad Institute's web service Oncotator (http://www.broadinstitute.org/oncotator/), which also incorporates cancer-specific annotations such as observed cancer mutation frequency annotations from COSMIC [32] and cancer variant annotations from ClinVar [33].

```
[...]SCVTACPYKYLSTDVGS[...]
      SCVTACPYN
       CVTACPYNY
        VTACPYNYL
         TACPYNYLS
          ACPYNYLST
           CPYNYLSTD
            PYNYLSTDV
             YNYLSTDVG
              NYLSTDVGS
```

Fig. 2 Extraction of all possible 9-mer peptides from a region with a single nucleotide variation

Once protein sequence mutations are located, every peptide containing a given variation must be extracted by applying a sliding window of the desired peptide length, i.e., 8–11 residues for HLA class binding predictions and 12–22 for HLA class II binding predictions (Fig. 2). Potential T cell epitopes can be predicted using a number of methods. T cell recognition of neoepitopes is determined by a number of rate-limiting steps in peptide preprocessing, transportation to cell surface, HLA binding, followed by recognition and binding by the TCR on circulating T cells. A large number of algorithms have been developed to predict the outcome of these steps, and it is beyond the scope of this chapter to review them all. Below we list a few of the best performing algorithms and discuss their utility in the prediction pipeline. The performance of prediction methods is often assessed by constructing a receiver operating characteristics (ROC) curve and calculating the area under the curve (AUC), as this is a nonparametric approach and therefore not biased by arbitrary thresholds. In the following sections, I will use AUC as a performance metric. As a rough guide, an AUC value of 1.0 represents a perfect prediction, but an algorithm achieving an AUC above 0.9 is generally considered highly accurate. AUCs of 0.8–0.9 can be interpreted as good performance, 0.7 to 0.8 is marginal performance, and 0.5–0.7 represents poor performance, whereas an AUC of 0.5 represents random assignment [34].

2.5.1 Prediction of Peptide Preprocessing

Preprocessing of epitopes starts with the proteasome cleaving intracellular proteins into smaller pieces, which can be predicted using a number of different algorithms such as NetChop [35]. NetChop achieves an AUC of 0.81 and captures approximately 70% of peptide C-terminus cleavage sites [36]. Some of the products from proteasomal cleavage are transported to the ER by the transporter associated with antigen processing (TAP) protein, where a subset binds the HLA, and are presented on the cell surface. TAP transport can also be predicted using, for example, PRED^{TAP} [37], which performs reasonably well with an AUC of 0.8. If one wishes to utilize cleavage prediction, TAP transport prediction, and HLA binding predictions, NetCTL [38] combines these three predictions to give broader prediction of antigen presentation. Although these methods can help filter out some false-positive predictions, it is generally accepted that HLA binding predictions alone are superior in accuracy, and the results from preprocessing prediction algorithms should be interpreted conservatively.

2.5.2 Prediction of HLA Binding

The biggest success in immunological bioinformatics is the prediction of HLA class I and II peptide binding, for which a number of highly accurate algorithms exist. Binders to the HLA class I molecule are 8–11 amino acids in length, although 9-mers are the most abundant class I epitope size [39]. Prediction of class I binders is more advanced than that for class II, due to a more stringent definition of the peptide-binding groove.

Currently, two of the best performing class I binding prediction algorithms are the artificial neural network-based methods NetMHC [39] and NetMHCpan [40]. NetMHC and NetMHCpan both perform very well with an AUC above 0.9 for a number of common HLA alleles. The primary difference between NetMHC and NetMHCpan is that NetMHC is trained solely on peptides with known HLA binding affinity, whereas NetMHCpan is trained on both peptides and HLA sequence. As such, the latter enables pan-specific prediction for any sequenced HLA allele, although care should be taken when predicting binding to rare alleles, as the less data there is available, the poorer the performance generally is. As additional experimental data is generated and models retrained, the predictive performance is known to fluctuate slightly. A number of popular HLA class I binding predicting algorithms are benchmarked weekly on epitopes from the IEDB [41] and hosted at the IEDB (http://tools.iedb.org/auto_bench/mhci/weekly/) [42].

HLA class II binding algorithms are not as accurate as those for HLA class I. In a static benchmark from 2008, the best performing algorithm was NetMHCIIpan [43] with an AUC of 0.82 (averaged over 11 sequenced alleles), which was updated recently to give an AUC of 0.875 averaged over 37 sequenced alleles [44]. HLA class II molecules are only expressed by certain cell types (professional antigen-presenting cells, such as B cells and dendritic cells). Depending on the tumor type, MHC class II molecules might not be expressed, making binding predictions irrelevant. For this reason the main focus of most studies remain class I epitopes.

All of the abovementioned algorithms are capable of predicting IC50 binding affinity. Generally, thresholds of log(IC50) <500 nM and log(IC50) <50 nM are used to denote weak and strong binders, respectively. However, different HLA alleles exhibit binding at different log(IC50) values (see http://help.iedb.org/entries/23854373 for a list of HLA class I IC50 cutoffs), and thus the recommended practice is a rank-based cutoff, where the top 1% of class I peptides and top 10% of class II peptides (based on predicted IC50) can be considered binders to a given HLA allele [45].

2.5.3 Prediction of Post-HLA binding Events

Although the rate-limiting steps of antigen presentation can all be predicted with reasonable accuracy, it is often observed that even peptides binding the HLA fail to activate an immune response. Multiple studies have attempted to explain and model the phenomenon, and different theories have emerged as a result.

The dissociation rate or stability of the peptide-HLA complex has been suggested as an important factor—that is, the longer a peptide is bound to an HLA, the more likely it is that binding will lead to activation of CTLs [46]. The peptide-HLA stability can be predicted using NetMHCstab [47], which in itself performs reasonably well in distinguishing HLA ligands from CTL epitopes (AUC = 0.86), but combined with HLA binding predictions, the predictive performance slightly exceeds those of the tools individually.

Another aspect of CTL activation is the ability of the T cell receptor (TCR) to bind the peptide-HLA complex. It has been suggested that this is primarily facilitated by residues 4, 5, and 6 in a 9-mer peptide [48, 49], while these positions also have the least impact on HLA class I binding affinity. This concept was used to train an algorithm predicting the T cell propensity, efforts which also lead to the conclusion that residues with large aromatic side chains on these positions increased immunogenicity. The resulting algorithm shows that immunogenicity can be predicted to some extent (AUC = 0.61) [50] but leaves ample room for improvement. Finally the predictor NetTepi [51] combines MHC class I binding affinity predictions with stability predictions and T cell propensity calculation to predict which MHC binding peptides are most likely to be T cell epitopes.

2.5.4 Integrated Pipelines

Due to the recent successes achieved using cancer immunotherapy, there is a strong interest in neoepitope predictions, which in turn has led to the recent development of complete pipelines to predict neoepitopes. Currently there are already a few pipelines available, e.g., MuPeXI [52] and pVAC-Seq [53], and we expect this number to increase in the future. Here we will focus on MuPeXI since this tool is available as web service and offers detailed results annotation. The input to MuPeXI is a file with somatic mutation calls, the HLA types, and optionally a gene expression profile (derived from RNA sequencing). MuPeXI will then return a list of tumor-specific peptides that is sorted by a priority score that is intended to predict the immunogenicity of the peptides. The priority score takes into account the ability of the peptides to bind MHC molecules, their similarity to self-peptides, and the gene expression level. To arrive at a list of potential neoepitopes, several analysis steps are necessary.

2.6 Selecting Predicted Epitopes for Therapy

Even after stringent variant calling and HLA affinity prediction, it is not unlikely to get a large number of potential neoepitopes. Filtering by HLA binding predictions alone, approximately every third mutation will result in a peptide predicted to bind 1 of the 12 HLA supertypes [54]. When designing personalized vaccines, time is often of the essence, and it is desirable to reduce the number of false-positive neoepitopes by ranking predicted epitopes by the probability that they will provide a therapeutic advantage.

It has generally been accepted that the stronger a peptide binds the HLA, the more likely it is to elicit an immune response [55], but even if this holds true, only a fraction of high-affinity binders are naturally processed to elicit a response. In a study of vaccinia virus, it was shown that only 2.5% of 9–10 mer peptides are high-affinity binders to a given HLA, only half of these could elicit a CTL response, and, out of these, only 15% were naturally processed [56]. The effect of natural processing of peptides is highlighted in the case of neoepitopes, where the binding of the cognate native peptide is often predicted to bind with similar affinity, even though these peptides do not elicit response [57]. This suggests that some manner of self-tolerance is enforced by the immune system, and although many have attempted to model this phenomenon, no one has yet provided a convincing predictive method. The general consensus is therefore to sort potential neoepitopes by predicted binding affinity and possibly additionally sorting by HLA allele, as predictive performance for common alleles is generally higher than that for rare alleles [58]. Newer tetramer-based validation systems provide means to test a large number of predicted binders at the same time [59], allowing for a more conservative filtering before testing.

Reported epitopes are often deposited in public databases, which provide a useful resource for querying previous experimental validation of predicted binders. The largest public repositories of reported tumor T cell epitopes are TANTIGEN [60, 61], SYFPEITHI [62], and the database of T cell-defined tumor antigens [63].

2.7 Expression Analysis

In order for the immune system to respond to a potential neoepitope, it is of course a prerequisite that the gene harboring the mutation is transcribed to mRNA and translated to protein at sufficient levels in the tumor cells. If using RNA sequencing, mRNA expression can be derived from the sequencing data, whereas if using WGS or WES for variant calling, this information must be gathered in parallel using either RNA sequencing or mRNA expression microarrays. In a 2013 study, Schumacher and colleagues measured gene expression using RNA sequencing and reported that the reactive neoepitope they discovered was ranked in the top 4% of binders to HLA-A*03:01 and was found in a gene (ATR) ranking among the top 28% of expressed genes [3]. A retrospective study of HLA ligands showed similar results; namely, that of the 2.5% most abundantly expressed mRNAs, 41% of the corresponding proteins contained HLA ligands [64]. On a side note, the latter study also revealed that HLA class I ligands tend to be located in intracellular proteins, whereas HLA class II ligands gravitated more toward membrane proteins. Finally, a recent study on a larger data set [65] concluded that expression level is an important factor and significantly higher in source proteins of HLA ligands, but there are also highly expressed proteins that do not contribute HLA ligands, indicating that expression level alone does not predict a proteins' ability to generate HLA ligands. Another conclusion from this study is that there are hot spots of HLA presentation in the proteome, and only 10% of the protein-coding exome was observed to be presented by the 27 MHC alleles studied. It can therefore be of value to measure mRNA expression to rank potential protein antigens, although it should be noted that no large-scale study has confirmed correlation between mRNA expression and naturally processed epitopes yet.

2.8 Recommended Tools

Having given a broad introduction to required and optional computational steps for identification of neoepitopes, it is time to revisit the workflow presented in Fig. 1 and provide recommendations for tools for each task. Recommended tools for each step are provided in Table 1, along with references and URLs.

3 Future Challenges

As mentioned a couple of times already, certain biological features of tumors can affect the clinical efficacy of discovered neoepitopes. A major challenge is tumor heterogeneity, which means that even effective neoepitope therapies can be rendered useless over time as subclonal tumor cell populations lacking the neoepitope are under heavy selective pressure during treatment—a process known as immunoediting [66]. The promise of single-cell sequencing may in the future enable parallel sequencing of a large number of subclones, which could resolve not only the issue of finding broadly expressed neoepitopes but also address the issue of tissue admixture [67].

Another issue touched upon in this chapter is the computational prediction of immunogenic HLA binders. Although HLA binding is a rate-limiting step in T cell recognition, most studies

Table 1
Recommended tools for core tasks in the workflow

Task	Description	Recommended tool	Type	URL	Ref
Base calling	Inferring the nucleotide bases from intensity signals	AYB	Local installation	http://www.ebi.ac.uk/goldman-srv/AYB/	[11]
Quality control	Assessing biases, errors, adapter contamination, etc.	FastQC	Local installation	http://www.bioinformatics.babraham.ac.uk/projects/fastqc/	–
Read trimming	Trim adapter sequences or regions of poor quality	Cutadapt	Local installation	https://cutadapt.readthedocs.org/	–
Read mapping	Mapping of reads to reference genome	BWA	Local installation	http://bio-bwa.sourceforge.net/	[18]
Variant calling	Calling somatic mutations in tumor tissue	VarScan 2	Local installation	http://massgenomics.org/varscan/	[22]
HLA typing	Prediction of HLA haplotype	OptiType	Local installation	https://github.com/FRED-2/OptiType/	[28]
Annotate mutations	Extract nonsynonymous mutations and indels	Oncotator	Web service	http://www.broadinstitute.org/oncotator/	–
Prediction of HLA-I epitopes	Prediction of peptide binding to HLA class I	NetMHCpan	Web service	http://www.cbs.dtu.dk/services/NetMHCpan/	[38]
Prediction of HLA-II epitopes	Prediction of peptide binding to HLA class II	NetMHCIIpan	Web service	http://www.cbs.dtu.dk/services/NetMHCIIpan/	[42]
Neoepitope prediction	Prediction of neoepitopes based on somatic mutation calls, HLA types, and gene expression profile	MuPeXI	Web service	http://www.cbs.dtu.dk/services/MuPeXI/	[52]

suffer from no or low response to even the strongest predicted HLA binders. For example, van Rooij et al. [3] predicted almost 500 potential epitopes using HLA binding prediction algorithms but found that only a single peptide led to a major response. Recently a growing number of studies use mass spectrometry to identify peptides presented by MHC molecules [65, 68, 69]. This type of experiment produces large amounts of peptides that have been subjected to processing and presentation pathway; by training predictors on this type of data, the restrictions caused by the processing and presentation pathway are automatically included in the model [70].

In addition to improving predictions of peptide presentation by MHC molecules, scientists are also working on predicting the specificity of T cells. In the past it has not been possible to train a T cell specificity predictor since there was not enough data available linking sequenced T cell receptors to the peptide-MHC complex they recognize. Lately high-throughput screens have been developed [71, 72] to generate these kinds of data sets, and first publications report that it is possible to cluster T cell receptors into epitope-specific clusters [73, 74]. This challenge remains to be solved either computationally through refined prediction algorithms or technically by high-throughput T cell response assays.

There are many more challenges to T cell-based immunotherapy that have not been covered in this chapter (comprehensively reviewed in [75, 76]), for example, overcoming modes of immune suppression employed by tumor cells using immune checkpoint blockade therapies. However, even in the light of these challenges, the future has never looked brighter for cancer immunotherapy.

References

1. Lennerz V, Fatho M, Gentilini C et al (2005) The response of autologous T cells to a human melanoma is dominated by mutated neoantigens. Proc Natl Acad Sci U S A 102:16013–16018. https://doi.org/10.1073/pnas.0500090102

2. Zhou J, Dudley ME, Rosenberg SA, Robbins PF (2005) Persistence of multiple tumor-specific T-cell clones is associated with complete tumor regression in a melanoma patient receiving adoptive cell transfer therapy. J Immunother 28:53–62. https://doi.org/10.2964/jsik.kuni0223

3. van Rooij N, van Buuren MM, Philips D et al (2013) Tumor exome analysis reveals neoantigen-specific T-cell reactivity in an ipilimumab-responsive melanoma. J Clin Oncol 31:e439–e442. https://doi.org/10.1200/JCO.2012.47.7521

4. Rajasagi M, Shukla SA, Fritsch EF et al (2014) Systematic identification of personal tumor-specific neoantigens in chronic lymphocytic leukemia. Blood 124:453–462. https://doi.org/10.1182/blood-2014-04-567933

5. Olsen LR, Campos B, Winther O et al (2014) Tumor antigens as proteogenomic biomarkers in invasive ductal carcinomas. BMC Med Genet 15:1–10

6. Rooney MS, Shukla SA, Wu CJ et al (2015) Molecular and genetic properties of tumors associated with local immune cytolytic activity. Cell 160:48–61. https://doi.org/10.1016/j.cell.2014.12.033

7. Olsen LR, Campos B, Barnkob MS et al (2014) Bioinformatics for cancer immunotherapy target discovery. Cancer Immunol Immunother. https://doi.org/10.1007/s00262-014-1627-7

8. Botstein D, Risch N (2003) Discovering genotypes underlying human phenotypes: past successes for mendelian disease, future approaches for complex disease. Nat Genet 33 (Suppl):228–237. https://doi.org/10.1038/ng1090

9. Reuter JA, Spacek DV, Snyder MP (2015) High-throughput sequencing technologies. Mol Cell 58:586–597. https://doi.org/10.1016/j.molcel.2015.05.004

10. Guo J, Xu N, Li Z et al (2008) Four-color DNA sequencing with 3′-O-modified nucleotide reversible terminators and chemically cleavable fluorescent dideoxynucleotides. Proc

Natl Acad Sci U S A 105:9145–9150. https://doi.org/10.1073/pnas.0804023105
11. Massingham T, Goldman N (2012) All your base: a fast and accurate probabilistic approach to base calling. Genome Biol 13:R13. https://doi.org/10.1186/gb-2012-13-2-r13
12. Kircher M, Stenzel U, Kelso J (2009) Improved base calling for the Illumina genome analyzer using machine learning strategies. Genome Biol 10:R83. https://doi.org/10.1186/gb-2009-10-8-r83
13. Renaud G, Kircher M, Stenzel U, Kelso J (2013) freeIbis: an efficient basecaller with calibrated quality scores for Illumina sequencers. Bioinformatics 29:1208–1209. https://doi.org/10.1093/bioinformatics/btt117
14. Cacho A, Smirnova E, Huzurbazar S, Cui X (2015) A comparison of base-calling algorithms for Illumina sequencing technology. Brief Bioinform 17(5):786–795. https://doi.org/10.1093/bib/bbv088
15. Del Fabbro C, Scalabrin S, Morgante M, Giorgi FM (2013) An extensive evaluation of read trimming effects on illumina NGS data analysis. PLoS One 8:1–13. https://doi.org/10.1371/journal.pone.0085024
16. Aronesty E (2013) Comparison of sequencing utility programs. Open Bioinform J 7:1–8. https://doi.org/10.2174/1875036201307010001
17. Reinert K, Langmead B, Weese D, Evers DJ (2015) Alignment of next-generation sequencing reads. Annu Rev Genomics Hum Genet 16:133–151. https://doi.org/10.1146/annurev-genom-090413-025358
18. Li H, Durbin R (2009) Fast and accurate short read alignment with Burrows-Wheeler transform. Bioinformatics 25:1754–1760. https://doi.org/10.1093/bioinformatics/btp324
19. Langmead B, Salzberg SL (2012) Fast gapped-read alignment with Bowtie 2. Nat Methods 9:357–359. https://doi.org/10.1038/nmeth.1923
20. Kim D, Pertea G, Trapnell C et al (2013) TopHat2: accurate alignment of transcriptomes in the presence of insertions, deletions and gene fusions. Genome Biol 14:R36. https://doi.org/10.1186/gb-2013-14-4-r36
21. Bray NL, Pimentel H, Melsted P, Pachter L (2016) Near-optimal probabilistic RNA-seq quantification. Nat Biotechnol 34:525–527. https://doi.org/10.1038/nbt.3519
22. Wang Q, Jia P, Li F et al (2013) Detecting somatic point mutations in cancer genome sequencing data: a comparison of mutation callers. Genome Med 5:91. https://doi.org/10.1186/gm495
23. Koboldt DC, Zhang Q, Larson DE et al (2012) VarScan 2: somatic mutation and copy number alteration discovery in cancer by exome sequencing. Genome Res 22:568–576. https://doi.org/10.1101/gr.129684.111
24. Cibulskis K, Lawrence MS, Carter SL et al (2013) Sensitive detection of somatic point mutations in impure and heterogeneous cancer samples. Nat Biotechnol 31:213–219. https://doi.org/10.1038/nbt.2514
25. Castle JC, Kreiter S, Diekmann J et al (2012) Exploiting the mutanome for tumor vaccination. Cancer Res 72:1081–1091. https://doi.org/10.1158/0008-5472.CAN-11-3722
26. Robinson J, Halliwell JA, Hayhurst JD et al (2015) The IPD and IMGT/HLA database: allele variant databases. Nucleic Acids Res 43:D423–D431. https://doi.org/10.1093/nar/gku1161
27. Middleton D, Gonzalez F, Fernandez-Vina M et al (2009) A bioinformatics approach to ascertaining the rarity of HLA alleles. Tissue Antigens 74:480–485. https://doi.org/10.1111/j.1399-0039.2009.01361.x
28. Mack SJ, Cano P, Hollenbach JA et al (2013) Common and well-documented HLA alleles: 2012 update to the CWD catalogue. Tissue Antigens 81:194–203. https://doi.org/10.1111/tan.12093
29. Szolek A, Schubert B, Mohr C et al (2014) OptiType: precision HLA typing from next-generation sequencing data. Bioinformatics 30:3310–3316. https://doi.org/10.1093/bioinformatics/btu548
30. Harrow J, Frankish A, Gonzalez JM et al (2012) GENCODE: the reference human genome annotation for the ENCODE project. Genome Res 22:1760–1774. https://doi.org/10.1101/gr.135350.111
31. Wang K, Li M, Hakonarson H (2010) ANNOVAR: functional annotation of genetic variants from high-throughput sequencing data. Nucleic Acids Res 38:e164. https://doi.org/10.1093/nar/gkq603
32. Forbes SA, Beare D, Gunasekaran P et al (2015) COSMIC: exploring the world's knowledge of somatic mutations in human cancer. Nucleic Acids Res 43:D805–D811. https://doi.org/10.1093/nar/gku1075
33. Landrum MJ, Lee JM, Riley GR et al (2014) ClinVar: public archive of relationships among sequence variation and human phenotype. Nucleic Acids Res 42:D980–D985. https://doi.org/10.1093/nar/gkt1113
34. Swets JA (1988) Measuring the accuracy of diagnostic systems. Science 240:1285–1293

35. Nielsen M, Lundegaard C, Lund O, Keşmir C (2005) The role of the proteasome in generating cytotoxic T-cell epitopes: insights obtained from improved predictions of proteasomal cleavage. Immunogenetics 57:33–41. https://doi.org/10.1007/s00251-005-0781-7

36. Saxová P, Buus S, Brunak S, Keşmir C (2003) Predicting proteasomal cleavage sites: a comparison of available methods. Int Immunol 15:781–787. https://doi.org/10.1093/intimm/dxg084

37. Zhang GL, Petrovsky N, Kwoh CK et al (2006) PRED(TAP): a system for prediction of peptide binding to the human transporter associated with antigen processing. Immunome Res 2:3. https://doi.org/10.1186/1745-7580-2-3

38. Larsen MV, Lundegaard C, Lamberth K et al (2007) Large-scale validation of methods for cytotoxic T-lymphocyte epitope prediction. BMC Bioinformatics 8:424. https://doi.org/10.1186/1471-2105-8-424

39. Andreatta M, Nielsen M (2015) Gapped sequence alignment using artificial neural networks: application to the MHC class I system. Bioinformatics 32(4):511–517. https://doi.org/10.1093/bioinformatics/btv639

40. Nielsen M, Andreatta M (2016) NetMHCpan-3.0; improved prediction of binding to MHC class I molecules integrating information from multiple receptor and peptide length datasets. Genome Med 8:33. https://doi.org/10.1186/s13073-016-0288-x

41. Vita R, Overton JA, Greenbaum JA et al (2015) The immune epitope database (IEDB) 3.0. Nucleic Acids Res 43:D405–D412. https://doi.org/10.1093/nar/gku938

42. Trolle T, Metushi IG, Greenbaum JA et al (2015) Automated benchmarking of peptide-MHC class I binding predictions. Bioinformatics 31(13):2174–2181. https://doi.org/10.1093/bioinformatics/btv123

43. Nielsen M, Lundegaard C, Blicher T et al (2008) Quantitative predictions of peptide binding to any HLA-DR molecule of known sequence: NetMHCIIpan. PLoS Comput Biol 4:e1000107. https://doi.org/10.1371/journal.pcbi.1000107

44. Andreatta M, Jurtz VI, Kaever T et al (2017) Machine learning reveals a non-canonical mode of peptide binding to MHC class II molecules. Immunology 152:255–264. https://doi.org/10.1111/imm.12763

45. Paul S, Weiskopf D, Angelo MA, et al. (2013) HLA class I alleles are associated with peptide-binding repertoires of different size, affinity, and immunogenicity. J Immunol 191:5831–9. https://doi.org/10.4049/jimmunol.1302101

46. van der Burg SH, Visseren MJ, Brandt RM et al (1996) Immunogenicity of peptides bound to MHC class I molecules depends on the MHC-peptide complex stability. J Immunol 156:3308–3314

47. Jørgensen KW, Rasmussen M, Buus S, Nielsen M (2014) NetMHCstab - predicting stability of peptide-MHC-I complexes; impacts for cytotoxic T lymphocyte epitope discovery. Immunology 141:18–26. https://doi.org/10.1111/imm.12160

48. Lee JK, Stewart-Jones G, Dong T et al (2004) T cell cross-reactivity and conformational changes during TCR engagement. J Exp Med 200:1455–1466. https://doi.org/10.1084/jem.20041251

49. Frankild S, de Boer RJ, Lund O et al (2008) Amino acid similarity accounts for T cell cross-reactivity and for "holes" in the T cell repertoire. PLoS One 3:e1831. https://doi.org/10.1371/journal.pone.0001831

50. Calis JJA, Maybeno M, Greenbaum JA et al (2013) Properties of MHC class I presented peptides that enhance immunogenicity. PLoS Comput Biol. https://doi.org/10.1371/journal.pcbi.1003266

51. Trolle T, Nielsen M (2014) NetTepi: an integrated method for the prediction of T cell epitopes. Immunogenetics 66:449–456. https://doi.org/10.1007/s00251-014-0779-0

52. Bjerregaard A-M, Nielsen M, Hadrup SR et al (2017) MuPeXI: prediction of neo-epitopes from tumor sequencing data. Cancer Immunol Immunother 66:1123–1130. https://doi.org/10.1007/s00262-017-2001-3

53. Hundal J, Carreno BM, Petti AA et al (2016) pVAC-Seq: a genome-guided in silico approach to identifying tumor neoantigens. Genome Med 8:11. https://doi.org/10.1186/s13073-016-0264-5

54. Sidney J, Peters B, Frahm N et al (2008) HLA class I supertypes: a revised and updated classification. BMC Immunol 9:1. https://doi.org/10.1186/1471-2172-9-1

55. Engels B, Engelhard VH, Sidney J et al (2013) Relapse or eradication of cancer is predicted by peptide-major histocompatibility complex affinity. Cancer Cell 23:516–526. https://doi.org/10.1016/j.ccr.2013.03.018

56. Assarsson E, Sidney J, Oseroff C et al (2007) A quantitative analysis of the variables affecting the repertoire of T cell specificities recognized after vaccinia virus infection. J Immunol 178:7890–7901

57. Fritsch EF, Rajasagi M, Ott PA et al (2014) HLA-binding properties of tumor neoepitopes in humans. Cancer Immunol Res 2:522–529. https://doi.org/10.1158/2326-6066.CIR-13-0227

58. Kim Y, Sidney J, Buus S et al (2014) Dataset size and composition impact the reliability of performance benchmarks for peptide-MHC binding predictions. BMC Bioinformatics 15:241. https://doi.org/10.1186/1471-2105-15-241

59. Andersen RS, Kvistborg P, Frøsig TM et al (2012) Parallel detection of antigen-specific T cell responses by combinatorial encoding of MHC multimers. Nat Protoc 7:891–902. https://doi.org/10.1038/nprot.2012.037

60. Olsen LR, Johan Kudahl U, Winther O, Brusic V (2013) Literature classification for semi-automated updating of biological knowledge-bases. BMC Genomics 14(Suppl 5):S14. https://doi.org/10.1186/1471-2164-14-S5-S14

61. Olsen LR, Tongchusak S, Lin H et al (2017) TANTIGEN: a comprehensive database of tumor T cell antigens. Cancer Immunol Immunother 66:731–735. https://doi.org/10.1007/s00262-017-1978-y

62. Rammensee H, Bachmann J, Emmerich NP et al (1999) SYFPEITHI: database for MHC ligands and peptide motifs. Immunogenetics 50:213–219

63. van der Bruggen P, Stroobant V, Vigneron N, Van den Eynde B (2013) Peptide database: T cell-defined tumor antigens. Cancer Immun

64. Juncker AS, Larsen MV, Weinhold N et al (2009) Systematic characterisation of cellular localisation and expression profiles of proteins containing MHC ligands. PLoS One 4:e7448. https://doi.org/10.1371/journal.pone.0007448

65. Pearson H, Daouda T, Granados DP et al (2016) MHC class I–associated peptides derive from selective regions of the human genome. J Clin Invest 126:4690–4701. https://doi.org/10.1172/JCI88590

66. Matsushita H, Vesely MD, Koboldt DC et al (2012) Cancer exome analysis reveals a T-cell-dependent mechanism of cancer immunoediting. Nature 482:400–404. https://doi.org/10.1038/nature10755

67. Navin N, Kendall J, Troge J et al (2011) Tumour evolution inferred by single-cell sequencing. Nature 472:90–94. https://doi.org/10.1038/nature09807

68. Abelin JG, Keskin DB, Sarkizova S et al (2017) Mass spectrometry profiling of HLA-associated peptidomes in mono-allelic cells enables more accurate epitope prediction. Immunity 46:315–326. https://doi.org/10.1016/j.immuni.2017.02.007

69. Bassani-Sternberg M, Chong C, Guillaume P et al (2017) Deciphering HLA-I motifs across HLA peptidomes improves neo-antigen predictions and identifies allostery regulating HLA specificity. PLoS Comput Biol 13:e1005725. https://doi.org/10.1371/journal.pcbi.1005725

70. Jurtz VI, Paul S, Andreatta M et al (2017) NetMHCpan 4.0: improved peptide-MHC class I interaction predictions integrating eluted ligand and peptide binding affinity data. https://doi.org/10.4049/jimmunol.1700893

71. Klinger M, Pepin F, Wilkins J et al (2015) Multiplex identification of antigen-specific T cell receptors using a combination of immune assays and immune receptor sequencing. PLoS One 10:e0141561. https://doi.org/10.1371/journal.pone.0141561

72. Bentzen AK, Marquard AM, Lyngaa R et al (2016) Large-scale detection of antigen-specific T cells using peptide-MHC-I multimers labeled with DNA barcodes. Nat Biotechnol 34:1037–1045. https://doi.org/10.1038/nbt.3662

73. Dash P, Fiore-Gartland AJ, Hertz T et al (2017) Quantifiable predictive features define epitope-specific T cell receptor repertoires. Nature 547:89–93. https://doi.org/10.1038/nature22383

74. Glanville J, Huang H, Nau A et al (2017) Identifying specificity groups in the T cell receptor repertoire. Nature 547:94–98. https://doi.org/10.1038/nature22976

75. de Aquino MTP, Malhotra A, Mishra MK, Shanker A (2015) Challenges and future perspectives of T cell immunotherapy in cancer. Immunol Lett 166:117–133. https://doi.org/10.1016/j.imlet.2015.05.018

76. Fesnak AD, June CH, Levine BL (2016) Engineered T cells: the promise and challenges of cancer immunotherapy. Nat Rev Cancer 16:566–581. https://doi.org/10.1038/nrc.2016.97

Chapter 10

Computational and Statistical Analysis of Array-Based DNA Methylation Data

Jessica Nordlund, Christofer Bäcklin, and Amanda Raine

Abstract

The characterization of aberrant DNA methylation is emerging as a key part of the study of cancer development and phenotype. The technical advancements and decreasing costs of methods for high-throughput profiling of DNA methylation have brought about a high interest in the use of such methods in disease association studies. Here we discuss the principles for DNA methylation analysis using data from the Infinium DNA methylation BeadChip assays and describe the computational steps and statistical considerations going from processing of the raw array data to analysis of differential methylation. Moreover, we provide detailed guidelines on how to perform tumor subtype classification based on DNA methylation signatures.

Key words DNA methylation, Epigenetics, Cancer, Classification, Subtyping, BeadChip Assay, 450k array

1 Introduction

Aberrant DNA methylation is a widespread and common feature of human cancers [1]. DNA methylation is by far the most well-characterized epigenetic modification, which is involved in the regulation of gene expression, genome stability, and developmental processes. Aberrant DNA methylation has been observed in nearly all cancer types studied, and there are many distinct subgroups of tumors that share similarities in DNA methylation patterns [2–5]. Moreover, aberrant DNA methylation may be a promising molecular biomarker for early cancer detection and diagnostic subtype detection [6–9].

Methods for measuring DNA methylation can be divided into three broad classes: those involving enrichment-based methods, digestion with methylation-sensitive restriction enzymes, and methods using bisulfite (BS) treatment. Here, we summarize methodologies we have been using for genome-wide DNA methylation analysis with BS treatment, with the focus on the analysis of array-based differential DNA methylation in relation to cancer phenotype data.

The Infinium BeadChip assays (Illumina) are widely considered the gold standard method for DNA methylation analysis as they have been used in the vast majority of large-scale methylome studies to date. The Infinium BeadChip assays are a cost-efficient, high-throughput method and require moderate quantities of DNA (~200–500 ng). The Infinium BeadChip assays offer quantitative measurement of DNA methylation levels a predetermined set of cytosine residues by genotyping cytosine or thymine (methylated vs unmethylated cytosine residues) in a microarray format. Infinium BeadChip assays with increasing numbers of target CpG sites over have been launched over the last decade, starting with the HumanMethylation 27 K BeadChip (27k array) that mostly targeted CpG islands [10]. The next generation of BeadChips, the HumanMethylation 450 K (450k array) [11], and the most recent iteration, the Infinium MethylationEPIC (850k array) [12], in addition to CpG islands, also assay CpG island shores, gene bodies, enhancers, and other noncoding genomic regions. The BeadChip assays provide a user-friendly and straightforward approach for analyzing hundreds of thousands of CpG sites in many samples at a relatively low cost.

Starting with raw data, herein we describe the computational steps to go from raw single-CpG DNA methylation levels to cancer phenotype-associated signatures. Although the methods described herein are focused toward array-based data primarily on the 450k array, data derived from the EPIC array and next-generation sequencing (NGS)-derived DNA methylation data with CpG site resolution and adequate biological replicates can also be analyzed using the practices described here.

2 Methods

There are several assays and methods now available for simultaneously measuring genome-wide DNA methylation in few to thousands of samples [13, 14]. With these methods, the central idea is to measure DNA methylation quantitatively at single-CpG site resolution. BS treatment of DNA causes deamination of unmethylated cytosine residues to uracil, while methylated cytosine residues are protected from conversion and remain as cytosine residues, thus allowing for CpG-specific discrimination between methylated and unmethylated sites. In the case of microarrays, predefined CpG sites are measured fluorescently for proportion of methylated to unmethylated cytosine signals using one or two color probe designs. The 450k array from Illumina Inc. has been the most commonly used platform for array-based DNA methylation analysis [15] (*see* **Note 1**). In the case of NGS, the DNA methylation status is determined by directly sequencing and digitally counting the number of methylated to unmethylated CpG sites in the reads [16]. Bioinformatic analysis of genome-wide DNA methylation data remains a complex task [17]; however there are now several different analysis packages freely available, which aid in the steps required for processing of array-based DNA methylation data described here. The data analysis consists of the following steps:

1. Preprocessing of the DNA methylation dataset
2. Probe filtering
3. Unsupervised exploratory analyses to identify biological structure and outlier samples
4. Differential DNA methylation analysis
5. Annotation and biological interpretation of differentially methylated CpG sites
6. Tumor subtype classification

2.1 Preprocessing

The basic preprocessing for the 450k array comprises the following steps, typically performed using the Genome Studio DNA methylation module (Illumina) or one of the various R packages that use raw IDAT files: bead-level signal extraction, signal intensity adjustment, calculation of detection *P*-value, and normalization. The same software can produce the DNA methylation β-values (Eq. 1) or *M*-values (Subheading 2.4) typically used for exploratory analyses (Subheading 2.3) and differential methylation analysis (Subheading 2.4).

$$\beta = \frac{A}{A + B + \alpha}$$

Equation 1 : *The degree of methylation of a CpG site is defined as a β-value. A and B represent the methylated and unmethylated signal intensities, and α is a small positive constant that prevents division with 0 (which would otherwise happen if both A and B are lower than the array's background signal intensity and therefore truncated to 0). Thus, $\beta = 0$ corresponds to 0% methylation, and $\beta \approx 1$ corresponds to 100% methylation*

The 450k array is comprised of two different Infinium bead types associated to two different chemical assays, Infinium type I and Infinium type II [18]. The difference between these bead types has been extensively reviewed elsewhere [14, 15, 19, 20]. Briefly, approximately 30% of the probes on the 450k array are Infinium I, which are based on allele-specific hybridization followed by single-base extension with fluorescently labeled nucleotides that measure the methylation status of CpG sites with two different bead types (methylated and unmethylated) in one color channel. The type I probe design assumes adjacent CpG sites under the probe sequence have the same methylation status as the interrogated CpG site. The remaining Infinium II probes are based on allele-specific base

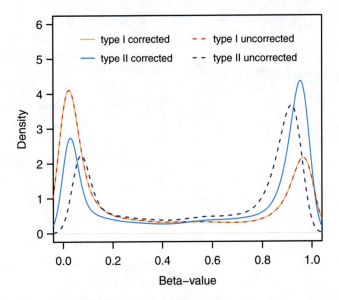

Fig. 1 Probe bias correction. The DNA methylation level (beta-value) distribution is plotted separately for Infinium type I and type II probes, before (dashed lines) and after (solid lines) peak-based correction

extension by fluorescently labeled nucleotides. Infinium II probes are measured in two color channels, one color for methylated and the other for unmethylated cytosines on one bead type. Different genomic elements (CpG islands, promoters, gene bodies, etc.) have different relative fraction of Infinium I or Infinium II probes. Because of this, there is a bias in the DNA methylation beta-value (β-value) distribution between the different Infinium probe types, which leads to compression or narrowing of the β-value distribution of Infinium II probes (Fig. 1). To date, several methods have been introduced to correct for probe-type bias that include peak-based correction [19], the Subset-quantile Within Array Normalization (SWAN) method [21], and beta-mixture quantile normalization [22]. The performance of the different normalization methods has been summarized elsewhere [23, 24]. Algorithms for reducing probe design bias are available through several user-friendly R packages such as Minfi [25], ChAMP [26], and RnBeads [27]. These R packages also provide different levels of functionality for high-level DNA methylation analysis, including batch correction, data visualization, quality control, differential DNA methylation analysis, etc. In our experience, the decision to use a normalization method at all or which method to use depends greatly on the source of material and the β-value distribution of the samples in the dataset. It has been shown, however, that in datasets with strong biological signal, the choice of normalization method makes little impact on the result, whereas in experiments with little signal, the normalization method makes a bigger impact on the final results [24]. Adjusting for the probe design bias using the methods mentioned above may be unnecessary when analyzing 450k array data on a CpG-by-CpG basis, because the comparisons will be made at the individual probe level [28]. However, if implementing a group-wise cutoff for differences in methylation levels (as discussed in Subheading 2.3), it is advisable to correct for probe biases so that the same stringency is applied for both type I and type II probes. For the examples given in this chapter, peak-based correction was implemented as it performed well for primary leukemia samples of high (>90%) tumor purity from GEO dataset GSE49031 [29].

2.2 Probe Filtering

Probes with unspecific genomic alignment or common genetic variants in the probe-binding site should be excluded since they may affect the hybridization reaction and may introduce variation the signal on the 450k array that does not reflect the DNA methylation levels that they are intended to measure [30, 31]. We previously presented an experimentally validated list of such probes [29]. Briefly, several probes on the 450k array overlap single nucleotide polymorphisms (SNPs) and/or small insertion/deletions (indels) according to the dbSNP database, which may affect the reported β-values. In the case of variants underlying the probe design, individuals with non-reference alleles will have a mismatch base that may affect probe hybridization or primer extension, particularly those variants located toward the 3' end of the probe. In order to find a threshold for filtering probes with variants under the probe design, we studied the standard deviation (SD) of β-values in non-cancer samples in relation to the location of annotated variants within the probe design in a stepwise fashion. This experiment showed that probes with an annotated variant within the CpG site to two bases from the 3' end of the probe displayed higher variability in β-values than probes without any annotated variants (Fig. 2a). It should be noted that probes with known variants between three and five bases from the 3' end of the probe may also affect β-value measurements, but the effect size is much smaller. In a similar fashion, we realigned the probe sequences to human genome build 37 with BWA [32], and probes that mapped to multiple sites were indicated by a BWA mapping score <37. By comparing the SD across non-cancer samples for probes that mapped to multiple positions to probes that mapped to a single position, we found that the multiple mapping probes with non-unique alignments displayed significantly greater variance in β-values than uniquely mapping probes (Fig. 2b). Our probe-filtering list is available in Supplementary Table 1 in Nordlund et al. [29] and within the "RnBeads" package [27]. A summary of the number of probes removed by each filter is shown in Table 1.

Probes that perform poorly in a given dataset should be removed. Each CpG site in each individual sample has an associated

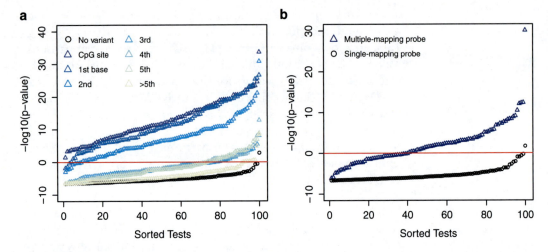

Fig. 2 Probes that stand a high chance of confounding DNA methylation measurements. In 100 iterations, the standard deviation across non-cancer samples was calculated for 100 randomly selected probes that either contained an annotated variant or mapped to multiple positions and compared those SDs to the SDs in 100 probes without known variants that mapped to a single location. Each point represents the corrected Wilcox rank-sum P-value derived from comparing the standard deviations. (**a**) Probes are classified by having a common variant with allele frequency >0.05 in dbSNP in the CpG site or in the bases from the 3' end of the probe sequence (colored points) or probes having no known variant underlying the probe sequence (black). Probes with variants in the CpG site or first two bases from the 3' end of the probe stand a high chance of influencing beta-values. (**b**) Probes that map to multiple places in the genome (blue) compared to probes with only one mapping position (black)

Table 1
Probe filtering

Variant type	N Probes
CNV probes	9702
CpG SNP	6901
Base 1 SNP	14,920
Base 2 SNP	7646
Base 3 SNP	2248
Base 4 SNP	2559
Base 5 SNP	2359
No SNP	332,464

with detection P-value, which compares the intensity of the CpG probe to that of the intensities of negative control probes on the array. Two strategies can be used here; either probes with a detection P-value of >0.01 in any sample can be removed entirely from the dataset or they can be masked with "NA" in the samples not meeting the detection *P*-value cutoff. If many samples are analyzed, the former strategy might result in an unnecessarily high number of probes removed, so a more pragmatic approach would use the masking procedure and only remove probes that are masked in 10–20% of the samples. How to handle masked values in downstream analyses depends on the choice of statistical test and computational methods used.

X-chromosome inactivation and lack of the Y chromosome in females can also lead to a bias in differentially methylated probes on the sex chromosomes if males and females are analyzed together. For simplicity, we typically remove probes from the X and Y chromosomes from differential methylation and subtyping analysis. However, these probes may be useful for identification of sample mix-ups (*see* Subheading 2.3). An additional 65 probes identified by their reference SNP (rs) numbers are also useful for controlling the identity of paired samples. These 65 SNPs should be removed before differential methylation or subtyping analysis, since they reflect SNP alleles instead of β-values.

After removing all probes with SNPs within the CpG site or 2 bp from the 3' end of the probe, probes that map to multiple regions of the genome, sex chromosomes, and the 65 genotyping probes, using our filtering 435,941 probes, are left for downstream analyses. Similar approaches to probe filtering can be implemented in most of the popular aforementioned R packages for analysis of 450k DNA methylation data.

2.3 Exploratory Analyses

Global changes in DNA methylation can often be identified by visual inspection of the normalized and quality-controlled DNA methylation data before in-depth analysis of differential DNA methylation. In the case of quantitative DNA methylation data in the context of cancer, clustering is an indispensable technique used for identification of subtype structure in the dataset. Prior to analyzing the dataset for biologically distinct subgroups, initial exploratory analyses can be helpful for detecting outlier samples and sample mix-ups. Hierarchical clustering, heat maps of the CpG sites with β-values that vary the most across samples, and dimension reduction using principal component analysis (PCA) provide a global assessment of sample structure in the dataset. Hierarchical agglomerative clustering implemented using the "hclust" function and principal component analysis (PCA) implemented using the "prcomp" function, both in the base package in R, can be used to describe the dominating structures in the DNA methylation dataset. This is especially important in clinical sample data where low tumor purity and sample mix-ups may occur.

One of the X chromosomes in females is inactivated by DNA methylation. This information can be leveraged to quickly check that the sex of the individual samples matches the DNA methylation patterns (Fig. 3a). This is very accurate for the majority of

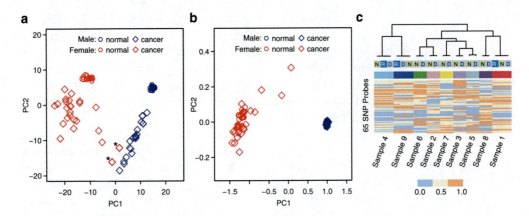

Fig. 3 Quality control. (**a**) Principal component analysis (PCA) of the β-values of CpG sites across the X chromosome. The first two principal components in male (blue) and female (red) samples are plotted. The samples are clearly divided by the sex of the individual along the first principal component. Two of the female cancer samples (highlighted by asterisks) cluster nearby the male cancer samples. (**b**) PCA of the β-values of 14 CpG sites on the X chromosome identified by classification that give the best separation between male and female samples. (**c**) Hierarchical clustering of paired diagnostic "D," normal "N," and relapse "R" samples from 9 individuals based on the values calculated for the 65 genotyping probes on the 450k array

samples; however in cancer and leukemia especially, whole chromosomes including chromosome X can be lost in tumor samples. As can be seen by the example PCA plot in Fig. 3, which is based on the β-values of all probes on the X chromosome, two cancer samples from female patients cluster close to the male patients. In both of these cancer samples, loss of one copy of the X chromosome was observed in routine karyotyping at the time of leukemia diagnosis. Therefore, in cancer samples that are known to display whole chromosome aneuploidies including those of the X chromosome, one should be cautious not to erroneously exclude samples/patients due to this. An alternative method to detect sex in DNA methylation data by classification as discussed in Subheading 2.6 is not as sensitive to deletion of X chromosomes in cancer samples because the classifier is trained on patients including those with deleted X chromosomes. To visualize this, we also plot the same patients based on the methylation status of 14 CpG sites that we previously identified [7] that provide the best separation of male and female samples (Fig. 3b).

Some experimental designs rely on analyzing paired samples, for example, tumor-normal or diagnosis-relapse pairs. Clustering of the patients based on the values of 65 genotyping probes is a very useful approach to quality control paired samples prior to downstream analyses (Fig. 3c).

Finally, once the samples are quality controlled, exploratory analysis of structure in the DNA methylation dataset can be performed. In an example of such an analysis, PCA was performed on the entire 450k dataset of filtered probes (Chr 1:22) for

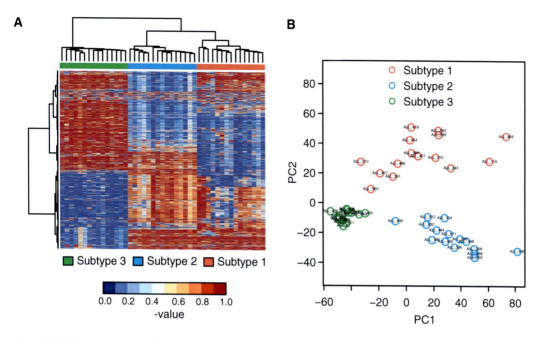

Fig. 4 Global assessment of sample structure in the dataset. (**a**) Hierarchical clustering of 45 primary pediatric ALL samples belonging to 3 distinct subtypes (15 samples each) based on the β-values of the filtered probe set of all CpG sites on chromosomes 1:22. The β-values of the 1000 most variable probes in the dataset are plotted in the heat map. Red indicates high methylation levels and blue low methylation levels. (**b**) Principal component analysis (PCA) based on the β-values of the filtered probe set of all CpG sites on chromosomes 1:22

45 diagnostic acute pediatric acute lymphoblastic leukemia (ALL) samples belonging to 3 distinct subgroups defined by recurrent cytogenetic aberrations denoted here as subtypes 1, 2, and 3 (Fig. 4a). The data was downloaded from publically available 450k data under series GSE49031 from the Gene Expression Omnibus [29]. A clustering heat map depicting the β-values of the 1000 most variable CpG sites demonstrates the large variability in DNA methylation between these 3 groups (Fig. 4b).

2.4 Differential DNA Methylation Analysis

The ultimate goal of most experiments is to identify DNA methylation changes that correlate with the phenotype of interest, for example, by comparing cases and controls or different cancer subtypes to each other. The appropriate statistical test must be applied. It is important to note that the DNA methylation β-values for individual CpG sites are, by definition, not normally distributed since they are limited to the interval between 0 and 1 (0–100% methylated) and are often bimodal or skewed. Thus, we prefer to use nonparametric tests, which are typically better suited than their parametric counterparts when working with β-values.

The first and very simple approach consists in the calculation of the difference between the median β-values of two experimental

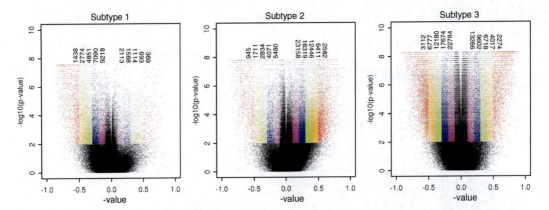

Fig. 5 Volcano plots of differentially methylated CpG sites. In each panel, the $\Delta\beta$-value is plotted along the x-axis, and the FDR-corrected P-value is plotted on the y-axis. The numbers of differentially methylated CpG sites for each subtype detected at $\Delta\beta$-value cutoffs ranging from 0.1 to 0.5 are shown on the top of each panel separately for hypo- and hypermethylated CpG sites

groups ($\Delta\beta$) for each CpG site. To test for a difference in distribution between two groups of unpaired observations (cancer type 1 and type 2), we use the nonparametric Wilcoxon rank-sum test by applying "wilcox.test" function in R. The P-values for each CpG site are subsequently corrected for multiple testing using the false discovery rate (FDR) method using the "p.adjust" function in R with the argument "method='fdr.'" To further decrease the false-positive rate and enrich for biologically meaningful differentially methylated sites, we implement a second threshold on the effect size. Requiring a $\Delta\beta$-value of 0.2 or 20% or greater should be considered. This threshold corresponds to the recommended difference that can be detected with >99% confidence [15]. Additionally, the biological and clinical relevance of smaller methylation changes ($\Delta\beta < 0.1$), especially in cancer studies, can also be questioned. An example of the number of differentially methylated CpG sites and their effect size between the 3 biologically distinct classes of pediatric leukemia (publically available at GEO: GSE49031) with 15 biological replicates in each group is illustrated in Fig. 5.

When analyzing quantitative phenotypes, rather than comparing discrete groups, regression models are typically used. It is important to be aware that many regression techniques assume that the independent variables are homoscedastic, which isn't fulfilled by β-values since their variance is much smaller close to 0 and 1 compared to 0.5 [33]. It is therefore advisable to carry out such analyses on M-values rather than β-values (Eq. 2).

$$M = \log_2 \left(\frac{\max(A, 0) + \alpha}{\max(B, 0) + \alpha} \right)$$

Equation 2 : *The degree of methylation at a CpG site defined as an M-value. A and B represent the unmethylated and methylated signal intensities, and α is a* small positive constant (typically 100) that guards against division by 0. Thus, $M <0$ corresponds to no methylation, $M >0$ to complete methylation, and M near 0 to intermediate methylation

M-values do not suffer from the severe heteroscedasticity of the β-values, expanding the range of analytical techniques that can be applied to them. However, M-values are still not normally distributed but merely related to β-values through a nonlinear monotonic transformation (Eq. 3).

$$M = \log_2\left(\frac{\beta}{1-\beta}\right); \quad \beta = \frac{2^M}{2^M + 1}$$

Equation 3 : *The relationship between β-values and M-values*

For statistical testing, this implies that nonparametric tests will give the exact same result for both β- and M-values and that parametric tests should be avoided for both. Changes in M-values are also considerably more difficult to interpret changes in β-values. Detection of differentially methylated CpG sites according to the procedures outlined above can also be performed within several of the popular R packages for analysis of 450k array data reviewed elsewhere [28].

2.5 Annotation and Biological Interpretation of Differentially Methylated CpG Sites

A central goal of studying cancer phenotypes is identifying related sets of genes and the perturbed underlying molecular pathways. As the functional annotation of the human genome steadily increases, also more in-depth annotation of differentially methylated CpG sites or regions correlated with phenotypic changes is becoming possible.

The easiest approach is to use the CpG site annotations to RefSeq genes and CpG islands according to HumanMethylation450 BeadChip manifest file, which can be downloaded from Illumina's website. It should be noted that the annotations using the 450k array manifest file are in some cases incomplete. Therefore, we strongly suggest that additional annotation is performed.

There are a plethora of additional databases that can be used for more advanced CpG site annotation. Data from the NIH Roadmap Epigenomics Mapping project [34] and ENCODE [35] can provide annotations from chromatin marks in various cell types. Comprehensive gene annotation can be downloaded from the GENCODE project [36]. Also, GENCODE annotation files, CpG islands, transcription factor binding sites, repetitive elements, etc. can also be downloaded directly from the UCSC Genome Browser using the Table Browser tool [37]. Enhancer annotations can be downloaded from the FANTOM5 data resources [38]. Annotation of the different genomic elements from the databases mentioned above can be extracted using a combination of awk one-liners and BEDTools (*see* **Note 2**). CpG sites can then be annotated to genomic features by comparing their chromosomal coordinates to annotation files, which can also be performed using BEDTools.

When analyzing functional annotation data, it may be advisable to split the differentially methylated CpG sites into two sets, one for CpGs that increase in DNA methylation (hypermethylated) and a second for those that decrease in methylation (hypomethylated). We prefer this method, since when screening for enrichment in a dataset, hypomethylated differentially methylated sites may be enriched toward one functional category, while the hypermethylated sites are not, and thus the signal will be diluted if they are analyzed together.

For annotation purposes, when a CpG site has more than one functional-level annotation, for example, present in both the transcription start site and a first exon, the CpG site is counted in both annotation categories. To determine enrichment of differentially methylated sites to a specific functional category, a fisher's exact test is used to calculate an enrichment P-value for the number of differentially methylated sites compared to the "array background," i.e., the number of sites in that functional category that were assayed on the array. Here it is important that only the CpG sites used for the differential methylation analysis are tested against; thus if filtering has been performed, the annotation of the filtered dataset should be used for the background.

Another popular form of annotation is pathway analysis, that is, the characterization of the function of the genes in which the individual or groups of differentially methylated sites are located. There are several R packages freely available to do this. Popular freely available alternatives are gene set enrichment analysis (GSEA) [39] and the gene ontology (GO), which provides detailed information on the functional relationships between various biological processes and molecular functions [40].

2.6 Subtype Classification

The field of machine learning offers many methods that can be used for cancer subtype classification, such as support vector machines [41], random forests [42], nearest shrunken centroids [43], and elastic net [44]. Combined with different techniques for preprocessing and feature selection, a plethora of possible modeling procedures can be conceived. Our preferred algorithm is described in Subheading 2.6.1 and general principles for performance evaluation in Subheading 2.6.2, and a complete implementation is outlined in Subheading 2.6.3.

2.6.1 The Nearest Shrunken Centroid Algorithm

The nearest shrunken centroid (NSC) classification method was originally designed for multiple tumor-type classification and prediction from array-based gene expression data but has been successfully applied to DNA methylation data [7, 45, 46]. We have shown that this method is extremely robust for identifying subtype-specific signatures in groups with as few as eight biological replicates [7]. It may be possible to create classifiers based on fewer samples as long as there is a clear differential DNA methylation patter in the subtype or class of interest.

The central idea of NSC is to represent each subtype by its average DNA methylation profile, called *class-wise centroid*, and assign previously unseen samples to the subtypes whose centroids they are the closest to in spatial context. Since some CpG sites are better subtype predictors than others, NSC only takes a relevant subset of all CpG sites into account when calculating the distances between samples and centroids. This subset is selected during classifiers training by moving, or *shrinking*, the class-wise centroids toward the *overall centroid* (the mean of all training samples) using soft thresholding. When more shrinkage is applied, fewer CpG sites are included in the model. Cross-validation is used to estimate the classification performance associated with different amounts of shrinkage. The best performing shrinkage is selected for use in future predictions. NSC classification is implemented in the "pamr" package in R (*see* **Note 3**).

Reasons for why we believe NSC to be a useful algorithm for DNA methylation array data include that it performs well when the number of samples is small compared to the number of CpG sites; it computes faster than more complex models (like support vector machines and random forests), thus allowing the user to calculate many cross-validation replicates (Subheading 2.6.2), and the resulting models are easy to interpret due to their linear and sparse nature. A potential drawback of NSC is its inability to capture nonlinear interactions between CpG sites. To assess whether or not this is an issue for a particular application, one can also build support vector machines or random forests and compare their performance to NSC. If the more complex models do not yield better classification, it is preferable to stick to the more simplistic NSC approach.

2.6.2 Performance Evaluation

In order to trust the predictions of a classifier, it is necessary to test its performance on data that has not been part of the process for creating it. Thus, a portion of the dataset should be withheld from the classifier training for evaluation. The importance of this principle cannot be stressed enough, and failure to adhere to it may produce severely over optimistic results.

Less obvious biases can occur when coupling classifier training to additional preprocessing steps. Consider the scenario where PCA (Subheading 2.3) is used for dimensionality reduction followed by the training of a quadratic discriminant classifier based on the first three principal components. If the entire dataset is used for PCA, instead of just the training set, the test set might influence the component definition strongly enough to give the classifier an unfair advantage when later applied for classification to that very same test set. This may happen even though PCA does not involve the class membership information and even if the test set was not allowed to be part of the discriminant training.

Another subtle matter of performance evaluation is that the size of test sets greatly affects the variance of the resulting performance estimates. Studies with small sample sizes will inevitably have small test sets and therefore risk obtaining markedly different performance estimates depending on which samples were used for training and testing. To study this variability, it is advisable to repeat the classifier training and testing multiple times with different partitions of samples into training and test sets, for example, by using cross-validation (CV) or repeated holdout, and report the mean and variance (*see* **Note 4**). To subject the previous example to CV, both PCA and classifier training must be performed separately for each training set. The repetitive nature of this approach lends itself well to automation, which can be considerably facilitated by readily available packages, e.g., the "emil" package for R (*see* **Note 5**) [47].

Ideally, one would also like to incorporate raw data processing and dataset normalization into the cross-validation procedure for the highest possible statistical rigor, but this is usually not practically feasible. One should still be aware of this issue and reflect on the potential biases of excluding each preprocessing step from CV. In the case of DNA methylation arrays, it should be safe to assume that the raw data processing in Genome Studio and peak-based normalization described above have very little influence on downstream classification analyses.

2.6.3 An Example of a Complete Subtype Classification Procedure

The subtype classification scheme that we apply [7] involves a slightly more elaborate setup than described above (Fig. 6). Instead of using NSC for simultaneous multi-class classification, as in the original publication [43], a compound classifier is created wherein the subtypes are modeled as a series of binary "one-vs-the-rest" problems. To identify CpG sites that are both excellent subtype predictors and robust to outliers in the training set, we train 25 NSC sub-classifiers for each subtype on different subsets in the dataset. CpG sites selected by $\tau = 17/25$ or more sub-classifiers are retained in the final model. In our example, the performance of the final classifier is essentially unaffected by the choice of τ. The τ of 17 was chosen in order to retain enough CpG sites to provide robustness through redundancy and the fewest number for practical reasons, for example, to keep down costs if the classification would be tested using a different technology. If the performance were to vary a lot with τ, this parameter would need to be treated as an additional complexity parameter and should be tuned with an additional layer of CV.

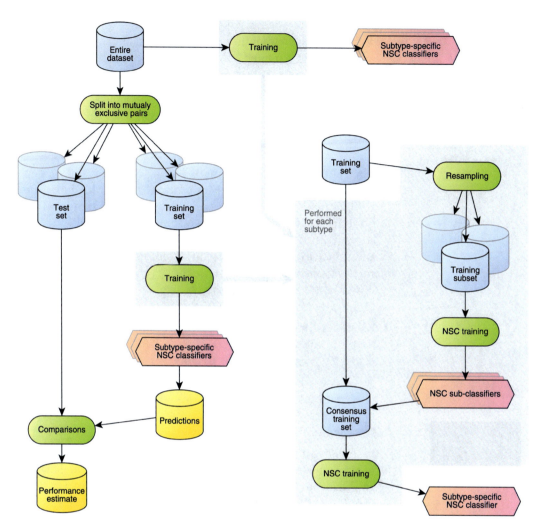

Fig. 6 Schematic overview of an example classifier training procedure. **Top**: A set of subtype-specific nearest shrunken centroid (NSC) classifiers are trained on the entire dataset, to be used for predicting the subtypes of future samples. This set of classifiers together constitutes the final compound classifier. **Right**: When training the compound classifier mentioned above, each subtype is modeled as a binary one-vs-the-rest problem (gray box). Using resampling, 25 subsets of the training set are produced, onto which 25 NSC sub-classifiers are fitted. CpG sites that are selected by at least τ (folds) in sub-classifiers are defined as the consensus sites for each class. A subtype-specific NSC classifier is then trained using the consensus sites of the entire training set. **Left**: Cross-validation is performed to assess the performance of the compound classifier and choose a suitable value of the parameter τ. Multiple mutually exclusive pairs of training and test sets are generated and used to fit classifiers and evaluate the performance at different values of τ. The procedure for fitting each classifier is identical to the procedure used to fit the compound classifier in the top of the figure (gray box)

Prior to each NSC classifier fitting, a preprocessing step is included that discards CpG sites with more than 10% missing values (NAs) and CpG sites with a difference in class-wise mean β-value <20%. This is done to remove CpG sites with many missing values in the sample set and to remove CpG sites with small methylation differences. We use five replicates of fivefold CV to assess the performance of the compound NSC classifiers, after which a single final classifier can be trained on all data. The final classifier can then be validated on external samples, which have not previously been used in the classifier design process.

3 Notes

1. The Human450k DNA methylation BeadChip has been replaced by the Infinium MethylationEPIC BeadChip. The EPIC array is based on the same chemistry and design using both Infinium type I and type II probes. The EPIC array contains 90% of the same content as on the 450k array with additional extended content in transcription factor binding sites, enhancers, and other regulatory regions. Therefore, the normalization and filtering approaches are expected to be similar for processing both array types.

2. Examples for extracting GENCODE annotation files can be found in the GitBook *DNA Methylation Sequencing Analysis*: https://www.gitbook.com/@ycl6.

3. Additional information and instructions for downloading and implementing the "pamR" package in R can be found here: http://statweb.stanford.edu/~tibs/PAM/Rdist/doc/readme.html.

4. If the intention of a study is to produce a classifier for future use, a final classifier should ultimately be trained with all available data in order to maximize its future performance. CV should still be performed to assess what performance can be expected of classifiers generated by the training procedure and dataset at hand, but technically such an estimate is not an estimate of the actual final classifiers' true performance. However, since the final classifier is trained on more data than the classifiers trained during CV, it is reasonable to assume that the final classifier will perform equally well or better.

5. The "emil" package can be downloaded from http://molmed.github.io/emil/.

References

1. Sandoval J, Esteller M (2012) Cancer epigenomics: beyond genomics. Curr Opin Genet Dev 22(1):50–55. https://doi.org/10.1016/j.gde.2012.02.008
2. Hansen KD, Timp W, Bravo HC, Sabunciyan S, Langmead B, McDonald OG, Wen B, Wu H, Liu Y, Diep D, Briem E, Zhang K, Irizarry RA, Feinberg AP (2011) Increased methylation variation in epigenetic domains across cancer types. Nat Genet 43(8):768–775. https://doi.org/10.1038/ng.865
3. Weisenberger DJ (2014) Characterizing DNA methylation alterations from the cancer genome atlas. J Clin Invest 124(1):17–23. https://doi.org/10.1172/JCI69740

4. Timp W, Bravo HC, McDonald OG, Goggins M, Umbricht C, Zeiger M, Feinberg AP, Irizarry RA (2014) Large hypomethylated blocks as a universal defining epigenetic alteration in human solid tumors. Genome Med 6 (8):61. https://doi.org/10.1186/s13073-014-0061-y

5. Nordlund J, Syvanen AC (2017) Epigenetics in pediatric acute lymphoblastic leukemia. Semin Cancer Biol. https://doi.org/10.1016/j.semcancer.2017.09.001

6. Witte T, Plass C, Gerhauser C (2014) Pan-cancer patterns of DNA methylation. Genome Med 6(8):66. https://doi.org/10.1186/s13073-014-0066-6

7. Nordlund J, Backlin CL, Zachariadis V, Cavelier L, Dahlberg J, Ofverholm I, Barbany G, Nordgren A, Overnas E, Abrahamsson J, Flaegstad T, Heyman MM, Jonsson OG, Kanerva J, Larsson R, Palle J, Schmiegelow K, Gustafsson MG, Lonnerholm G, Forestier E, Syvanen AC (2015) DNA methylation-based subtype prediction for pediatric acute lymphoblastic leukemia. Clin Epigenetics 7(1):11. https://doi.org/10.1186/s13148-014-0039-z

8. Danielsson A, Nemes S, Tisell M, Lannering B, Nordborg C, Sabel M, Caren H (2015) MethPed: a DNA methylation classifier tool for the identification of pediatric brain tumor subtypes. Clin Epigenetics 7(1):62. https://doi.org/10.1186/s13148-015-0103-3

9. Teschendorff AE, Widschwendter M (2012) Differential variability improves the identification of cancer risk markers in DNA methylation studies profiling precursor cancer lesions. Bioinformatics 28(11):1487–1494. https://doi.org/10.1093/bioinformatics/bts170

10. Bibikova M, Le J, Barnes B, Saedinia-Melnyk S, Zhou LX, Shen R, Gunderson KL (2009) Genome-wide DNA methylation profiling using Infinium (R) assay. Epigenomics 1 (1):177–200. https://doi.org/10.2217/EPI.09.14

11. Sandoval J, Heyn H, Moran S, Serra-Musach J, Pujana MA, Bibikova M, Esteller M (2011) Validation of a DNA methylation microarray for 450,000 CpG sites in the human genome. Epigenetics 6(6):692–702

12. Pidsley R, Zotenko E, Peters TJ, Lawrence MG, Risbridger GP, Molloy P, Van Djik S, Muhlhausler B, Stirzaker C, Clark SJ (2016) Critical evaluation of the Illumina MethylationEPIC BeadChip microarray for whole-genome DNA methylation profiling. Genome Biol 17(1):208. https://doi.org/10.1186/s13059-016-1066-1

13. Walker DL, Bhagwate AV, Baheti S, Smalley RL, Hilker CA, Sun Z, Cunningham JM (2015) DNA methylation profiling: comparison of genome-wide sequencing methods and the Infinium Human Methylation 450 Bead Chip. Epigenomics 1–16. doi:https://doi.org/10.2217/EPI.15.64

14. Marabita F, Tegnér J, Gomez-Cabrero D (2015) Introduction to data types in epigenomics. In: Teschendorff AE (ed) Computational and statistical Epigenomics, Translational bioinformatics, vol 7. Springer, Netherlands, pp 3–34. https://doi.org/10.1007/978-94-017-9927-0_1

15. Bibikova M, Barnes B, Tsan C, Ho V, Klotzle B, Le JM, Delano D, Zhang L, Schroth GP, Gunderson KL, Fan JB, Shen R (2011) High density DNA methylation array with single CpG site resolution. Genomics 98 (4):288–295. https://doi.org/10.1016/j.ygeno.2011.07.007

16. Lister R, Pelizzola M, Dowen RH, Hawkins RD, Hon G, Tonti-Filippini J, Nery JR, Lee L, Ye Z, Ngo QM, Edsall L, Antosiewicz-Bourget J, Stewart R, Ruotti V, Millar AH, Thomson JA, Ren B, Ecker JR (2009) Human DNA methylomes at base resolution show widespread epigenomic differences. Nature 462(7271):315–322. https://doi.org/10.1038/nature08514

17. Bock C (2012) Analysing and interpreting DNA methylation data. Nat Rev Genet 13 (10):705–719. https://doi.org/10.1038/nrg3273

18. Gunderson KL, Steemers FJ, Lee G, Mendoza LG, Chee MS (2005) A genome-wide scalable SNP genotyping assay using microarray technology. Nat Genet 37(5):549–554. https://doi.org/10.1038/ng1547

19. Dedeurwaerder S, Defrance M, Calonne E, Denis H, Sotiriou C, Fuks F (2011) Evaluation of the Infinium Methylation 450K technology. Epigenomics 3(6):771–784. https://doi.org/10.2217/epi.11.105

20. Sun Z, Cunningham J, Slager S, Kocher JP (2015) Base resolution methylome profiling: considerations in platform selection, data preprocessing and analysis. Epigenomics. https://doi.org/10.2217/epi.15.21

21. Maksimovic J, Gordon L, Oshlack A (2012) SWAN: subset-quantile within array normalization for Illumina Infinium HumanMethylation450 BeadChips. Genome Biol 13(6):R44. https://doi.org/10.1186/Gb-2012-13-6-R44

22. Teschendorff AE, Marabita F, Lechner M, Bartlett T, Tegner J, Gomez-Cabrero D, Beck S (2013) A beta-mixture quantile

normalization method for correcting probe design bias in Illumina Infinium 450 k DNA methylation data. Bioinformatics 29(2):189–196. https://doi.org/10.1093/bioinformatics/bts680

23. Marabita F, Almgren M, Lindholm ME, Ruhrmann S, Fagerstrom-Billai F, Jagodic M, Sundberg CJ, Ekstrom TJ, Teschendorff AE, Tegner J, Gomez-Cabrero D (2013) An evaluation of analysis pipelines for DNA methylation profiling using the Illumina HumanMethylation450 BeadChip platform. Epigenetics 8(3):333–346. https://doi.org/10.4161/epi.24008

24. Wu MC, Joubert BR, Kuan PF, Haberg SE, Nystad W, Peddada SD, London SJ (2014) A systematic assessment of normalization approaches for the Infinium 450K methylation platform. Epigenetics 9(2):318–329. https://doi.org/10.4161/epi.27119

25. Aryee MJ, Jaffe AE, Corrada-Bravo H, Ladd-Acosta C, Feinberg AP, Hansen KD, Irizarry RA (2014) Minfi: a flexible and comprehensive bioconductor package for the analysis of Infinium DNA methylation microarrays. Bioinformatics 30(10):1363–1369. https://doi.org/10.1093/bioinformatics/btu049

26. Morris TJ, Butcher LM, Feber A, Teschendorff AE, Chakravarthy AR, Wojdacz TK, Beck S (2014) ChAMP: 450k Chip analysis methylation pipeline. Bioinformatics 30(3):428–430. https://doi.org/10.1093/bioinformatics/btt684

27. Assenov Y, Muller F, Lutsik P, Walter J, Lengauer T, Bock C (2014) Comprehensive analysis of DNA methylation data with RnBeads. Nat Methods 11(11):1138–1140. https://doi.org/10.1038/nmeth.3115

28. Wilhelm-Benartzi CS, Koestler DC, Karagas MR, Flanagan JM, Christensen BC, Kelsey KT, Marsit CJ, Houseman EA, Brown R (2013) Review of processing and analysis methods for DNA methylation array data. Br J Cancer 109(6):1394–1402. https://doi.org/10.1038/bjc.2013.496

29. Nordlund J, Backlin CL, Wahlberg P, Busche S, Berglund EC, Eloranta ML, Flaegstad T, Forestier E, Frost BM, Harila-Saari A, Heyman M, Jonsson OG, Larsson R, Palle J, Ronnblom L, Schmiegelow K, Sinnett D, Soderhall S, Pastinen T, Gustafsson MG, Lonnerholm G, Syvanen AC (2013) Genome-wide signatures of differential DNA methylation in pediatric acute lymphoblastic leukemia. Genome Biol 14(9):r105. https://doi.org/10.1186/gb-2013-14-9-r105

30. Naeem H, Wong NC, Chatterton Z, Hong MK, Pedersen JS, Corcoran NM, Hovens CM, Macintyre G (2014) Reducing the risk of false discovery enabling identification of biologically significant genome-wide methylation status using the HumanMethylation450 array. BMC Genomics 15:51. https://doi.org/10.1186/1471-2164-15-51

31. Chen YA, Lemire M, Choufani S, Butcher DT, Grafodatskaya D, Zanke BW, Gallinger S, Hudson TJ, Weksberg R (2013) Discovery of cross-reactive probes and polymorphic CpGs in the Illumina Infinium HumanMethylation450 microarray. Epigenetics 8(2):203–209. https://doi.org/10.4161/epi.23470

32. Li H, Durbin R (2009) Fast and accurate short read alignment with Burrows-Wheeler transform. Bioinformatics 25(14):1754–1760. https://doi.org/10.1093/bioinformatics/btp324

33. Du P, Zhang X, Huang CC, Jafari N, Kibbe WA, Hou L, Lin SM (2010) Comparison of Beta-value and M-value methods for quantifying methylation levels by microarray analysis. BMC Bioinformatics 11:587. https://doi.org/10.1186/1471-2105-11-587

34. Bernstein BE, Stamatoyannopoulos JA, Costello JF, Ren B, Milosavljevic A, Meissner A, Kellis M, Marra MA, Beaudet AL, Ecker JR, Farnham PJ, Hirst M, Lander ES, Mikkelsen TS, Thomson JA (2010) The NIH roadmap epigenomics mapping consortium. Nat Biotechnol 28(10):1045–1048. https://doi.org/10.1038/nbt1010-1045

35. Consortium EP (2012) An integrated encyclopedia of DNA elements in the human genome. Nature 489(7414):57–74. https://doi.org/10.1038/nature11247

36. Harrow J, Frankish A, Gonzalez JM, Tapanari E, Diekhans M, Kokocinski F, Aken BL, Barrell D, Zadissa A, Searle S, Barnes I, Bignell A, Boychenko V, Hunt T, Kay M, Mukherjee G, Rajan J, Despacio-Reyes G, Saunders G, Steward C, Harte R, Lin M, Howald C, Tanzer A, Derrien T, Chrast J, Walters N, Balasubramanian S, Pei B, Tress M, Rodriguez JM, Ezkurdia I, van Baren J, Brent M, Haussler D, Kellis M, Valencia A, Reymond A, Gerstein M, Guigo R, Hubbard TJ (2012) GENCODE: the reference human genome annotation for The ENCODE Project. Genome Res 22(9):1760–1774. https://doi.org/10.1101/gr.135350.111

37. Kuhn RM, Haussler D, Kent WJ (2013) The UCSC genome browser and associated tools. Brief Bioinform 14(2):144–161. https://doi.org/10.1093/bib/bbs038

38. Andersson R, Gebhard C, Miguel-Escalada I, Hoof I, Bornholdt J, Boyd M, Chen Y, Zhao X,

Schmidl C, Suzuki T, Ntini E, Arner E, Valen E, Li K, Schwarzfischer L, Glatz D, Raithel J, Lilje B, Rapin N, Bagger FO, Jorgensen M, Andersen PR, Bertin N, Rackham O, Burroughs AM, Baillie JK, Ishizu Y, Shimizu Y, Furuhata E, Maeda S, Negishi Y, Mungall CJ, Meehan TF, Lassmann T, Itoh M, Kawaji H, Kondo N, Kawai J, Lennartsson A, Daub CO, Heutink P, Hume DA, Jensen TH, Suzuki H, Hayashizaki Y, Muller F, Consortium F, Forrest AR, Carninci P, Rehli M, Sandelin A (2014) An atlas of active enhancers across human cell types and tissues. Nature 507(7493):455–461. https://doi.org/10.1038/nature12787

39. Subramanian A, Tamayo P, Mootha VK, Mukherjee S, Ebert BL, Gillette MA, Paulovich A, Pomeroy SL, Golub TR, Lander ES, Mesirov JP (2005) Gene set enrichment analysis: a knowledge-based approach for interpreting genome-wide expression profiles. Proc Natl Acad Sci U S A 102(43):15545–15550. https://doi.org/10.1073/pnas.0506580102

40. Balakrishnan R, Harris MA, Huntley R, Van Auken K, Cherry JM (2013) A guide to best practices for gene ontology (GO) manual annotation. Database 2013:bat054. https://doi.org/10.1093/database/bat054

41. Cortes C, Vapnik V (1995) Support-vector networks. Mach Learn 20(3):273–297. https://doi.org/10.1007/BF00994018

42. Breiman L (2001) Random forests. Mach Learn 45(1):5–32. https://doi.org/10.1023/A:1010933404324

43. Tibshirani R, Hastie T, Narasimhan B, Chu G (2002) Diagnosis of multiple cancer types by shrunken centroids of gene expression. Proc Natl Acad Sci U S A 99(10):6567–6572. https://doi.org/10.1073/pnas.082099299

44. Zou H, Hastie T (2005) Regularization and variable selection via the elastic net. J R Stat Soc Series B Stat Methodol 67(2):301–320. https://doi.org/10.1111/j.1467-9868.2005.00503.x

45. Milani L, Lundmark A, Kiialainen A, Nordlund J, Flaegstad T, Forestier E, Heyman M, Jonmundsson G, Kanerva J, Schmiegelow K, Soderhall S, Gustafsson MG, Lonnerholm G, Syvanen AC (2010) DNA methylation for subtype classification and prediction of treatment outcome in patients with childhood acute lymphoblastic leukemia. Blood 115(6):1214–1225. https://doi.org/10.1182/blood-2009-04-214668

46. Stefansson OA, Moran S, Gomez A, Sayols S, Arribas-Jorba C, Sandoval J, Hilmarsdottir H, Olafsdottir E, Tryggvadottir L, Jonasson JG, Eyfjord J, Esteller M (2015) A DNA methylation-based definition of biologically distinct breast cancer subtypes. Mol Oncol 9 (3):555–568. https://doi.org/10.1016/j.molonc.2014.10.012

47. Backlin CL, Gustafsson MG (2018) Developer friendly and computationally efficient predictive modeling without information leakage: the emil package for R. J Stat Softw, 85(13). https://doi.org/10.18637/jss.v085.i13, https://www.jstatsoft.org/v085/i13

Chapter 11

Computational Methods for Subtyping of Tumors and Their Applications for Deciphering Tumor Heterogeneity

Shihua Zhang

Abstract

With the rapid development of deep sequencing technologies, many programs are generating multi-platform genomic profiles (e.g., somatic mutation, DNA methylation, and gene expression) for a large number of tumors. This activity has provided unique opportunities and challenges to stratify tumors and decipher tumor heterogeneity. In this chapter, we summarize several computational methods to address the challenge of tumor stratification with different types of genomic data. We further introduce their applications in emerging large-scale genomic data to show their effectiveness in deciphering tumor heterogeneity and clinical relevance.

Key words Bioinformatics, Cancer genomics, Cancer subtype, Cancer stratification, Machine learning, Model and algorithm

1 Introduction

Cancer genome aberrations observed through basic research have been used to categorize patients in an effort to improve clinical decision-making and develop more effective treatments. Although such grouping methods have improved treatment efficacy of many different cancers, overcoming heterogeneity within these populations is a major challenge. With the advent of high-throughput genomic technologies, many molecular-based diagnostics have been developed, and several have recently gained regulatory approval. Many of these diagnostics are applicable to diverse cancers, suggesting that individual molecular diagnostics for therapeutic strategies may provide objective and precise prediction of clinical outcomes.

Cancer is no longer viewed as a single disease; rather, it is heterogeneous consisting of different subtypes on the molecular, histopathological, and clinical level with different prognostic and therapeutic implications. For example, gene expression profiling has classified breast cancer into five biologically distinct intrinsic subtypes: luminal A, luminal B, HER2-enriched (HER2+), basal-like, and normal-like [1]. Parker et al. [1] developed an efficient classifier PAM50 to distinguish these five intrinsic subtypes using the expression of 50 "classifier genes." In a more recent study, a large breast cancer patient cohort (~2000) was clustered into 10 molecularly defined subgroups with apparently distinct biological and disease-specific survival characteristics [2]. The molecular heterogeneity among breast tumors suggests that respective stratified therapy and clinical prediction of prognosis would be beneficial. In an effort to guide the selection of the most appropriate therapy for individual patients, numerous prognostic gene expression signatures have been reported [3].

With the fast development of deep sequencing technologies, it is becoming possible to characterize large samples of biological systems on multiple levels simultaneously. For example, The Cancer Genome Atlas (TCGA) project aims to generate multidimensional genomic profiles for a set of patient samples including more than 20 types of tumors [4].

This emerging activity has provided unique opportunities and challenges to stratify tumors and explore tumor subtype-specific biological mechanisms. Shen et al. [5] proposed a joint clustering model for multiple genomic datasets, but it was designed for sample clustering and subtype discovery and cannot identify modules comprising correlated variables. Zhang et al. [6, 7] proposed a powerful nonnegative matrix factorization framework [6] and a semi-supervised variant [7], and Li et al. [8] developed an extended partial least square method to identify correlative relationships in multidimensional genomic data, which can be used to reveal significantly disrupted pathways and stratify patients into clinically distinct groups.

In this chapter, we summarize several computational methods to address the challenge of tumor stratification. We survey the intrinsic subtyping tools (PAM50 and AIMS) using gene expression and a network-based stratification (NBS) from mutations. We further introduce their applications in emerging large-scale genomic data to show their effectiveness in deciphering tumor heterogeneity and clinical relevance.

2 Methods

2.1 PAM50 and AIMS

Computational analyses of gene expression profiles provided the so-called intrinsic subtyping scheme [1, 9], which can also be similarly adopted for diverse genomic data. For example, Parker et al. [1] developed an efficient classifier PAM50 to distinguish five intrinsic subtypes of breast cancer using the expression of 50 "classifier genes." However, typical subtyping tools like PAM50 have severe shortcomings [9], which can lead to different subtype classifications for patients, due to the application of various normalization procedures and gene-centering techniques. Recently, Paquet and Hallett [9] presented a new bioinformatics approach named Absolute Intrinsic Molecular Subtyping (AIMS) for estimating patient subtype. This method can accurately assign a subtype to a single patient but is insensitive to changes in normalization procedures or relative frequencies of different types of patients. Here, we briefly introduce PAM50 and AIMS, respectively.

We first describe a typical procedure to identify tumor subtypes using gene expression or other molecular profiling data as used in [10]. It first employs a hierarchical clustering using agglomerative average linkage and a distance metric defined by one minus the Pearson's correlation coefficient (or other clustering methods) as the basis for consensus clustering to detect robust clusters. This procedure is run over a given number of iterations (e.g., 1000) and a subsampling ratio (e.g., 0.8) with 1740 reliably expressed genes. SigClust is performed to establish the significance of the clusters in a pairwise fashion. The "core" members of each subtype can be calculated using silhouette width values for all samples with positive silhouette values. It applies significance analysis of microarrays and receiver operating characteristic curve methods to identify marker genes of each subtype. Each class is compared to the other classes combined, and each class is compared to the other three individual classes in a pairwise manner. A nearest centroid-based classification algorithm is used to find signatures of each class to assess class cross validation error and to predict subtype in the validation set.

Accordingly, PAM50 first identifies prototypical intrinsic subtype samples and genes. Specifically, it employs a method to objectively select prototype samples for training and then predicts subtypes independent of clustering. To identify prototypic tumor samples, it expands an intrinsic gene set comprised of 1906 genes found in four previous studies. As the typical procedure, it clusters the expression data by hierarchical clustering (median centered by feature/gene, Pearson's correlation, average linkage), and the sample dendrogram is analyzed using SigClust to extract significant clusters representing the intrinsic subtypes. It further obtains a minimized gene set with 50 genes using prototype samples to assess the robustness of the minimized gene sets. The 50 genes are assessed for reproducibility of classification using several methods including Prediction Analysis of Microarray (PAM) with the distances calculated using Spearman's rank correlation.

AIMS is designed to identify a small set of rules of the form "if expression of gene A is less than expression of gene B, then tend to classify the patient as subtype X." These rules only examine the expression of genes A and B within the specific patient, and the expression of any other genes within any other patients is not used to make such a decision. AIMS adopts a standard machine learning approach—a single naïve Bayes classifier to combine the results of all the individual rules supporting or denying the inclusion in one of the subtypes. Thus, the decision-making is performed entirely within the expression profile of a single patient and not relative to a large cohort of expression profiles as other typical methods do. AIMS package is available at http://www.bci.mcgill.ca/AIMS/.

Specifically, AIMS is used to analyze a given combined matrix of the unnormalized, untransformed expression values for all the datasets focusing on the prior intrinsic genes. AIMS employs k-top scoring-pairs strategy with k representing the number of rules to be selected for each subtype. In other words, each rule represents a binary classification marker that distinguishes the specific subtype from remaining ones. Then, AIMS creates an indicator matrix denoting all the k rules of each subtype to train one naïve Bayes classifier. AIMS employs a cross-validation stratification to select the optimal k. However, AIMS requires a gold standard dataset of patients with subtype assignments for its training. For example, they adopted the PAM50 subtype assignment as a gold standard in their study [9]. For some cancer type or new data types, AIMS needs to be used together with other techniques.

2.2 An Application of PAM50

Given the limited patient number for many studies, the Molecular Taxonomy of Breast Cancer International Consortium (METABRIC) provides an unprecedented resource [2], which contains a large breast cancer patient cohort of ~2000 samples with detailed clinical measurements and genome-wide molecular profiles including gene expression and copy number variation data. Sage Bionetworks launched a competition called DREAM Breast Cancer Prognosis Challenge to assess the accuracy of computational models, like METABRIC, that use comprehensive molecular profiling data and clinical information to predict patient survival.

However, Liu et al. [11] found that the molecular features such as gene expression only moderately improve the clinical prediction with regard to the whole cancer cohort. Taking into account the heterogeneity of breast cancers and the subtype-specific molecular signatures, Liu et al. [11] hypothesized that making clinical predictions for five subtypes separately would provide diverse prediction performance. They adopted the heterogeneous PAM50 breast cancer subtypes of METABRIC expression data and systematically evaluated patient survival prediction performance on these subgroups using both clinical observations and the gene expression profiles of the METABRIC dataset. Then, they also applied a network module-based cancer prognostic signature identification method on each subtype to search for network biomarkers to further demonstrate the differences of prediction performance.

To this end, they adopted the five PAM50 tumor groups defined in the METABRIC dataset for analysis. The dataset was composed of 328 basal-like tumors, 238 HER2+ tumors, 719 luminal A, 490 luminal B, 200 normal-like tumors, and 6 samples with unclear category. They applied the Cox model to gene expression covariates, clinical feature covariates, or the combination of these two for each of the five intrinsic subtypes and the METABRIC whole dataset, respectively [11].

2.2.1 Breast Cancer Subtypes Show Different Prognostic Performance

As mentioned above, after defining the subgroups, they applied the multivariate Cox proportional hazards (multivariate Cox PH) model on different breast cancer subtypes. This analysis revealed significant differences in prognostic performance (Fig. 1a), confirmed by a different machine learning model—random survival forest model. First, consistent with the DREAM Breast Cancer Prognosis Challenge, the multivariate Cox PH model using clinical feature covariates alone demonstrated performance comparable to the combination of clinical feature and gene expression data based on the whole population. Generally, the clinical feature covariates were more informative for predicting patient survival time than the gene expression covariates on the five breast cancer subtype datasets and the whole dataset. The exception, however, was the normal-like tumor subtype. In addition, the predictive power of using both covariates together versus clinical features was increased slightly except for HER2+ (0.597 vs.0.625) and luminal A (0.712 vs.0.715) tumors. These data suggest that the inclusion of gene expression only improves the prediction performance very limitedly.

Both the basal-like and HER2+ subgroups had poor survival prediction performance, while the luminal A and normal-like breast cancer subgroups demonstrated better performance. The clinical outcomes of luminal A and normal-like subtypes, based on genetic and clinical covariates, were more predictable than the other three subgroups. Particularly, all three Cox models underperformed when applied to basal-like breast cancer. This observation is consistent with previous studies that the basal-like tumor subtype, referred to as triple-negative breast cancer in some literature, is associated with a particularly poor prognosis. Compared with the basal-like subgroup, the HER2+ subgroup had a relatively weak prognosis without significance for all three models. In addition, the concordance index (CI) dropped when including the three gene principal components (PCs) to the clinical covariates on the Cox model. It is possible that the three PCs are not representative of the survival-related information hidden in the expression matrix for this subgroup.

Compared with luminal A tumors, luminal B breast cancer was associated with a worse outcome, which is consistent with published results. The ER-positive and histological low-grade luminal A tumors have the highest significant averaged CIs using either

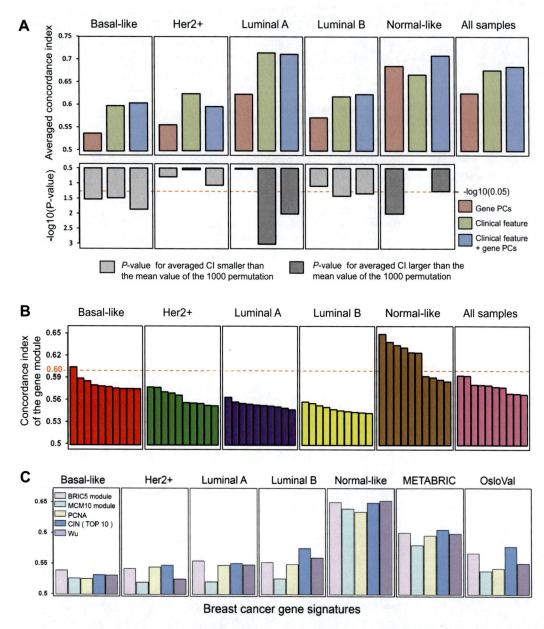

Fig. 1 (**a**) Breast cancer subtypes show different prediction performances. Bar graphs show averaged CIs of the three cases of multivariate Cox PH model on the five breast cancer subtypes and the METABRIC whole dataset. *P* values are from the permutation test. (**b**) The CIs of the top 10 prognostic network modules from five distinct subtypes and the METABRIC whole dataset. The modules generated from each dataset were ranked according to their CIs, which were calculated based on the averaged gene expression value of each module and survival time of corresponding patient cohorts. The dashed red line denotes CI = 0.60. (**c**) Comparison of breast cancer prognostic gene signatures. CIs of the five breast cancer signatures on the five subtypes, the METABRIC dataset, and another dataset (OsloVal)

clinical covariates alone (0.715, *P* value = 0.01) or combined with gene expression covariates (0.712, *P* value = 0.001). This result suggests that the clinical features of luminal A breast cancer are most relevant to patient survival time among the five subgroups and have the best prognostic power.

The normal-like breast cancer subtype ($n = 200$) was of particular interest because of the high expression-based model score (0.686, P value=0.01) compared to the other four subtypes and the METABRIC whole dataset. In addition, unlike the other subgroups, gene expression covariate analysis of normal-like breast cancer was more predictive of patient survival than clinical features covariate analysis (0.667 vs. 0.686).

Taken together, these results demonstrate that (1) the predictive ability of the same method on different cancer subtypes is diverse, (2) gene expression data can improve the predictive performance to different degrees, and (3) the predictive power of gene expression covariates on the normal-like subtype is more informative than that on other subgroups, suggesting that gene expression data of normal-like subgroup contain more prognostic value than that of other breast cancer subtypes. Further research should be conducted on this promising subtype-specific molecular dataset with the purpose of providing effective and reliable support for clinical diagnosis and personalized medicine treatment.

2.2.2 Identifying Subgroup-Specific Prognostic Network Gene Modules

They further hypothesized that the functional network of biomarkers defined for breast cancer is only biologically meaningful for a set of tumor subgroups. To verify this hypothesis, they applied a method to the current five PAM50 subtypes and the METABRIC whole dataset to identify network biomarkers or gene modules that were significantly correlated with patient survival. They found that six network modules obtained from the normal-like subgroup had CIs greater than 0.6, while only one in the basal-like tumors had a CI of 0.605. In addition, no modules satisfied this for all other subtypes and the whole tumor dataset (Fig. 1b). (Each module was named in terms of the name of the gene having the highest CI in the module.) The BIRC5 module consisting of 25 genes generated from the normal-like subtype achieved the highest CI of 0.650. The second one (MCM10 module) from normal-like subtype was comprised of 18 genes and had a CI of 0.640. Moreover, the BRIC5 module was only detected in the normal-like tumors, and it was highly correlated with its overall patient survival.

2.2.3 Previous Gene Signatures Show Similar Subtype Specificity with the BRIC5 Module

They further found that a 31-gene signature discovered using five independent datasets had a strong overlap with the BIRC5 module obtained from normal-like tumors. These two modules had 11 genes in common, among which, 6 were in the top 9 BIRC5 module genes with CIs larger than 0.60. Moreover, the BIRC5 gene was also found to be the most prognostic in this signature.

They also found that mitotic CIN attractor metagene (one of the three universal signatures called attractor metagenes used by the winners of the Breast Cancer Prognosis Challenge) is the most prognostic of the METABRIC and OsloVal datasets. It also has the significant overlap with the BRIC5 module. Fourteen of the 25 genes in the BRIC5 module were in the top 100 genes of the CIN attractor.

Another study observed that many published breast cancer gene signatures have strong correlation to a cell proliferation-related gene set called meta-PCNA. This gene set contains 131 genes whose expression levels were correlated most positively with the proliferation marker PCNA. Liu et al. [11] found that the meta-PCNA signature significantly overlapped with the BIRC5 module and the MCM10 module, which are the top two prognostic modules obtained from the normal-like tumors. In this comparison, 7 of the 25 BIRC5 module genes and 10 of the 18 MCM10 module genes were among the meta-PCNA signature, respectively. Notably, all three of these gene signatures were defined based on whole breast cancer or multicancer datasets without considering tumor heterogeneity. Interestingly, they tend to share a significant number of genes with the modules found to be the most prognostic for the normal-like tumor subgroup.

Given this correlation, Liu et al. [11] deduced that these previously defined gene signatures were also tumor subtype-specific and had significantly high prognostic performance for the normal-like tumor subgroup. To confirm this, they calculated corresponding CIs for each of the five subgroups, the METABRIC whole dataset and the OsloVal dataset by the similar strategy applied for the identified gene modules (Fig. 1c). This analysis revealed that all these gene signatures had the highest CIs for the normal-like breast cancer subgroup, and CIs on METABRIC dataset were also larger than those on other four subgroups. In addition to the BIRC5 module, CIN attractor and Wu's signature had comparable performances with subtle differences on the normal-like subtype and METABRIC dataset.

2.3 NBS

Cancer is a complex and heterogeneous disease, which is driven by a combination of genes with great variety between patients. Hofree et al. [12] proposed the network-based stratification (NBS) approach by integrating tumor somatic mutation profiles with knowledge of the molecular network architecture of human cells. The key underlying idea is that it is widely appreciated that cancer is a disease not of individual mutations or genes but of gene combinations acting in molecular networks corresponding to hallmark processes. They assumed that two tumors may not have any mutations in common, but they may share the networks affected by these mutations.

2.3.1 The NBS Method

The NBS integrates genome-scale somatic mutation profiles of a large number of tumor patients with a gene interaction network to produce a robust classification of patients into a given number of subtypes (Fig. 2a). Briefly, somatic mutations for each patient are represented as a profile of binary states (1, 0) across a number of genes, in which "1" indicates the gene is mutated in the patient. For each patient, NBS projects the mutation profiles onto a prior human gene interaction network. Next, NBS adopts the network propagation technique to spread the influence of each mutation over its network neighborhoods (Fig. 2a). Then each gene obtains a network-smoothed mutation score ranging from 0 to 1, which reflects its network proximity to the mutated genes in that patient. Using this smoothed mutation profile, NBS clusters all patients into a predefined number of subtypes ($k = 2, 3, \ldots$) using a variant of nonnegative matrix factorization (NMF). A network-regularized NMF is adopted to encourage the selection of gene sets relating to each subtype with high modular characteristics. Lastly, NBS uses the consensus clustering technique to promote robust cluster assignments by repeating this procedure for 1000 different subsamples of 80% of patients and genes drawn randomly. NBS aggregates all 1000 runs into a (patient × patient) co-occurrence matrix, which summarizes the frequency that each pair of patients has co-clustered into the same class. This co-occurrence matrix is then clustered a second time to recover a final stratification of the patients into subtypes (Fig. 2d). The implementation of the NBS method is available as a Matlab package from http://idekerlab.ucsd.edu/software/NBS/.

2.4 Application of NBS for Pan-Cancer Stratifications

Recently, Liu et al. [13] adopted the NBS procedure to integrate genome-scale alteration profiles of 3299 tumor patients from 12 cancer types with a gene interaction network to produce robust classifications of patients (Fig. 2b). They employed NBS to stratify samples into k ($k = 3 \sim 15$) clusters (Fig. 2c). All other parameters were set as defaults. They adopted the Pearson's chi-squared test to determine the enrichment significance of a certain tumor type or subtype in a cluster. All P values were corrected for the FDR q values.

They obtained 479 selected functional events (SFEs) (including 116 copy number gains, 151 copy number losses, 199 recurrently mutated genes, and 13 epigenetically silenced genes recorded across 3299 tumor samples from 12 cancer types) that were filtered by statistical and functional significant analysis from thousands of genomic and epigenetic changes [14, 15]. After mapping to genes, this resulted in a binary matrix of 3299 samples with 1750 genes, where "1" means the gene has been altered by some kind of genomic or epigenetic change. Finally, genes were projected onto a biological network STRING v.9.

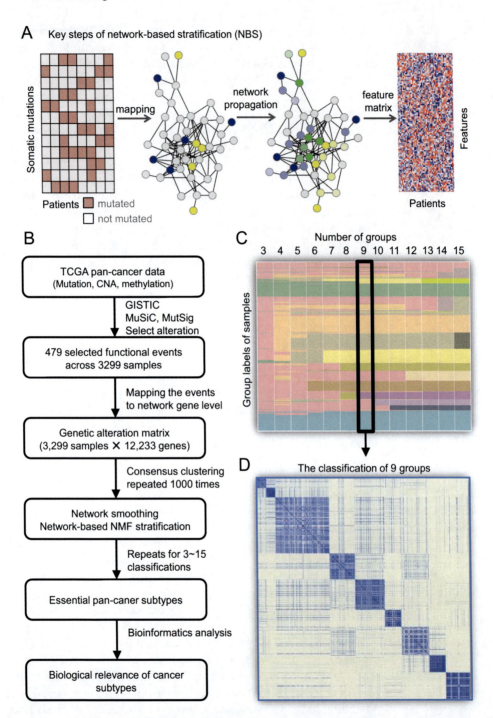

Fig. 2 Overview of the network-based stratification (NBS) tool and its application for pan-cancer stratification analysis. (**a**) Illustration of key steps of NBS for classifying cancer samples using mutation data. (**b**) Flowchart of the main computational steps for pan-cancer stratification analysis. (**c**) The landscape of pan-cancer subgroups with $k = 3$–15 classes obtained from the consensus NBS clustering. Each row denotes a sample, and each column presents a classification. Different colors in each column denote different subgroups. (**d**) The heat map of the co-clustering matrix for nine subgroups obtained from the consensus NBS clustering

2.4.1 Overview of the Pan-Cancer Stratification Analysis

They adopted the NBS to reveal pan-cancer subgroups with similar molecular features and observed clear consistency between every successive two classifications (e.g., $k = 6$ versus $k = 7$) of the samples (Fig. 2c). In particular, two patient subgroups were consistently identified across all 3–15 classes (samples denoted by light blue and green in Fig. 2c). One subgroup was dominated by KIRC tumors, which have been reported to have the strongest exclusivity from the other 11 cancer types with a high frequency of exclusive von Hippel-Lindau (VHL) mutation. The other subgroup consists of subsets of GBM, BLCA, LUSC, and HNSC tumors. The similarity of these tumors has been implicated in the mutation or amplification of ERBB2-HER2. The remaining patients were progressively subdivided into new subgroups as the number of classes got larger. They further explored those representative subgroups in terms of macroscale (with $k = 3$) and microscale (with $k = 9$ and Fig. 2d) classes.

2.4.2 Macroscale Pan-Cancer Subgroups Reveal Clinical Relevance

They found that the unsupervised macroscale pan-cancer subgroups (with $k = 3$) reveal distinct clinical relevance across diverse cancer types. They first observed that each cancer type was significantly clustered into one of the three pan-cancer subgroups. They further found that the significantly enriched patients of five cancer types demonstrated significantly different survival rates compared to the remaining patients of the same cancer types, respectively. In particular, the patients for OV and LAML in subgroup 1 were associated with long survival time, and those for HNSC, LUAD, and LUSC in subgroup 3 were correlated with bad survival outcomes. More intriguingly, they found that patients in subgroup 3 tended to have relatively poorer survival for almost all cancer types, and COADREAD and UCEC subgroup 3 patients also showed statistically significant shorter survival time (log-rank P value <0.05). Similarly, subgroup 1 patients were associated with better survival outcomes for almost all cancer types, and HNSC, LUAD, and LUSC showed statistical significance. Lastly, they found that a large fraction of KIRC tumors and a subset of UCEC tumors were significantly enriched in subgroup 2. Those KIRC tumors and UCEC tumors in subgroup 2 tended to be patients at early tumor stage and low grade. More than half of the KIRC tumors in subgroup 2 were at Stage I, and no UCEC tumor in subgroup 2 was at Stage IV and high grade. All these observations demonstrate that the pan-cancer macroscale stratification reveals strong clinical relevance and shows consistent clinical tendency in some cancer types, implying distinct pan-cancer heterogeneity as well as oncogenic mechanisms. This pan-cancer macroscale stratification divides almost all cancers into subgroups with consistent good or poor survival rates, revealing underlying pan-cancer similarities among cancer types and providing valuable information for patient clinical assessments and stratified therapeutic strategies.

2.4.3 Microscale Pan-Cancer Subgroups Reveal Abundant Cross-Cancer Similarities

Further, they found that the microscale pan-cancer subgroups (e.g., with $k = 9$) reveal heterogeneous aberration patterns across diverse cancer types. (For convenience, all subgroups were named as PC9 subgroup-X, $X = 1\ldots 9$, or subgroup-X for short.) They observed that most of the 12 cancer types and their subtypes were significantly clustered into at least one of the 9 pan-cancer subgroups.

They first found that 94.4% of the tumors in subgroup 5 were KIRC types, making this subgroup highly exclusive to a single cancer type, and more than half of tumors (56.8%) in subgroup 4 were BRCA types. In contrast to these two subgroups dominated by individual cancer type, other subgroups consisted of multiple cancer types. For example, subgroup 7 was significantly enriched with a large fraction of GBM (60.6%), HNSC, LUSC, and BLCA tumors. In subgroup 6, 59.1% of LAML tumors and three molecule-defined COADREAD subtypes were clustered together, indicating potential commonalities between solid and liquid tumors.

2.4.4 Microscale Pan-Cancer Subgroups Demonstrate Distinct Subgroup-Specific Patterns

More importantly, genes from each gene set with high aberration frequencies among corresponding subgroups indeed show significantly distinct patterns among the 9 subgroups (Fig. 3). These observations imply that diverse carcinogenic implementations and functional genetic alteration events exist in different pan-cancer subgroups, depicting essential tumor heterogeneity. More

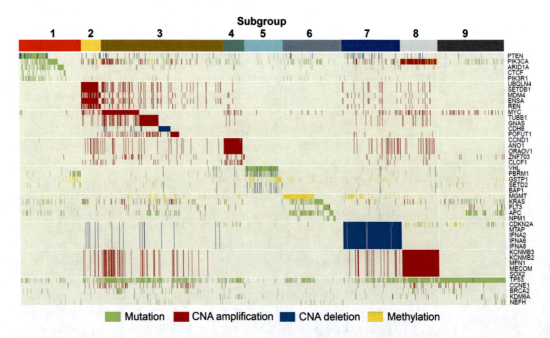

Fig. 3 Landscape of genomic alteration patterns of each pan-cancer subgroup with $k = 9$. Each row denotes a gene and each column indicates a sample

specifically, the KIRC-specific subgroup 5 possesses exclusive somatic mutation of the tumor suppressor gene VHL with a mutation rate of 81.8% in subgroup 5 (Fig. 3). The relationship between mutations of VHL and KIRC has been established for decades, and the association between VHL and tumor stage, tumor cell proliferation, and patient prognosis has also been well studied. Besides VHL, other genetic alterations in subgroup 5 involve the mutation of the chromatin remodeling gene PBRM1 and the mutation of the histone methyltransferase gene SETD2, which has been identified as a tumor suppressor in KIRC and high methylation rate of GSTP1 (Fig. 3). Moreover, VHL, SETD2, PBRM1, and others display significant low expression in this subgroup compared to the remaining ones. These genomic alterations in this subgroup are exclusive to KIRC, marking it highly exclusive from other cancer types.

Multiple cancer types or subtypes including COADREAD-ultra and UCEC as well as BRCA-luminal A tumors were significantly enriched in pan-cancer subgroup 1. This subgroup was marked by mutations of multiple genes that exhibited a mutually exclusive pattern in this cohort (Fig. 3). Both PTEN and PIK3CA alterations have been reported to have strong relationships with UCEC and COADREAD, and the loss of PTEN expression is also observed to be associated with PIK3CA mutations in metastatic colorectal cancer. Subgroup 6 was mainly characterized by frequent promoter hypermethylation of MGMT and mutations of APC, KRAS, FLT3, and NPM1 (Fig. 3). Patients in this subgroup contained 40.6% COADREAD and 59.1% LAML as well as sporadic samples from other types.

Subgroup 7 was characterized by the copy number deletion on chromosome 9p21 (98.4% CNA deletion; Fig. 3). Genes located in this region include CDKN2A, CDKN2B, KLHL9, and MTAP as well as the IFNA gene family. More than half of GBM (60.6%) were clustered in subgroup 7 with other significant enriched cancer types of HNSC, LUSC, and BLCA. This subgroup demonstrates a typical cross-cancer similarity phenomenon that subsets of samples from different tumor types are characterized by the same genomic alterations on chromosome 9. Subgroup 2 mainly consists of LUAD and BRCA tumors, which were characterized by the amplifications on chromosome 1 involving UBQLN4, SETDB1, MDM4, ENSA, and so forth. The largest patient group, subgroup 3 enriched with BRCA-basal, UCEC-serous, and OV tumors, was characterized by multiple recurrent chromosomal gains and losses.

3 Conclusion

Human cancers frequently display substantial tumor heterogeneity in all distinguishable phenotypic features. This has profound implications both for tumor development and therapeutic outcomes. In this chapter, we aim to present several computational methods to address the challenge of tumor stratification. Specifically, we survey a typical intrinsic subtyping tool PAM50 and a recent one AIMS using gene expression. We also present a network-based stratification (NBS) from mutations by incorporating a gene interaction network. We further introduce their applications in emerging large-scale genomic data to show their effectiveness in deciphering tumor heterogeneity and clinical relevance.

One application of PAM50 subtypes is to explore diverse prognostic performance of standard prediction tools by applying genetic and clinical characteristics to breast cancer subtypes individually. This study observed that prediction tools show distinct diversity of survival prediction ability when applied to breast cancer subtypes individually compared to whole breast cancer data. They found that prognostic network biomarkers for the normal-like subtype had significant overlap with cancer signatures previously defined for whole breast cancer, suggesting that the high prognostic ability of these gene signatures on the whole breast cancer samples likely results from their relative higher prognostic power on the normal-like subtype. The gene-based signatures derived from all breast tumors have an extremely diverse clinical predictive ability when applied to intrinsic subtypes, and breast cancer heterogeneity greatly affects clinical prediction tasks. Developing computational methods based on genomic profiling to improve clinical diagnosis and survival prediction is an increasingly important issue in computational biology. This study supports the notion of considering tumor heterogeneity when using gene expression data to predict patient survival and opens new avenues for this type of analysis.

One application of NBS is to reveal essential pan-cancer heterogeneity among diverse cancers without considering the origin organ of primary tumor. The uncovered similarities among cancers of different organs suggest important cross-cancer commonalities. These commonalities not only cover most of the recurrently reported cross-cancer similarities, but also identify several novel potential ones. The macroscale pan-cancer subgroups demonstrate strong clinical relevance and reveal consistent clinical risk tendency among cancer types. The microscale stratification shows essential pan-cancer heterogeneity with subgroup-specific genomic network characteristics and molecular implementations of oncogenesis. With the rapid accumulation of cancer genomic data, this pan-cancer subgrouping procedure can be adopted for a more comprehensive understanding of the pan-cancer heterogeneity.

Acknowledgment

This work has been supported by the National Natural Science Foundation of China [No. 11661141019, 61621003, 61422309 and 61379092], the Strategic Priority Research Program of the Chinese Academy of Sciences (CAS) [XDB13040600], and CAS Frontier Science Research Key Project for Top Young Scientist [No. QYZDB-SSW-SYS008].

References

1. Parker JS et al (2009) Supervised risk predictor of breast cancer based on intrinsic subtypes. J Clin Oncol 27:1160–1167
2. Curtis C et al (2012) The genomic and transcriptomic architecture of 2,000 breast tumours reveals novel subgroups. Nature 486:346–352
3. Wu G, Stein L (2012) A network module-based method for identifying cancer prognostic signatures. Genome Biol 13:R112
4. McLendon R et al (2008) Comprehensive genomic characterization defines human glioblastoma genes and core pathways. Nature 455:1061–1068
5. Shen R, Olshen AB, Ladanyi M (2009) Integrative Clustering of multiple genomic data types using a joint latent variable model with application to breast and lung cancer subtype analysis. Bioinformatics 25:2906–2912
6. Zhang S, Liu CC, Li W, Shen H, Laird PW, Zhou XJ (2012) Discovery of multi-dimensional modules by integrative analysis of cancer genomic data. Nucleic Acids Res 40:9379–9391
7. Zhang S, Li Q, Liu J, Zhou XJ (2011) A novel computational framework for simultaneous integration of multiple types of genomic data to identify microRNA-gene regulatory modules. Bioinformatics 27:i401–i409
8. Li W, Zhang S, Liu CC, Zhou XJ (2012) Identifying multi-layer gene regulatory modules from multi-dimensional genomic data. Bioinformatics 28:2458–2466
9. Paquet ER, Hallet MT (2015) Absolute assignment of breast cancer intrinsic molecular subtype. J Natl Cancer Inst 107:dju357. https://doi.org/10.1093/jnci/dju357
10. Verhaak RG et al (2010) Integrated genomic analysis identifies clinically relevant subtypes of glioblastoma characterized by abnormalities in PDGFRA, IDH1, EGFR, and NF1. Cancer Cell 17:98–110
11. Liu Z, Zhang XS, Zhang S (2014) Breast tumor subgroups reveal diverse clinical predictive power. Sci Rep 4:4002
12. Hofree M, Shen JP, Carter H, Gross A, Ideker T (2013) Network-based stratification of tumor mutations. Nat Methods 10:1108–1115
13. Liu Z, Zhang S (2015) Tumor characterization and stratification by integrated molecular profiles reveals essential pan-cancer features. BMC Genomics 16:503
14. Liu Z, Zhang S (2014) Toward a systematic understanding of cancers: a survey of the pan-cancer study. Front Genet 5:194
15. Ciriello G, Miller ML, Aksoy BA, Senbabaoglu Y, Schultz N, Sander C (2013) Emerging landscape of oncogenic signatures across human cancers. Nat Genet 45:1127–1133

Chapter 12

Statistically Supported Identification of Tumor Subtypes

Guoli Sun and Alexander Krasnitz

Abstract

Identification of biologically and clinically consequential subtypes within tumor types is a long-standing goal of cancer bioinformatics. Here we provide practical guidance to the use of a recently developed statistical subtyping tool, termed Tree Branches Evaluated Statistically for Tightness (TBEST), and its eponymous R language implementation. TBEST employs hierarchical clustering to partition the data at a user-specified level of significance. Functionalities of the package are illustrated using as an example a benchmark data set of mRNA expression levels in leukemia.

Key words Tumor subtypes, Unsupervised learning, Hierarchical clustering, Permutation tests

1 Introduction

Unsupervised learning of biologically and clinically meaningful subsets from high-dimensional data is a widely used methodology in computational biology of cancer. Hierarchical clustering (HC) has been by far the most popular learning tool employed for this purpose, starting with the pioneering work [1] on molecular subtypes of breast cancer. Among the advantages of HC are the simplicity of the algorithm and the ease with which the results can be visualized. Further, unlike other popular unsupervised methods, such as k-means, HC does not require the user to predetermine the number of types into which the data are to be partitioned. Instead, it is common practice to visualize the result of HC as a dendrogram, in combination with the data matrix displayed as a heat map, with the expectation that a meaningful partition of the data will be apparent to the observer. In doing so, one usually seeks to identify "tight" nodes (branches) of the hierarchical tree, i.e., those whose height is substantially less than that of the parent node.

Clearly, this popular approach to data partition using HC lacks mathematical and statistical rigor, and the resulting partitions generally are observer-dependent. In response, we introduced a computational tool termed Tree Branches Examined Statistically for Tightness (TBEST) [2]. Key to the method is a quantity called tightness, defined, for each node of the hierarchical tree, as 1-h/H where h and H, respectively, are the heights of the node and of its parent. Tightness of a node is then viewed as a statistic, and a permutation-based statistical test is conducted to assign statistical significance to the observed value. The principles underlying TBEST are explained in detail in our publication [2], where we also test the performance of the tool on a number of benchmark data sets originating from biology [3–7]. We find that TBEST outperforms other published subtype identification methods [8–10]. Here we focus on our implementation of TBEST as an eponymous R language package, available as open-source software from the Comprehensive R Archive Network (CRAN) [11], and provide a walk-through tutorial for this package using an example. Thus, in the language familiar to R users, this chapter may be termed a "vignette" for the TBEST package.

2 Methods

2.1 Overview of Features

The package TBEST contains functions to perform the following key operations:

1. Computation and statistical assessment of tightness for all nodes in a hierarchical tree (SigTree).

2. Data partition corresponding to tight branches of a tree (PartitionTree).

3. Graphical annotation of a dendrogram to indicate, for each node, its tightness and the associated statistical significance (plot.best).

The most likely use of TBEST would involve performing these operations, in the order as listed. The first of these is the crucial step in the analysis, and we now review the input parameters necessary to specify this step. These parameters fall into several distinct categories:

1. Input data: a matrix M with rows representing objects to be clustered, e.g., RNA expression profiles of individual tumors. The data may be floating point, numerical, or logical, as long as dissimilarity function can be defined for any pair of rows.

2. Specification of HC algorithm, consisting of two items:

    (a) A method to compute pairwise dissimilarities among the objects to be clustered. TBEST allows a broad choice of such methods. In addition to all the dissimilarity options defined in the core R function hclust(), TBEST admits correlation-based dissimilarities, defined, for any two rows X, Y of M, as $1 - Cor(X,Y)$, where Cor may be

Pearson, Spearman, or Kendall correlation. Finally, a user-defined dissimilarity function may be specified. The latter must result in an R object of class dist for any two rows X, Y of M.

(b) The linkage method for HC must be chosen as one of linkage options allowed by hclust(), e.g., "complete" or "average".

3. Specification of the null distribution for tightness. The underlying idea of TBEST is that the null distribution of tightness is obtained by computing tightness for nodes of the trees grown from all permutations of the data within a given class of permutations. Thus, the null distribution of tightness is defined by the class of permutations allowed for the data. TBEST currently implements one such class, wherein the data matrix M is partitioned into blocks of columns, with arbitrary row permutations allowed, independently in each block. The blocks are specified by a vector of factors, whose length is equal to the column dimension of M. By default, each column of M constitutes a block. In addition, a user-defined permutation method may be provided, with data matrices of equal dimensions as input and output.

4. An approximate method for estimating significance for each observed value of tightness must be specified. Here TBEST offers two options:

(a) A purely empirical estimate for the *P*-value, using a sample from the null distribution and applying Laplace's rule of succession: $P = (N_> + 1)/(N + 2)$, where $N_>$ is the number of times the sampled tightness exceeds the observed one and N is the sample size. While simple, this option may become prohibitively expensive computationally if the number of objects being clustered (the row dimension of M) is large, in order to overcome the multiplicity of hypotheses being tested. Indeed, tightness must be computed for any internal node of the HC tree, with the exception of the root node. The number of the null hypotheses being tested is therefore two less than the row dimension of M. *P*-values corresponding to statistically significant observations must therefore be much smaller than the reciprocal of this number, and therefore N must be much larger than this number itself.

(b) According to the extreme value theory, the null distribution of the values of tightness above a threshold is approximately of the generalized Pareto (GP) type if the threshold is sufficiently high. With this property in mind, TBEST offers an option to estimate the *P*-value by fitting the GP distribution to the empirical null sample of the excesses of tightness above threshold. This option potentially requires much smaller sample sizes than the purely empirical alternative. However, additional parameters must be specified. The first of these is the threshold to be exceeded. This threshold must be high enough for GP approximation to be valid but not too high so as to permit the number of excesses sufficient for a good fit. The second additional parameter is the fitting method, which must be one of the maximum likelihood (ML) or moments-based.

In addition to these input parameters, the current implementation of TBEST also allows the user to choose among several alternative measures of tightness, differing in terms of their dependence on the height of the parent node and that of one or both descendants. In this protocol, we will focus on the original definition above, which, in our experience, is sufficient for most purposes. This is achieved by setting the mystat parameter in the function SigTree and/or statname parameter to in the function ParitionTree to "fldc".

2.2 An Example of Subtype Discovery Using TBEST

We next use the Leukemia data set, included with the package, to illustrate the use of TBEST. The data form a matrix of 38 rows and 500 columns, wherein each row corresponds to a case of acute leukemia, belonging to one of the three subtypes: AML (myeloid), T-ALL (T-lymphocytic), or B-ALL (B-lymphocytic). Each column of the matrix corresponds to a gene, and the values represent normalized expression levels on a logarithmic scale. More details can be found at the package website [11]. Following the installation of TBEST and linking the corresponding library to an R session, the Leukemia data are loaded, and the SigTree function is executed (Fig. 1). In this example, hierarchical trees are grown using Euclidean distances among rows of the data matrix, either observed (leukemia) or randomized, and Ward linkage is adopted for agglomeration. Null distribution of tightness is generated from multiple randomizations of the input matrix by independent shuffles in each column. This choice of randomization is appropriate for gene expression data, where its effect is to diminish correlations among expression levels of genes. In order to reduce the execution time, a multicore parallelization option is chosen by setting the distrib parameter to Rparallel. As a result, functions from the core R package parallel will be invoked to set up a 10-core cluster on the host computer. Each core will perform an approximately equal share of randomizations. Finally, by setting Ptail parameter to TRUE (default), the generalized Pareto distribution is used to approximate the tail of the null distributions of tightness.

The output variable mytree is an object of class "best", essentially an R list comprised of three items. The first two of these are a

```
> data(leukemia)
> mytree<-SigTree(myinput=data.matrix(leukemia),mystat="fldc",
+ mymethod="ward.D2",mymetric="euclidean",rand.fun="shuffle.column",
+ distrib="Rparallel",njobs=10,Ptail=TRUE)
> class(mytree)
[1] "best"
> names(mytree)
[1] "Call"         "data"          "indextable"
```

Fig. 1 Illustration of use for function SigTree (lines 2–4), as applied to the Leukemia data set (line 1), distributed with the package. The data class and the item list of the output object are queried in the last two lines of code

```
> mypartition<-PartitionTree(x=mytree,siglevel=0.001,statname="fldc",
+ sigtype="raw")
> class(mypartition)
[1] "partition"
> names(mypartition)
[1] "Call"      "best"      "sigvalue"  "partition"
> mypartition$partition[1:4,]
                 ID index
1 ALL_19769_B.cell    34
2 ALL_23953_B.cell    34
3 ALL_28373_B.cell    34
4  ALL_9335_B.cell    34
> table(mypartition$partition[,"index"])

31 34 35
 8 20 10
```

Fig. 2 Illustration of use for function PartitionTree. An object of class "partition" is created by invoking the function (lines 1 and 2), with the tree object created by a prior call to function SigTree (Fig. 1). Next, the class and the item content of the output object are queried. In particular, the "partition" item is a data frame listing, for each leaf of the tree (left column) the part it belongs to. The sizes of parts in the partition can be queried by a call to the R core table function

character string containing the SigTree function call and the input data matrix. The key results are all tabulated in the third item, a matrix called indextable, with each row corresponding to a node of a hierarchical tree grown by SigTree. This matrix is formed by first binding the merge and height items of the standard R hclust object, with an additional column indicating, for each node, its leaf count. The final two columns tabulate, for each node, its tightness and the corresponding P-value, in this case estimated using extreme value theory.

Next, we use the function PartitonTree to explore whether the 38 cases in the Leukemia set fall into distinct subtypes. The function finds the most detailed partition of a hierarchical tree into tight branches, given a level of significance for tightness. The first argument x (Fig. 2) is an object of class "best", produced by a call to SigTree. The other notable arguments are siglevel, i.e., the significance level for tightness above which a node is considered tight, and sigtype to indicate how the significance level set by siglevel should be interpreted. Here the "raw" value of sigtype means that the siglevel value is to be used directly as a threshold on the P-values computed by SigTree. Other interpretable values of sigtype offer the user two different ways to account for the multiplicity of hypotheses which, in this case, is equal to the number of nodes in the tree. These are "corrected", meaning that the value of sigtype is a threshold on the Bonferroni-corrected P-values, and "fdr", to use this value as a threshold on false discovery rates.

The output of PartitonTree is an object of class "partition", in essence, an R list with four items. Of these, the first two echo the function call and the input object of the class "best". Next, sigvalue is a table of significance levels for each node of the tree, adjusted as determined by the sigtype argument. Finally, partition, an item of most interest for subtype analysis, tabulates, for each leaf of the tree, its subtype identity, as the number of the node which corresponds to the subtype. In the example above, the resulting partition is into three subtypes, with node numbers 31, 34, and 35, corresponding, respectively, to the T-ALL, B-ALL, and AML subtypes of acute leukemia. In deriving a partition, TBEST recursively examines the nodes of the tree, starting from the root node, as to whether at least one of the two descendant nodes is tight. If so, the node is considered split, and the same rule is applied to each of the two descendant nodes. The process terminates when no further splits are possible, i.e., when the most detailed partition has been found.

Next, we discuss how output of TBEST analysis can be visualized using the plot.best function. plot.best is a plot method for class "best", made by overloading the plot method for class "hclust". There are two principal ways to use plot.best, illustrated in the second and third lines in Fig. 3. The first of these serves to generate a dendrogram with TBEST-specific annotation, as shown in Fig. 4, and, therefore, it can be invoked as the plot function with the x argument of this class. A call to plot.best generates a dendrogram, annotated with significance estimates for tight branches and/or for branches that form a most detailed partition.

A dendrogram resulting from a call to plot.best in the second line in Fig. 3 is shown in Fig. 4. All nodes of the tree are enumerated in green, in the order of increasing height. In addition, the rounded permutation P-value for tightness is displayed in red for all nodes for which it is below the chosen threshold of 0.001. The user may choose other colors to annotate the dendrogram by specifying the col.best argument. Alternatively, if the tree partition into tight nodes is available to form a call to PartitionTree, the resulting object of the class "partition" may be supplied as an argument to plot.best. In this case the call, as shown in the third line of Fig. 3, will generate a dendrogram with the P-values displayed in red for the nodes forming the partition.

```
> ?plot.best
> plot(x=mytree,mystat="fldc",siglevel=0.001,sigtype="raw",hang=-1)
> plot(x=mytree,mystat="fldc",partition=mypartition,hang=-1)
```

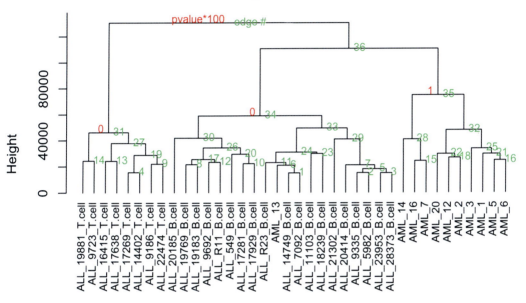

Fig. 3 Illustration of plot methods for objects "best" (line 2) and "partition" (line 3). The graphical output for the latter case is shown in the lower portion of the figure. All nodes of the tree are labeled in green, and all leaves are labeled below the dendrogram

```
> ?LeafContent
> LeafContent(myinput=mytree,mynode=c(1,28))
$`branch 1`
[1] "ALL_14749_B.cell" "ALL_7092_B.cell"

$`branch 28`
[1] "AML_14" "AML_16" "AML_7"
```

Fig. 4 Illustration of use for the utility function LeafContent

Finally, tree objects belonging to one of the classes "hclust", "best", or "partition" may be interrogated as to the leaf content of the nodes. This is accomplished by the utility function LeafContent, as illustrated in Fig. 4. This function is particularly useful in situations where the number of observations is large, making their labels hard to display clearly in the dendrogram. In the function call shown in Fig. 4, myinput is the tree object to be interrogated, and mynode is an integer vector of the numbers of nodes whose leaf content is desired.

In the example shown, labels of observations under branch 1 and 28 are listed. The branch number is always positive, between 1 and 28. A single-leaf node, however, is represented by a negative number, specifically, minus the row number of the observation corresponding to the leaf, represented in R. If we used "mynode = c(−1, −28)" in the example above, the output would be a character vector of length 2 containing the labels of the 1st and the 28th individual observations.

References

1. Sorlie T, Tibshirani R, Parker J, Hastie T, Marron JS, Nobel A, Deng S, Johnsen H, Pesich R, Geisler S, Demeter J, Perou CM, Lonning PE, Brown PO, Borresen-Dale AL, Botstein D (2003) Repeated observation of breast tumor subtypes in independent gene expression data sets. Proc Natl Acad Sci U S A 100 (14):8418–8423. https://doi.org/10.1073/pnas.0932692100

2. Sun G, Krasnitz A (2014) Significant distinct branches of hierarchical trees: a framework for statistical analysis and applications to biological data. BMC Genomics 15:1000. https://doi.org/10.1186/1471-2164-15-1000

3. Diaz-Romero J, Romeo S, Bovee JV, Hogendoorn PC, Heini PF, Mainil-Varlet P (2010) Hierarchical clustering of flow cytometry data for the study of conventional central chondrosarcoma. J Cell Physiol 225(2):601–611. https://doi.org/10.1002/jcp.22245

4. Golub TR, Slonim DK, Tamayo P, Huard C, Gaasenbeek M, Mesirov JP, Coller H, Loh ML, Downing JR, Caligiuri MA, Bloomfield CD, Lander ES (1999) Molecular classification of cancer: class discovery and class prediction by gene expression monitoring. Science 286 (5439):531–537

5. Kislinger T, Cox B, Kannan A, Chung C, Hu P, Ignatchenko A, Scott MS, Gramolini AO, Morris Q, Hallett MT, Rossant J, Hughes TR, Frey B, Emili A (2006) Global survey of organ and organelle protein expression in mouse: combined proteomic and transcriptomic profiling. Cell 125(1):173–186. https://doi.org/10.1016/j.cell.2006.01.044

6. Monti S, Tamayo P, Mesirov J, Golub T (2003) Consensus clustering: A resampling-based method for class discovery and visualization of gene expression microarray data. Mach Learn 52(1–2):91–118. https://doi.org/10.1023/A:1023949509487

7. Navin N, Kendall J, Troge J, Andrews P, Rodgers L, McIndoo J, Cook K, Stepansky A, Levy D, Esposito D, Muthuswamy L, Krasnitz A, McCombie WR, Hicks J, Wigler M (2011) Tumour evolution inferred by single-cell sequencing. Nature 472 (7341):90–94. https://doi.org/10.1038/nature09807

8. Munneke B, Schlauch KA, Simonsen KL, Beavis WD, Doerge RW (2005) Adding confidence to gene expression clustering. Genetics 170(4):2003–2011. https://doi.org/10.1534/Genetics.104.031500

9. Liu Y, Hayes DN, Nobel A, Marron JS (2008) Statistical significance of clustering for high-dimension, low-sample size data. J Am Stat Assoc 103(483):1281–1293. https://doi.org/10.1198/016214508000000454

10. Langfelder P, Zhang B, Horvath S (2008) Defining clusters from a hierarchical cluster tree: the Dynamic Tree Cut package for R. Bioinformatics 24(5):719–720. https://doi.org/10.1093/Bioinformatics/Btm563

11. Sun G, Krasnitz A (2013) TBEST: Tree branches evaluated statistically for tightness. The Comprehensive R Archive Network. http://cran.r-project.org/web/packages/TBEST/index.html

Chapter 13

Computational Methods for Analysis of Tumor Clonality and Evolutionary History

Gerald Goh, Nicholas McGranahan, and Gareth A. Wilson

Abstract

Cancer is an evolutionary process. Recent advances in sequencing technologies have allowed us to investigate intratumor heterogeneity at the single nucleotide level. Here, we describe computational methods that use sequencing data to identify genetically distinct tumor subclones and reconstruct tumor evolutionary histories.

Key words Cancer, Next-generation sequencing, Heterogeneity, Clonal, Evolution, Phylogeny

1 Introduction

In 1976, Peter Nowell proposed a clonal evolution model of cancer and described cancer as an evolutionary process driven by somatic cell mutations that were subject to selection pressures [1]. With the advent of next-generation sequencing, the extent of intratumor heterogeneity (ITH) has begun to be resolved at the single cell and single nucleotide level. Increasing evidence suggests that this genetic heterogeneity exists both in space and time and has implications for predictive biomarker strategies and may provide clues to attractive therapeutic targets [2–4]. Branched tumor evolution can give rise to multiple genetically distinct subclones, and sampling these different cell populations allows phylogenetic analysis that can help with reconstructing tumor evolutionary histories.

Here, we summarize methodologies that we have been using for investigating ITH and clonal evolution in cancer, with a focus on multi-region biopsy sequencing data and specific examples as applied in a recent study of esophageal cancer [5]. Starting with a set of variant calls, we use the information from whole-exome sequencing in order to identify tumor subclones, construct phylogenetic trees, and infer mutational timing and processes underlying tumorigenesis and tumor evolution.

2 Materials

2.1 Data Files

1. A list of somatic single nucleotide variant calls, from variant callers such as VarScan2 or MuTect [6, 7]. This should include variant allele frequencies and read depth information.
2. A list of somatic copy number alterations (sCNA) and an estimate of tumor purity, from callers such as Sequenza [8].

2.2 Software

1. MEDICC—software for phylogenetic reconstruction based on sCNA data, obtained at https://bitbucket.org/rfs/medicc [9].
2. phangorn—R package for phylogenetic analysis, obtained at https://cran.r-project.org/web/packages/phangorn/index.html [10].
3. deconstructSigs—R package for deconvolution of mutational signatures, obtained at https://cran.rstudio.com/web/packages/deconstructSigs/index.html [11].

3 Methods

3.1 Cancer Cell Fraction Estimation

The cancer cell fraction (CCF) of a variant represents the proportion of cancer cells within a sample carrying that variant. Therefore a clonal variant would be predicted to have a cancer cell fraction of 1 because 100% of the cancer cells contain this mutation. In contrast, subclonal variants will theoretically have a cancer cell fraction of less than 1.

3.1.1 Method for Estimating Cancer Cell Fraction

1. Extract the variant allele frequencies (VAF), the integer copy number, and tumor purity estimates for the given sample.
2. The CCF can be calculated using Eq. 1 below:

$$\text{Expected VAF (CCF)} = p \times \text{CCF}/\text{CPNnorm}\,(1-p) + p \times \text{CPNmut} \tag{1}$$

where p represents the tumor purity as estimated by Sequenza and CPNmut and CPNnorm are the local copy number of the tumor and the matched normal sample, respectively, again determined by Sequenza.

3. Given that the calculated value of CCF is unlikely to be exactly 1, there is a possibility of overestimating the subclonal fraction of mutations. One method for correcting for this bias is to calculate 95% confidence intervals around the CCF value. If the upper interval is greater than or equal to 1, the variant can be classed as clonal. Such correction is particularly relevant in samples with lower read depth. Confidence intervals can be determined by using a binomial distribution:

$$P(CCF) = \text{binom}(a|N, \text{VAF(CCF)}) \quad (2)$$

in which "a" represents the number of reads supporting the mutant allele and "N" the total number of reads for a given variant call. CCF values can then be determined and normalized for the range of CCF values (0.01–1).

3.1.2 Example for Cancer Cell Fraction Estimation

Variant A has a read depth (N) of 538 and variant read count (a) of 73, giving a VAF of 0.1356 (73/538). The local copy number of the tumor has been estimated as 1, while the matched normal copy number is 2. Sequenza has estimated the cellularity or purity as being 0.1788, meaning that only 17.88% of the cells within the sample were actual tumor cells. With this information and using Eq. 1, we can now generate a binomial distribution to estimate the probability of having a given cancer cell fraction, with the possible CCF values ranging from 0.01 to 1. For example, with a proposed CCF value of 0.98, the probability entered in the binomial distribution is:

$$(0.98 \times 0.1788)/((2 \times (1 - 0.1788)) + (0.1788 \times 1)) = 0.0962$$

giving:

$$P(CCF) = \text{binom}(73|538, \ 0.0962) = 0.00066$$

By repeating this process, for all values from 0.01 to 1, we obtain a list of 100 potential CCF values (x); from this we can generate a normalized set by simply dividing all values in x by the total sum of x (x/sum(x)), leading to a posterior distribution from which we can select the most likely CCF value and the 95% confidence intervals. In this example, our method leads to a clonal CCF of 1, with a lower 95% confidence interval of 0.9.

3.2 Identification of Tumor Subclones

Once the CCF has been calculated for all somatic mutation calls, it is possible to try to infer the clonal population structure of the tumor. There are a number of tools and methods available for this (*see* **Note 1**). We'll describe one such method as used in Murugaesu et al. [5] for analyzing multi-region exome data from esophageal tumor samples and then provide other options.

3.2.1 Method for Identifying Tumor Subclones

1. Using the CCF values calculated previously, generate a binary matrix in which each column represents a tumor region and each row a somatic variant. The contents of each element should indicate the presence (CCF $\geq$ 10%) or absence (<10%) of that variant in the specific tumor region.

2. Clusters can be easily defined by grouping on the binary profile generated. For example, if a tumor had six regions and mutation A was found in regions 1, 2, 5, and 6, the profile would be 110011. All mutations matching this profile would be clustered together.

3. Clusters containing fewer than five SNVs are removed.

4. By plotting the CCF of variants in one region against another and coloring by cluster, it is possible to visualize cases in which there is an illusion of clonality. This occurs when a mutation appears to be clonally dominant within one region but is not detectable or is subclonal within another (Fig. 1).

3.2.2 Tools for Identification of Tumor Subclones

In addition to the method described above, a number of software tools are available for subclonal classification. PyClone [12] uses a Bayesian Dirichlet clustering process on deeply sequenced ($>1000\times$) mutations to define the subclonal composition of a tumor. Another method, SciClone [13], takes a different approach, while still using a Bayesian clustering method, by focusing only on those variants in regions of the genome not impacted upon by copy number aberrations or loss of heterozygosity (LOH) events. Both SciClone and PyClone can be used on single-region and multi-region tumor datasets.

3.3 Phylogenetic Tree Construction Using Somatic Variants

As with the analyses described above, there are many different methods that could be used to build a phylogenetic tree from the somatic variant calls. We will focus on the method employed in Murugaesu et al. [5]. This method utilizes multi-region exome samples and treats each region as if it were a distinct entity in comparison with the others. This is clearly an oversimplification that does not take account of clonal/subclonal relationships and cellular intermingling between the regions. However, it does provide a good indication of the early and late events in tumor development.

3.3.1 Method for Phylogenetic Tree Construction

1. Obtain list of variants, filtered according to relevant quality criteria. For tree construction, while ensuring only high confidence variants are used for input, the genomic location of the variant is not important. The variant list should therefore include all high-quality mutation calls from exonic, intronic, and intergenic regions.

2. As when clustering the variants, a binary matrix should be constructed indicating the presence or absence of each variant in each tumor region by using a preset VAF or CCF threshold (e.g., CCF $\geq 10\%$ for presence or $<10\%$ indicating absence).

3. With the matrix constructed, a variety of tree generation methods can be used, a number of which can be accessed through the R software package "phangorn." The first stage is to generate a basic tree, for example, using the Unweighted Pair Group Method with Arithmetic Mean (UPGMA) method. The dist() function can be used to generate a distance matrix from the previously created binary matrix. This then serves as

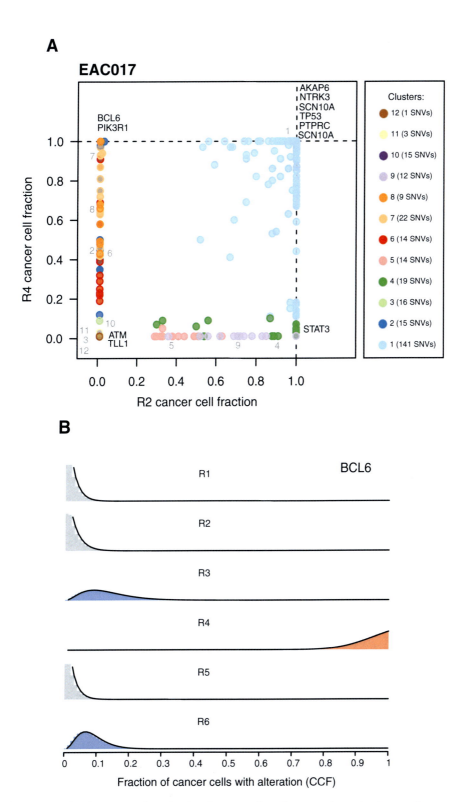

Fig. 1 Cancer cell fraction comparison for two tumor regions from esophageal adenocarcinoma sample EAC017 [5]. (**a**) Each SNV is plotted according to the cancer cell fraction within each tumor region and colored according to the cluster it is in. (**b**) Probability distributions over the cancer cell fraction for a mutation identified in *BCL6*. This mutation provides an example of the illusion of clonality as it is found to be clonal in a single region (R4) but absent in the majority of cells in the other tumor regions

the input into the upgma() function, additionally specifying "method=binary."

4. The UPGMA tree created above can be used as the finished tree; however other methods can also be applied to attempt to increase the accuracy of the tree. For these methods, data is required in "phyDat" format. This conversion can be accomplished using the phyDat() function with the binary matrix as input and setting the levels as being 0 or 1. The optim.parsimony() function can be used to try to identify the most parsimonious tree and then further refined using the parsimony ratchet method, pratchet().

5. The trees can be further annotated using the acctran function to estimate branch lengths. Bootstrapping can also be applied to indicate the degree of support for the final tree.

6. Finally the type of tree visualization can be defined, for example, phylogram or unrooted, using plot.phylo().

3.3.2 SNV Heterogeneity Driven by Copy Number Alterations

Occasionally apparent inconsistencies in the phylogenetic tree can be explained by a single copy number change rather than multiple single nucleotide variants. Variants impacted in this manner should be identified and removed from the phylogenetic analysis. The method is described below:

1. Identify genomic segments that display heterogeneous copy number values across the tumor regions, and extract the variants located in such regions.

2. Variants are further categorized according to the mutation cluster, as designated in Subheading 3.2.1.

3. Using a one-sided Wilcoxon test (when there are two potential copy number states in the tumor regions) or a one-sided Cochran-Armitage trend test (more than two copy number states), try to establish whether copy number loss is significantly associated with lower CCF values. Variants within clusters, for whom the test is significant, should be removed from the phylogenetic analysis.

4. Finally a regression analysis, using copy number and tumor region as the predictors or independent variables, can be performed to ensure that it is copy number driving the difference in CCF value.

3.4 Phylogenetic Tree Construction Using CNV Data

Aside from using somatic variant calls to build phylogenetic trees, copy number variant data can be used as well. This is especially helpful in cancers, such as high-grade serous ovarian cancer, that are driven largely by genomic aberrations and rearrangements rather than point mutations. One method that uses integer copy number profiles to generate phylogenetic inferences is MEDICC

(Minimum Event Distance for Intra-tumor Copy-number Comparisons) [9], which we will discuss in detail here (*see* **Note 2**).

1. To run MEDICC, the only arguments required are the description file and an output directory. This description file has three columns: chromosome name, major allele file, and minor allele file.

2. To create the major and minor allele files, you need the output from a copy number caller such as Sequenza, namely, the major and minor copy number states.

3. For each chromosome in each tumor region, determine the number of copy number states present. Compare across all the tumor regions in the sample, and generate a list of integer copy number states of the same length for each tumor region. Create these lists for both major and minor alleles in separate text files in the fasta file format, i.e., samples are denoted with the symbol ">," and a string of copy number states follow in the next line. Example files are available in the MEDICC installation folder.

4. After running MEDICC on the command line, the output files can be explored using the R library package MEDICCquant. Follow-up analyses include tests for molecular clock, phylogenetic structure, and quantification of clonal heterogeneity.

3.5 Temporal Dissection of Mutations

Mutational timing can help distinguish between driver and passenger mutations. Depending on the study design, whether single biopsies, multi-region biopsies, or temporally distinct biopsies such as primary-metastatic pairs, defining mutations as early or late events can also aid in the understanding of tumor evolution and disease progression.

3.5.1 Timing Mutations Using Phylogenetic Trees

If phylogenetic trees have been constructed as described in Subheading 3.3, classifying mutations as "early" or "late" is simply defined by where the mutation is located on the phylogenetic tree. All truncal mutations should be classified as "early" and all branch mutations classified as "late."

3.5.2 Timing Mutations in Single Samples

If only single samples are available and phylogenetic trees are not constructed, mutations can be classified as "early" or "late" based on their clonal status, utilizing cancer cell fraction (as estimated in Subheading 3.1) and the mutation copy number as determined by Sequenza (or any CNV caller of choice). Where possible, point mutations can also be timed relative to copy number events.

1. In regions with at least two copies of the major allele, mutations at mutation copy number >1 are classified as "before event," and mutations with a mutation copy number of 1 are classified as "after event."

224   Gerald Goh et al.

2. Combining this with our cancer cell fraction estimates and whether the mutation is clonal or subclonal (refer to Subheading 3.2), all clonal mutations that are not classified as "after event" can be aggregated as "early," and all subclonal or "after event" mutations can be aggregated as "late."

3.5.3 Exploring Temporal Dynamics of Mutational Processes

Classifying mutations temporally as "early" or "late" allows us to explore the mutational processes that vary during tumor evolution [14]. One way of doing this is to utilize previously identified mutational signatures and determine the contribution of each signature that gives rise to the spectrum of somatic mutations in each sample [15], utilizing the R package *deconstructSigs*.

1. Obtain list of somatic mutations for mutational signature analysis, consisting of genomic coordinates and reference and variant alleles. This analysis can be implemented separately on early and late mutations, as well as on all mutations.

2. Using the *mut.to.sigs.input* function in the R package *deconstructSigs*, generate a data frame of how frequently a mutation in each trinucleotide context is observed in your dataset.

3. Calculate the contribution of each signature to each cancer sample using the *whichSignatures* function in *deconstructSigs* (*see* **Note 3**).

4. The *makePie* function can be used to visualize the percentage contribution of each mutational process in every cancer sample (*see* **Note 4**). Alternatively, a barplot chart is useful for comparing the prevalence of mutational signatures across multiple samples. An example is shown in Fig. 2, where mutational signatures have been identified in a cohort of skin cutaneous

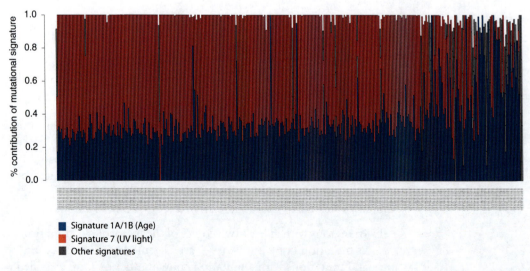

Fig. 2 Mutational signatures identified in skin cutaneous melanoma. Majority of the somatic mutations identified can be attributed to either signature 1 or 7, related to age and UV light, respectively

melanoma based upon data generated by the TCGA Research Network: http://cancergenome.nih.gov/.

5. To compare the prevalence of mutational signatures in early and late mutations, a paired Wilcoxon test can be used, comparing the proportion of early and late mutations that correspond to a given signature for each tumor (*see* **Note 5**).

4 Notes

1. Methods that attempt to utilize the output from the subclonal deconvolution, described in Subheading 3.2, to generate "clone trees," potentially providing a more accurate representation at the cellular level, are under active development. Examples include SubcloneSeeker [16], BitPhylogeny [17], PhyloWGS [18], and LICHeE [19].

2. MEDICC has a maximum total copy number of 2K in a diploid genome, where K is the maximum haploid copy number and 2K = 8 by default, which is the upper end of the dynamic range of SNP arrays.

3. When using the *whichSignatures* function, the output is often improved if the mutational signatures being assigned are limited based on prior knowledge of the tumor type.

4. Tumors can be classified as harboring a mutational signature if at least 25% of mutations or over 100 mutations were found to belong to a given signature, as defined in the paper by Alexandrov et al. (2013).

5. When comparing the prevalence of mutational signatures, only samples that harbor at least 30 mutations in total, with 10 early and 10 late mutations, should be included, as performed in McGranahan et al. [14].

References

1. Nowell PC (1976) The clonal evolution of tumor cell populations. Science 194(4260):23–28
2. Burrell RA, Swanton C (2014) The evolution of the unstable cancer genome. Curr Opin Genet Dev 24:61–67. https://doi.org/10.1016/j.gde.2013.11.011
3. Lee AJ, Swanton C (2012) Tumour heterogeneity and drug resistance: personalising cancer medicine through functional genomics. Biochem Pharmacol 83(8):1013–1020. https://doi.org/10.1016/j.bcp.2011.12.008
4. Swanton C (2012) Intratumor heterogeneity: evolution through space and time. Cancer Res 72(19):4875–4882. https://doi.org/10.1158/0008-5472.CAN-12-2217
5. Murugaesu N, Wilson GA, Birkbak NJ, Watkins TB, McGranahan N, Kumar S et al (2015) Tracking the genomic evolution of esophageal adenocarcinoma through neoadjuvant chemotherapy. Cancer Discov 5(8):821–831. https://doi.org/10.1158/2159-8290.CD-15-0412
6. Cibulskis K, Lawrence MS, Carter SL, Sivachenko A, Jaffe D, Sougnez C et al (2013) Sensitive detection of somatic point mutations in impure and heterogeneous cancer samples. Nat Biotechnol 31(3):213–219. https://doi.org/10.1038/nbt.2514

7. Koboldt DC, Zhang Q, Larson DE, Shen D, McLellan MD, Lin L et al (2012) VarScan 2: somatic mutation and copy number alteration discovery in cancer by exome sequencing. Genome Res 22(3):568–576. https://doi.org/10.1101/gr.129684.111

8. Favero F, Joshi T, Marquard AM, Birkbak NJ, Krzystanek M, Li Q et al (2015) Sequenza: allele-specific copy number and mutation profiles from tumor sequencing data. Ann Oncol 26(1):64–70. https://doi.org/10.1093/annonc/mdu479

9. Schwarz RF, Trinh A, Sipos B, Brenton JD, Goldman N, Markowetz F (2014) Phylogenetic quantification of intra-tumour heterogeneity. PLoS Comput Biol 10(4):e1003535. https://doi.org/10.1371/journal.pcbi.1003535

10. Schliep KP (2011) phangorn: phylogenetic analysis in R. Bioinformatics 27(4):592–593. https://doi.org/10.1093/bioinformatics/btq706

11. Rosenthal R, McGranahan N, Herrero J, Taylor BS, Swanton C (2016) deconstructSigs: delineating mutational processes in single tumors distinguishes DNA repair deficiencies and patterns of carcinoma evolution. Genome Biol 17(1):31. https://doi.org/10.1186/s13059-016-0893-4

12. Roth A, Khattra J, Yap D, Wan A, Laks E, Biele J et al (2014) PyClone: statistical inference of clonal population structure in cancer. Nat Methods 11(4):396–398. https://doi.org/10.1038/nmeth.2883

13. Miller CA, White BS, Dees ND, Griffith M, Welch JS, Griffith OL et al (2014) SciClone: inferring clonal architecture and tracking the spatial and temporal patterns of tumor evolution. PLoS Comput Biol 10(8):e1003665. https://doi.org/10.1371/journal.pcbi.1003665

14. McGranahan N, Favero F, de Bruin EC, Birkbak NJ, Szallasi Z, Swanton C (2015) Clonal status of actionable driver events and the timing of mutational processes in cancer evolution. Sci Transl Med 7(283):283ra54. https://doi.org/10.1126/scitranslmed.aaa1408

15. Alexandrov LB, Nik-Zainal S, Wedge DC, Aparicio SA, Behjati S, Biankin AV et al (2013) Signatures of mutational processes in human cancer. Nature 500(7463):415–421. https://doi.org/10.1038/nature12477

16. Qiao Y, Quinlan AR, Jazaeri AA, Verhaak RG, Wheeler DA, Marth GT (2014) SubcloneSeeker: a computational framework for reconstructing tumor clone structure for cancer variant interpretation and prioritization. Genome Biol 15(8):443. https://doi.org/10.1186/s13059-014-0443-x

17. Yuan K, Sakoparnig T, Markowetz F, Beerenwinkel N (2015) BitPhylogeny: a probabilistic framework for reconstructing intra-tumor phylogenies. Genome Biol 16:36. https://doi.org/10.1186/s13059-015-0592-6

18. Deshwar AG, Vembu S, Yung CK, Jang GH, Stein L, Morris Q (2015) PhyloWGS: reconstructing subclonal composition and evolution from whole-genome sequencing of tumors. Genome Biol 16:35. https://doi.org/10.1186/s13059-015-0602-8

19. Popic V, Salari R, Hajirasouliha I, Kashef-Haghighi D, West RB, Batzoglou S (2015) Fast and scalable inference of multi-sample cancer lineages. Genome Biol 16:91. https://doi.org/10.1186/s13059-015-0647-8

Chapter 14

Predictive Modeling of Anti-Cancer Drug Sensitivity from Genetic Characterizations

Raziur Rahman and Ranadip Pal

Abstract

Accurately predicting sensitivity of tumor cells to anti-cancer drugs based on genetic characterizations is a significant challenge for personalized cancer therapy. This chapter provides a computational procedure to design predictive models from individual genomic characterizations and combine them to arrive at an integrated predictive model. Integrated modeling employs the complementary information from heterogeneous genetic characterizations to improve the prediction error as well as lowering the error confidence interval.

Key words Integrated genomic modeling, Random Forests, Drug sensitivity prediction

1 Introduction

An important goal of systems medicine is to generate genomics informed personalized therapeutic regimes with higher efficacy. The ability of inferred models to accurately predict sensitivity of an individual tumor to a drug can assist in designing personalized cancer therapy treatments with expected effectiveness significantly higher than current standard of care approaches. Sensitivity prediction models are primarily designed by supervised training of drug responses based on genetic characterizations. The availability of multiple heterogeneous forms of genetic characterizations such as RNA expression, Protein Expression, Methylation, Single Nucleotide Polymorphisms (SNPs), etc. is expected to lower the mean prediction error as well as increase the robustness of prediction by reducing uncertainty.

Here we summarize methodology that we use to design drug sensitivity prediction models from heterogeneous genetic characterizations based on ensemble models. The methodology was a top performer in the NCI-DREAM drug sensitivity prediction challenge [1, 2].

2 Methods

A variety of techniques have been proposed for drug sensitivity prediction based on genetic characterizations. A common approach is to consider a training set of cell lines with experimentally measured genomic characterizations (RNA expression, Protein Expression, Methylation, SNPs, etc.) and response to different drugs, and design supervised predictive models for each individual drug based on one or more genomic characterizations. For instance, statistical tests have been used to show that genetic mutations can be predictive of the drug sensitivity in non-small cell lung cancers [3]. In [4], gene expression profiles have been used to predict the binarized efficacy of a drug over a cell line with an accuracy ranging from 64 to 92%. In [5], a co-expression extrapolation (COXEN) approach was used to predict the drug sensitivity for samples outside the training set with an accuracy of around 82 and 75% in predicting the binarized sensitivity of bladder and breast cancer cell lines, respectively. Tumor sensitivity prediction has also been considered as (a) a drug-induced topology alteration [6] using phosphor-proteomic signals and prior biological knowledge of generic pathway and (b) a molecular tumor profile based prediction [3, 7]. Drug sensitivity prediction using an elastic net regression analysis [8] over more than 100,000 genomic features (RNA expression, Mutational status of specific genes and SNPs) was considered in [9]. The correlation coefficients between the predicted and actual sensitivity over 450 cell lines using 10 fold cross validation ranged from 0.08 to 0.76 for different targeted drugs. Riddick et al. [10] used a Random Forest (RF) based approach to tumor prediction in the NCI 60 cell lines with performance exceeding multiple existing approaches. For the recently concluded NCI-DREAM Drug sensitivity prediction challenge [1], which was a crowd-sourced initiative to evaluate different predictive modeling approaches, designed from genomic characterizations (Gene Expression, Methylation, RNASeq, SNP6, Exome Sequencing, and RPPA), our methodology based on individual Random Forest models for each genomic characterization and integrating the prediction based on a linear regression model was a top performer [1, 2]. We present this methodology in detail in this chapter with emphasis on individual steps in the pipeline and the effect of various model parameters on the performance in different scenarios.

The steps involved in generating the integrated model are as follows:

1. **Data Preprocessing**: Process the data such that for a tumor culture, a numerical vector can represent each type of genomic characterization.

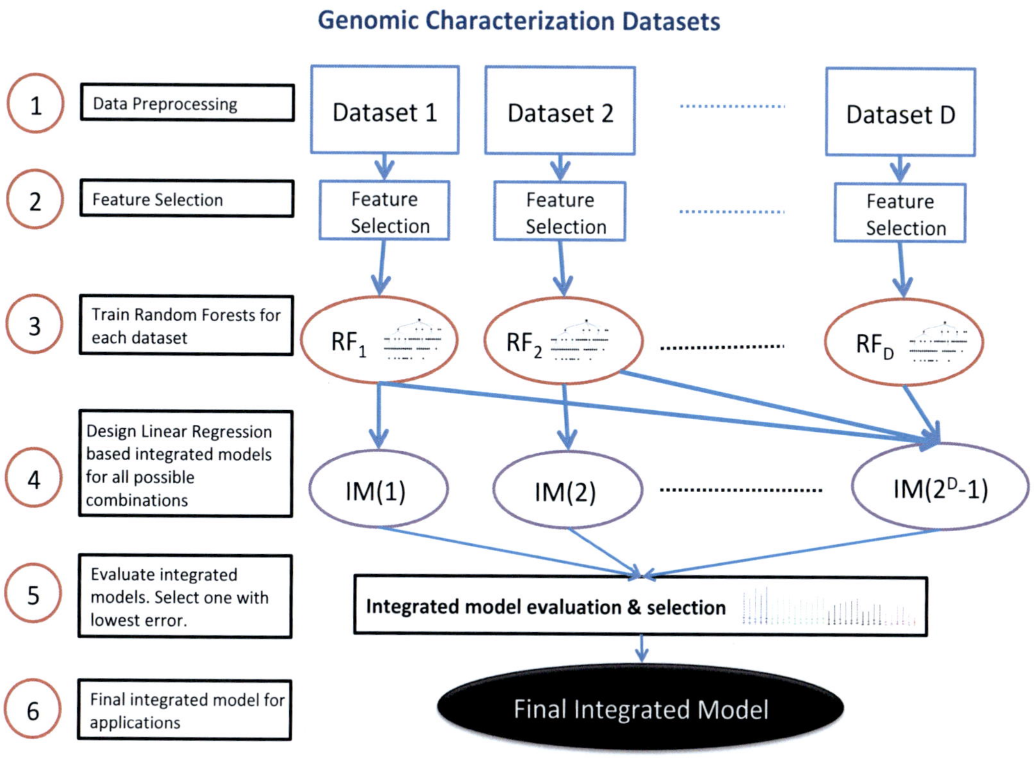

Genomic Characterization Datasets

Fig. 1 Flowchart for Integrated Model Generation

2. **Feature Selection**: Use feature selection to reduce the starting number of features for model generation.
3. **Train Random Forest**: Train ensemble of regression trees for each genetic characterization.
4. **Generate Regression Models**: Design Linear Regression based integrated models for all possible combinations.
5. **Evaluate Integrated Models**: Select the model with lowest error.
6. **Final Integrated Model**: Use the final integrated model for applications and further validation.

The flowchart for the steps to generate the integrated model is shown in Fig. 1.

2.1 Data Preprocessing

Genetic characterization data can be derived from diverse levels of the cell such as the genome, transcriptome, proteome, or metabolome. The different levels can provide diverse set of information such as mutations in the genome or altered transcriptional behavior that can assist in predicting the sensitivity of the tumor to a drug. A brief description of the various levels along with commonly used data quantification approaches for sensitivity prediction is provided next:

(a) **DNA Level**: At the DNA level, Single Nucleotide Polymorphism (SNPs) and Copy Number Variations (CNVs) are generally measured using Genome Wide arrays such as the *Affymetrix Genome-Wide Human SNP Array 6.0* and further analyzed using software platforms such as http://aroma-project.org [11]. Following normalization, the copy number variations as compared to normal cell lines are calculated for each segment (in the form of start of segment in base pair, end of segment in base pair, mean copy number of the segment). For our purposes, it is preferable to have the genomic information as a numerical feature vector for each cell line and characterization type. Since the start and stop segments can vary between different cell lines, it is advisable to convert the CNV information of start and stop parts of a segments to gene level variations which makes it seamless to map different cell lines. One potential program to achieve the conversion is using **R** Package *CNTools*. Another common approach for measuring variations in DNA level is through Exome Sequencing (such as using *Agilent SureSelect*) that measures the variations in the coding regions of the genome. Similar to whole genome sequencing SNPs, the mismatch at different parts of the genes observed through exome sequencing has to be converted to a common set of features for all tumor cell lines.

(b) **Epigenetic Level**: At the epigenetic level, DNA methylation is process of methyl groups attaching to DNA that can alter the transcription process. It is usually measured using arrays such as *Illumina Human Methylation Bead Array* where the proportion of methylated groups is generated based on the intensities of methylated and unmethylated probes.

(c) **Transcriptomic Level**: At the transcriptomic level, RNA expression is frequently measured using DNA microarrays or recently developed technique of RNA-seq. Microarrays are able to provide the average expression of each RNA for a cell line using the individual processing software of the platform such as *Affymetrix Human Transcriptome Arrays*. The conversion of RNA-seq raw data calculated from whole transcriptome shotgun sequencing can be conducted using available software such as *Alexa-seq* and numerous others [12–14].

(d) **Proteome Level**: Measurement of protein expressions for drug sensitivity studies normally employ Reverse protein lysate array (RPPA) as in NCI-DREAM drug sensitivity prediction challenge dataset [1] or *Liquid Chromatograph Mass Spectrometry* (LC-MS) [15]. RPPA data can provide measurements for native proteins as well as phosphorylated isoforms. For our

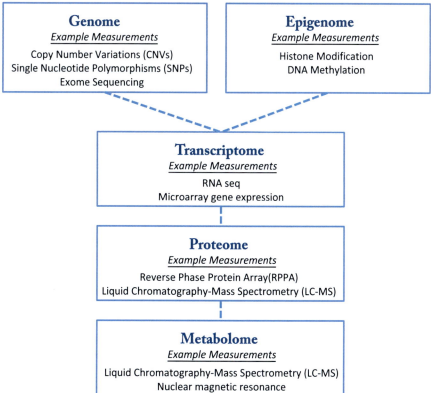

Fig. 2 Flowchart for genetic characterizations

subsequent analysis, we consider that the same set of protein features are maintained for all cell lines.

(e) **Metabolome Level**: Metabolites in a cell before or after drug application can be measured using techniques such as *Liquid Chromatography Mass Spectrometry* (LCMS) [16]. Since metabolism of cancerous cells is different from normal cells, the metabolic profiles of cancerous cells can provide unique insights on the potential sensitivity of drugs.

Examples of quantification techniques at various genetic levels are represented as a flowchart in Fig. 2.

Missing Value Estimation: *The genetic characterizations can have missing values due to experimental uncertainties that are provided in the form of variables such as level of background noise for RNA expression, cross-reactivity for proteins, or average base quality for exome sequencing. Features with missing values either need to be removed from the analysis or the missing values have to be estimated for continuing with the subsequent analysis steps. One of the basic techniques for missing value estimation is to approximate it based on the weighted average of closely*

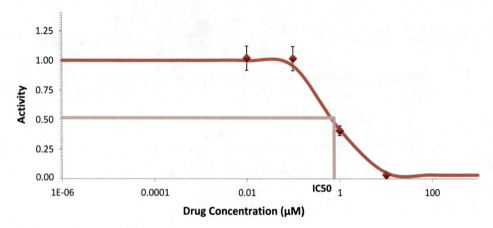

Fig. 3 Example Dose Response Curve

related cell lines. The weights are inversely proportional to the Euclidean distance of the cell line containing the missing feature to cell lines with the feature present [17].

Drug Response: *The drug responses are usually observed using pharmacological assays that measure metabolic activity in terms of reductase-enzyme product or energy-transfer molecule ATP levels following 72–84 h of drug delivery. A dose response curve for each cell line and specific drug is generated by observing the cell viability at different drug concentrations and fitting a curve through the observations (see **Note** 1) as shown in Fig. 3. Commonly used univariate features to represent dose response curve includes IC_{50} (drug concentration required to reduce cell viability to 50%) and AUC (area under the dose response curve). The IC_{50}'s are usually converted to sensitivities between 0 and 1 using a logarithmic mapping function such as $y = 1 - \frac{\log(IC_{50})}{\log(MaxDose)}$ [18, 19].*

2.2 Feature Selection

In the drug sensitivity-modeling context, feature selection is the process of selecting relevant features to potentially avoid over-fitting and reduce training time. Some of the modeling techniques such as Elastic Net [8] or Random Forests (as used in our methodology) are traditionally well suited for large number of features and can produce good performance even without the feature selection process. However, Random Forests (RFs) will require a large number of trees when working with all the available features and the feature importance measure of Random Forests will provide poor performance when there are too many features. Usually, the starting number of features in each genetic characterization can be in the thousands such as $\geq 10,000$ for gene expression. We use feature selection to reduce them to the range of ≤ 1000 features. Note that feature selection is applied separately for each genetic characterization data and some genetic characterization datasets may not require feature selection if we have only few hundred features in the dataset.

We apply *RReliefF* feature selection algorithm [20] with *K* neighbors using **Matlab** *relief* function or **R** *relief* function in *FSelector* package. We select the number of neighbors *K* to be 5 or 10. RReliefF computes the weights (in the range of −1 to 1 with large positive weights denoting important features) of features for input data matrix *X* and response vector *Y*. The *Regression ReliefF* weights are calculated by an adaptation of the *ReliefF* for classification that approximated the difference in probabilities of *P(different value of f | nearest instance from different class) − P(different value of f | nearest instance from same class)* where *f* is the feature whose weight is being estimated [21].

Feature selection can also be applied based on prior biological knowledge such as when we select only the kinase producing genes (around 400–500 of them) for designing our RF models (*see* **Note** 2). The reasoning behind the choice is that most targeted drugs target the human kinome (the kinase producing genes) [22–24] and thus, those kinase producing genes might generate the biologically relevant models.

2.3 Train Random Forests

Random Forest (RF) regression refers to an ensemble of regression trees [25] where a set of *T* un-pruned regression trees are generated based on bootstrap sampling from the original training data. We usually consider $T = 200$ or $T = 500$. For each node, the optimal node splitting feature is selected from a set of *m* features that are picked randomly from the total *M* features. For $m \ll M$, the selection of the node splitting feature from a random set of features decreases the correlation between different trees and thus, the average response of multiple regression trees is expected to have lower variance than individual regression trees. Larger *m* can improve the predictive capability of individual trees but can also increase the correlation between trees and void any gains from averaging multiple predictions. The bootstrap resampling of the data for training each tree also increases the variation between the trees. We usually select $m = 10$.

Process of splitting a node: *Let* X (i, j) *and* Y (i) *(i = 1, ..., n, j = 1, ..., M) denote the training predictor features and output response samples, respectively. At any regression tree node* η_P, *the goal is to select a feature* j_s *from a random set of m features and a threshold z to partition the node to child nodes* η_L *(left node with samples satisfying* $x_{tr}(I \in \eta_P, j_s) \leq z$*) and* η_R *(right node with samples satisfying* $x_{tr}(i \in \eta_P, j_s) > z$*).*

We consider the node cost as sum of square differences:

$$D(\eta_P) = \sum_{i \in \eta_P} (y(i) - \mu(\eta_P))^2 \tag{1}$$

where $\mu(\eta_P)$ is the average value of Y (i) in node η_P. Thus the reduction in cost for partition ζ at node η_P is

$$C(\zeta, \eta_P) = D(\eta_P) - D(\eta_L) - D(\eta_R) \quad (2)$$

The partition ζ^* that maximizes C (γ, η_P) for all possible partitions is selected for node η_P. Note that for a continuous feature with n samples, a total of n partitions need to be checked. Thus, the computational complexity of each node split is O(mn). During the tree generation process, a node with less than n_{lmin} training samples is not partitioned any further. We usually consider $n_{lmin} = 5$. A very small n_{lmin} (≤ 3) can cause overfitting by creating extremely small partitions in the data space.

Forest Prediction: *Using the randomized feature selection process, we fit the tree based on the bootstrap sample $\{(X_1, Y_1), \ldots, (X_n, Y_n)\}$ generated from the training data.*

*Let us consider the prediction based on a test sample **x** for the tree Θ. Let $\eta(x, \Theta)$ be the partition containing **x**, the tree response takes the form [25–27]:*

$$y(\mathbf{x}, \Theta) = \sum_{i=1}^{n} w_i(\mathbf{x}, \Theta) y(i) \quad (3)$$

where the weights $w_i(\mathbf{x}, \Theta)$ are given by

$$w_i(\mathbf{x}, \Theta) = \frac{\mathbf{1}_{\{x_{tr}(i) \in \eta(\mathbf{x}, \Theta)\}}}{\{r : x_{tr}(i) \in \eta(x_{tr}(r), \Theta)\}} \quad (4)$$

Let the T trees of the Random forest be denoted by $\Theta_1, \ldots, \Theta_T$ and let $w_i(\mathbf{x})$ denote the average weights over the forest, i.e.

$$w_i(\mathbf{x}) = \frac{1}{T} \sum_{j=1}^{T} w_i(\mathbf{x}, \Theta_j). \quad (5)$$

*The Random Forest prediction for the test sample **x** is then given by*

$$\bar{y}(\mathbf{x}) = \sum_{i=1}^{n} w_i(\mathbf{x}) y(i) \quad (6)$$

The above process of generating a Random Forest is represented as a step diagram in Fig. 4.

2.4 Generate Regression Models

Once we have the random forests built for individual datasets in step 3, we can integrate the predictions from different datasets using linear least square regression. Note that other approaches such as linear regression with regularization or regression trees can also be applied for this integration but our simulation studies have shown that linear least square regression provides robust performance over multiple scenarios.

Least Square Regression: *Let $\bar{y}(x_{i,j})$ denote the prediction obtained by Random Forest approach for genomic characterization dataset G_i and*

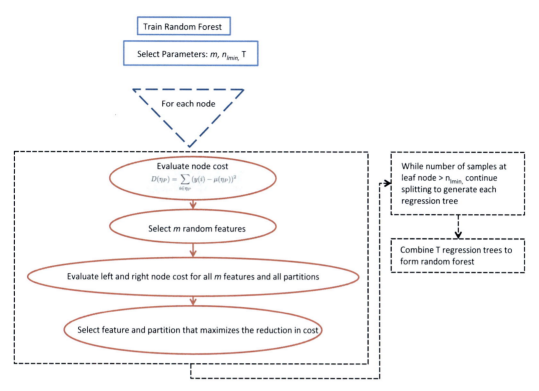

Fig. 4 Steps involved in Individual Random Forest generation

cell line j. To utilize the biological information in different datasets for prediction, we consider a linearly weighted combination model. We use linear least square regression to estimate the weights for each dataset G_i by minimizing

$$\sum_{j=1}^{n}\left(\Upsilon_j - \sum_{i=1}^{d}\alpha_i \bar{y}(\mathbf{x}_{i,j})\right)^2 \qquad (7)$$

where Y_j is the experimental drug response for cell line j, α_i is the corresponding weight of dataset G_i, and d is the number of genetic characterization datasets used for integrated model generation. The **Matlab** function fitlm or **R** function lm can be used to generate the linear regression model.

Considering D genetic characterization datasets, we can produce $2^D - 1$ different non-empty combinations of these datasets. Thus, **step 4** produces $2^D - 1$ integrated regression models that are evaluated in **step 5** for selecting the optimal integrated model.

2.5 Evaluate Integrated Models:

To evaluate the integrated models, we require an error estimation approach. Before estimating the error, we normalize the samples and decide on the type of error (*see* **Note 3**). Some common forms of error estimation approaches that are used are Leave One Out (LOO) error estimation and 0.632 Bootstrap error estimation.

Leave One Out Error: *In LOO error, all the cell lines are used for training except for one sample that is left out for testing. This is repeated n times where* n *is the number of samples. Let ε_j^{loo} denote the normalized error in prediction of cell line* j *and the average leave-one-out error across all cell lines for a drug is calculated as follows:*

$$\varepsilon^{loo} = \frac{1}{|x_i|} \sum_{j \in x_i} \varepsilon_j^{loo} \qquad (8)$$

Bootstrap Error: *Bootstrapping considers random sampling with replacement. On an average, 63.2% unique data samples are picked randomly while the rest 36.8% are repeated in bootstrapping. In bootstrap standard error calculations, the data samples that are picked by random sampling with replacement are used for training the model and the residual data are used to estimate the error of the model. Let* x_i *for* $i \in S$ *and* $S = [1, 2, \ldots, n]$ *denote the initial samples. Let the bootstrap samples be denoted by* x_{b_j} *for* $j = 1, \ldots, n$ *and* $b_j \in S_b$ *where* S_b *is a set of* n *numbers randomly selected from* S. *The testing set is denoted by* $S_T = S \setminus S_B$. *The bootstrap error* ε^{bsp} *is the average error over the testing data samples denoted by* ε_{x_i} *for sample* x_i.

$$\varepsilon^{bsp} = \frac{1}{|S_T|} \sum_{i \in S_T} \varepsilon_{x_i} \qquad (9)$$

This process is repeated for a user-defined number of times (see **Note** *4*) *and the average error is used to generate the final BSP error. The corresponding 0.632 bootstrap error can be computed as* $\varepsilon^{632bsp} = 0.632\varepsilon^{bsp} + 0.368\varepsilon^{resub}$, *where* ε^{resub} *denotes the re-substitution error. For re-substitution error calculations, all the samples are used for training and tested on the same set of training samples.*

For small samples in the dataset, LOO frequently provides better estimates as compared to 0.632 bootstrap error estimation as was observed in some of our drug sensitivity studies. For instance, consider the DREAM drug sensitivity prediction challenge dataset with $D = 5$ *and consider the various error estimates for* $^5 - 1 = 31$ *integrated models as shown in Fig. 5, the LOO error estimate was closer to validation error as compared to the other error estimates (see* **Note** *5). Validation error is considered to be the error of the model calculated from a set of holdout data that were never used earlier for model building or error estimation. In the DREAM Challenge dataset, there are 18 cell lines that are separated from the 35 cell lines that were used for training the model or estimating errors like bootstrap error or leave-one-out error. We consider the validation error as an estimate of the true error. True error denotes the error of a generated model over the whole data distribution. The validation set is used to represent the data distribution and thus a larger validation set increases the chances of the validation error being closer to the true error.*

Generate Error Confidence Interval Using Jackknife-After-Bootstrap: *The error estimation approaches mentioned above provide an estimate of mean error and we can calculate the uncertainties or*

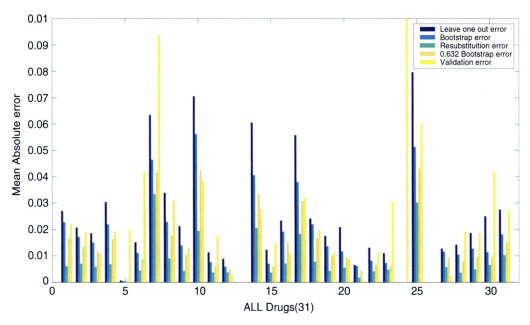

Fig. 5 Leave-one-out, Bootstrap, Re-substitution, 0.632 Bootstrap, and True error for all 31 drugs for NCI-Dream challenge Dataset. The prediction for drugs 13, 24, and 26 shows zero error as they contained minimal variations in sensitivity

confidence interval of the mean error using an approach described next. Jackknife-After-Bootstrap Approach is used for generating the confidence intervals of the 0.632 Bootstrap errors. Let N_k denote the set of bootstrap samples that do not contain sample X_k and the 0.632 bootstrap estimate computed from N_k is denoted by ε_k. The standard error can be computed as

$$s = \sqrt{\frac{n-1}{n} \sum_{k=1}^{n} (\varepsilon_k - \bar{\varepsilon})^2} \tag{10}$$

where $\bar{\varepsilon} = (1/n) \sum_{k=1}^{n} \varepsilon_k$. The $100(1-\alpha)\%$ prediction intervals for the true error can be computed as $[\bar{\varepsilon} - sz_{\alpha/2}, \bar{\varepsilon} + sz_{\alpha/2}]$ where z_α is the α quantile of the standard normal distribution. Since we consider the absolute error, the lower bound of the confidence interval is calculated as $\max[0, \bar{\varepsilon} - sz_{\alpha/2}]$.

Figure 6 shows the 80% confidence interval for drug-15 in the DREAM Drug Sensitivity Prediction challenge dataset and it illustrates that the addition of datasets decreases the confidence interval. With single dataset, the confidence interval is highest (leftmost combinations) and the confidence interval decreases gradually with the integration of multiple genetic characterizations (going right). The rightmost bar represents the confidence interval of 0.632 bootstrap error with all 5 datasets, which has the lowest confidence interval among all combinations. In all the cases, the validation error denoted by cross is within 80% confidence interval.

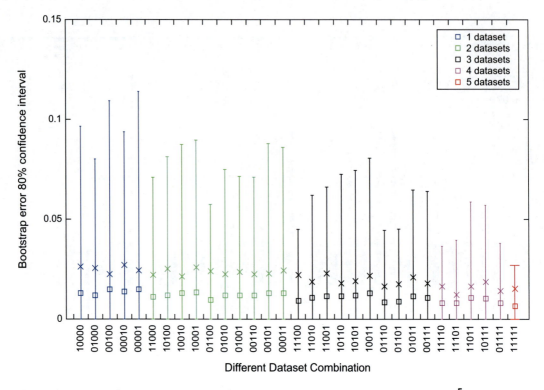

Fig. 6 Mean 0.632 Bootstrap error and 80% confidence intervals for Drug 15 for 31($=2^5 -1$) different dataset combinations. The datasets are denoted by binary digits with the following order: Gene Expression (most significant bit), Methylation, RNASeq, RPPA, and SNP6 (least significant bit). For instance, 01100 denotes Methylation and RNASeq data combination

2.6 Final Integrated Model

The final integrated model is selected based on the dataset combination producing the lowest error. As discussed earlier, either LOO or 0.632 Bootstrap can be used to estimate the integrated model error. The final integrated model for application to new samples is stored as a collection of d random forests RF(i) for $i = 1, \ldots, d$ whose combined prediction is given by a linear regression model with coefficients $\alpha_1, \ldots, \alpha_d$. Each Random Forest RF($i$) is a collection of T regression trees RT(i, j) for $j = 1, \ldots, T$. Each regression tree RT(i, j) is an ordered set of $\eta_{i,j,k}$ nodes where each node contains information on the node split feature and the threshold for splitting.

3 Notes

1. One of the models to fit observed drug responses in the cancer cell line encyclopedia study [9] was the following four parameter (A_t, A_B, H, EC_{50}) sigmoidal model

$$y = A_b + \frac{A_t - A_b}{1 + (\frac{x}{EC_{50}})^H} \qquad (11)$$

where A_t and A_b denote the top and bottom asymptotes of the response, respectively, H is the hill slope, and EC_{50} denotes the concentration at which the curve response is midway between A_b and A_t.

2. The list of kinases can be obtained from the supplementary information of the article [24].

3. Following the generation of predictions from our integrated random forest approach, we normalize the predicted and experimental drug sensitivities between 0.0 and 1.0 by min-max normalization [28]. The normalized prediction $\hat{\Upsilon}_C(j)$ and actual drug response $\hat{Y}_j$ are calculated as follows:

$$\hat{\Upsilon}_C(j) = \frac{\Upsilon_C(j) - min_{j\in\Pi}(\Upsilon_C(j), \Upsilon_j)}{max_{j\in\Pi}(\Upsilon_C(j), \Upsilon_j) - min_{j\in\Pi}(\Upsilon_C(j), \Upsilon_j)}.$$

$$\hat{Y}_j = \frac{\Upsilon_j - min_{j\in\Pi}(\Upsilon_C(j), \Upsilon_j)}{max_{j\in\Pi}(\Upsilon_C(j), \Upsilon_j) - min_{j\in\Pi}(\Upsilon_C(j), \Upsilon_j)}.$$

where Π denotes the set of all available cell lines. After normalization, the corresponding error ε_j of cell line j is generated as the absolute error $|\hat{\Upsilon}_C(j) - \hat{Y}_j|$. The *Mean Absolute Error* (MAE) is used for further error calculations.

4. We usually repeat it 50–100 number of times.

5. The closer approximation of true error by the LOO error estimate as compared to 0.632 Bootstrap Error estimate need not hold for all studies but we observed it for smaller samples (< 100) in our CCLE and DREAM Challenge sensitivity studies.

References

1. Costello JC et al (2014) A community effort to assess and improve drug sensitivity prediction algorithms. Nat Biotechnol. https://doi.org/10.1038/nbt.2877

2. Wan Q, Pal R (2014) An ensemble based top performing approach for NCI-dream drug sensitivity prediction challenge. PLoS One 9(6): e101183

3. Sos ML, Michel K, Zander T, Weiss J, Frommolt P, Peifer M, Li D, Ullrich R, Koker M, Fischer F, Shimamura T, Rauh D, Mermel C, Fischer S, Stückrath I, Heynck S, Beroukhim R, Lin W, Winckler W, Shah K, LaFramboise T, Moriarty WF, Hanna M, Tolosi L, Rahnenführer J, Verhaak R, Chiang D, Getz G, Hellmich M, Wolf J, Girard L, Peyton M, Weir BA, Chen TH, Greulich H, Barretina J, Shapiro GI, Garraway LA, Gazdar AF, Minna JD, Meyerson M, Wong KK, Thomas RK (2009) Predicting drug susceptibility of non-small cell lung cancers based on genetic lesions. J Clin Invest 119 (6):1727–1740

4. Staunton JE, Slonim DK, Coller HA, Tamayo P, Angelo MJ, Park J, Scherf U, Lee JK, Reinhold WO, Weinstein JN, Mesirov JP, Lander ES, Golub TR (2001)

Chemosensitivity prediction by transcriptional profiling. Proc Natl Acad Sci 98:10787–10792

5. Lee JK, Havaleshko DM, Cho H, Weinstein JN, Kaldjian EP, Karpovich J, Grimshaw A, Theodorescu D (2007) A strategy for predicting the chemosensitivity of human cancers and its application to drug discovery. Proc Natl Acad Sci 104(32):13086–13091

6. Mitsos A, Melas IN, Siminelakis P, Chairakaki AD, Saez-Rodriguez J, Alexopoulos LG (2009) Identifying drug effects via pathway alterations using an integer linear programming optimization formulation on phosphoproteomic data. PLoS Comput Biol 5(12): e1000591+

7. Walther Z, Sklar J (2011) Molecular tumor profiling for prediction of response to anticancer therapies. Cancer J 17(2):71–79

8. Zou H, Hastie T (2005) Regularization and variable selection via the elastic net. J R Stat Soc Ser B 67:301–320

9. Barretina J et al (2012) The Cancer Cell Line Encyclopedia enables predictive modelling of anticancer drug sensitivity. Nature 483 (7391):603–607

10. Riddick G, Song H, Ahn S, Walling J, Borges-Rivera D, Zhang W, Fine HA (2011) Predicting in vitro drug sensitivity using Random Forests. Bioinformatics 27(2):220–224

11. Bengtsson H, Simpson K, Bullard J, Hansen K (2008) aroma.affymetrix: a generic framework in R for analyzing small to very large Affymetrix data sets in bounded memory. Tech. Rep. 745, Department of Statistics, University of California, Berkeley

12. Garber M, Grabherr MG, Guttman M, Trapnell C (2011) Computational methods for transcriptome annotation and quantification using RNA-seq. Nat Methods 8(6):469–477

13. Wilhelm BT, Landry JR (2009) RNA-seq-quantitative measurement of expression through massively parallel RNA-sequencing. Methods 48(3):249–257

14. Li S, Tighe SW, Nicolet CM, Grove D, Levy S, Farmerie W, Viale A, Wright C, Schweitzer PA, Gao Y, Kim D, Boland J, Hicks B, Kim R, Chhangawala S, Jafari N, Raghavachari N, Gandara J, Garcia-Reyero N, Hendrickson C, Roberson D, Rosenfeld J, Smith T, Underwood JG, Wang M, Zumbo P, Baldwin DA, Grills GS, Mason CE (2014) Multi-platform assessment of transcriptome profiling using RNA-seq in the ABRF next-generation sequencing study. Nat Biotechnol 32 (9):915–925

15. Xie F, Liu T, Qian WJ, Petyuk VA, Smith RD (2011) Liquid chromatography-mass spectrometry-based quantitative proteomics. J Biol Chem 286(29):25443–25449

16. Li F, Gonzalez FJ, Ma X (2012) LC–MS-based metabolomics in profiling of drug metabolism and bioactivation. Acta Pharm Sin B 2 (2):118–125. Drug Metabolism and Transport

17. Troyanskaya OG, Cantor MN, Sherlock G, Brown PO, Hastie T, Tibshirani R, Botstein D, Altman RB (2001) Missing value estimation methods for DNA microarrays. Bioinformatics 17(6):520–525

18. Berlow N, Haider S, Wan Q, Geltzeiler M, Davis LE, Keller C, Berlow RN (2014) An integrated approach to anti-cancer drugs sensitivity prediction. IEEE/ACM Trans Comput Biol Bioinform. https://doi.org/10.1155/2014/873436

19. Berlow N, Davis LE, Cantor EL, Seguin B, Keller C, Pal R (2013) A new approach for prediction of tumor sensitivity to targeted drugs based on functional data. BMC Bioinformatics 14:239

20. Robnik-Sikonja M, Kononenko I (1997) An adaptation of relief for attribute estimation in regression. In: Proceedings of the fourteenth international conference on machine learning (ICML '97). Morgan Kaufmann Publishers Inc, San Francisco, pp 296–304

21. Šikonja MR, Kononenko I (2003) Theoretical and empirical analysis of ReliefF and RReliefF. Mach Learn 53(1–2):23–69

22. Zarrinkar PP, Gunawardane RN, Cramer MD, Gardner MF, Brigham D, Belli B, Karaman MW, Pratz KW, Pallares G, Chao Q, Sprankle KG, Patel HK, Levis M, Armstrong RC, James J, Bhagwat SS (2009) AC220 is a uniquely potent and selective inhibitor of FLT3 for the treatment of acute myeloid leukemia (AML). Blood 114(14):2984–2992

23. Fabian MA, Biggs WH, Treiber DK, Atteridge CE, Azimioara MD, Benedetti MG, Carter TA, Ciceri P, Edeen PT, Floyd M, Ford JM, Galvin M, Gerlach JL, Grotzfeld RM, Herrgard S, Insko DE, Insko MA, Lai AG, Lelias JM, Mehta SA, Milanov ZV, Velasco AM, Wodicka LM, Patel HK, Zarrinkar PP, Lockhart DJ (2005) A small molecule-kinase interaction map for clinical kinase inhibitors. Nat Biotechnol 23(3):329–336

24. Karaman MW, Herrgard S, Treiber DK, Gallant P, Atteridge CE, Campbell BT, Chan KW, Ciceri P, Davis MI, Edeen PT, Faraoni R, Floyd M, Hunt JP, Lockhart DJ, Milanov ZV, Morrison MJ, Pallares G, Patel

HK, Pritchard S, Wodicka LM, Zarrinkar PP (2008) A quantitative analysis of kinase inhibitor selectivity. Nat Biotechnol 26(1):127–132

25. Breiman L (2001) Random forests. Mach Learn 45(1):5–32

26. Meinshausen N (2006) Quantile regression forests. J Mach Learn Res 7:983–999

27. Biau G (2012) Analysis of a random forests model. J Mach Learn Res 98888:1063–1095

28. Shalabi LA, Shaaban Z, Kasasbeh B (2006) Data mining: a preprocessing engine. J Comput Sci 2(9):735

Chapter 15

In Silico Oncology Drug Repositioning and Polypharmacology

Feixiong Cheng

Abstract

Network-aided in silico approaches have been widely used for prediction of drug-target interactions and evaluation of drug safety to increase the clinical efficiency and productivity during drug discovery and development. Here we review the advances and new progress in this field and summarize the translational applications of several new network-aided in silico approaches we developed recently. In addition, we describe the detailed protocols for a network-aided drug repositioning infrastructure for identification of new targets for old drugs, failed drugs in clinical trials, and new chemical entities. These state-of-the-art network-aided in silico approaches have been used for the discovery and development of broad-acting and targeted clinical therapies for various complex diseases, in particular for oncology drug repositioning. In this chapter, the described network-aided in silico protocols are appropriate for target-centric drug repositioning to various complex diseases, but expertise is still necessary to perform the specific oncology projects based on the cancer targets of interest.

Key words Drug-target interactions, Drug repositioning, Polypharmacology, Network-based inference, Systems biology, Systems pharmacology, Panomics, Cancer genomics, Precision oncology, Targeted therapy

1 Introduction

The term "polypharmacology" refers to the potential of a molecule to bind with multiple proteins, not a single protein [1]. Polypharmacology, focusing on designing novel therapeutics to target multiple proteins (e.g., receptors or enzymes) or disease pathways, has been found as a highly efficient paradigm in oncology drug discovery and development [2, 3]. However, it has been recognized that multiple "on-target" and "off-target" binding affinities often generate both beneficial therapeutic effects and harmful side effects for many drugs across a broad range of therapeutic fields, including cancer. In the past several decades, polypharmacology has shown various translational implications for oncology drug repositioning (finding new anticancer indication for the existing drugs that are

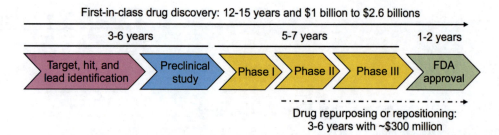

Fig. 1 Comparison of time cost and effort cost between the classic first-in-class drug discovery paradigm and drug repositioning

not approved originally for this cancer type), assessment of drug safety caused by the harmful off-target effects, and rational design of multiple-target oncology drugs or combinatorial therapies [1, 4].

Recent advances in high-throughput technologies, such as next-generation sequencing, have been widely used to catalog the genomic landscape in cancer [5, 6]. These efforts have generated over 500 cancer significantly mutated genes for over 20 cancer types/subtypes in several national or interactional projects, such as The Cancer Genome Atlas (TCGA) [7] and the International Cancer Genome Consortium (ICGC) [8]. However, the cost of oncology drug development continues to increase dramatically (Fig. 1) [9, 10]. In 2013, $91 billion were spent on oncology drugs in the United States, and the ten biggest-selling oncology drugs reached $43 billion. In addition, the cost of drug development, including the price of failure and the opportunity cost, has increased significantly in the past decade [9, 10]. It is a pressing need to develop innovative technologies for speeding up cancer therapies with a faster development while at low cost. Recently, oncology drug repositioning has revealed several notable advantages (Fig. 1), including the availability of the safety profiles (e.g., well-known pharmacokinetics and pharmacodynamics properties) already studied in its previous preclinical studies or clinical trials [11–14].

Faced with skyrocketing costs for developing new drugs via traditionally experimental technologies, computational approaches have suggested the great advantages for systematic identification of novel drug-target interactions (DTIs) to old drugs, failed drugs in clinical trials, and new chemical entries (NCEs) at proteome-wide scale for target-centric oncology drug repositioning [15]. There are several different categories for the computational drug repositioning approaches, including ligand-based [16], target-based [17, 18], chemogenomics-based [16], and network-aided approaches [19–22]. For example, machine learning-based models [16, 23, 24] or protein structure-based molecular docking approaches [25–27] have been widely used for prediction of DTIs

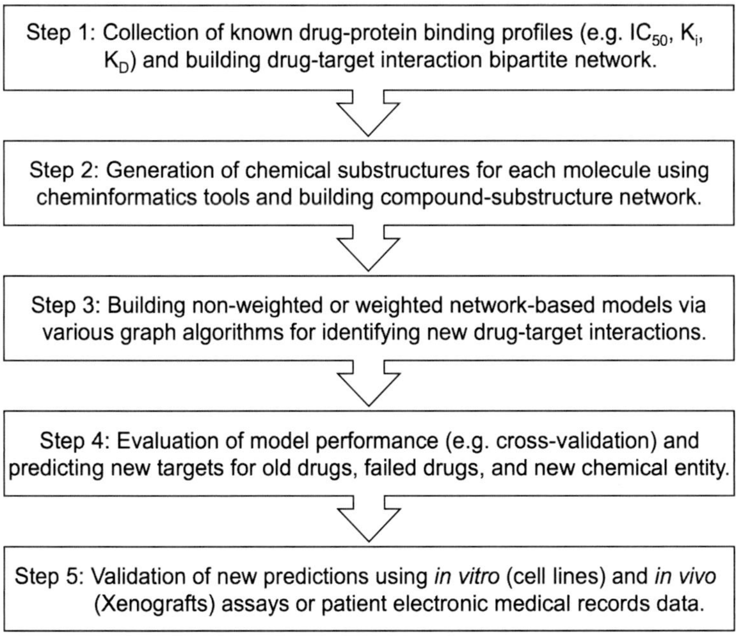

Step 1: Collection of known drug-protein binding profiles (e.g. IC_{50}, K_i, K_D) and building drug-target interaction bipartite network.

Step 2: Generation of chemical substructures for each molecule using cheminformatics tools and building compound-substructure network.

Step 3: Building non-weighted or weighted network-based models via various graph algorithms for identifying new drug-target interactions.

Step 4: Evaluation of model performance (e.g. cross-validation) and predicting new targets for old drugs, failed drugs, and new chemical entity.

Step 5: Validation of new predictions using *in vitro* (cell lines) and *in vivo* (Xenografts) assays or patient electronic medical records data.

Fig. 2 Flowchart showing the five-step network-aided drug repositioning infrastructure for identification of new targets for old drugs (Step 2 and Steps 3–5), failed drugs, and new chemical entities (Steps 1–5)

during oncology drug discovery and development. However, these approaches often have several potential pitfalls, such as lack of available high-quality protein three-dimensional structures or lack of gold-standard negative samples for building machine learning-based classification models [18, 23, 24, 28–30]. Recently, network-aided approaches derived from research fields of network science provide great opportunities for drug-target identification and prioritize DTIs for target-centric drug repositioning [15, 20, 21, 31–34]. Those network-aided computational approaches shed important lights on the topology of DTIs during oncology drug discovery and suggest that polypharmacological features of drugs play crucial roles for development of the highly efficient targeted cancer therapies under the systems pharmacology framework [35].

In this chapter, we primarily focused on introducing network-aided in silico approaches for target-centric drug repositioning. Specifically, we describe several state-of-the-art network-aided in silico approaches or tools (Fig. 2) that have been developed by our group for the development of target-centric drug repositioning and drug discovery for both approved drugs and NCEs. Finally, we will highlight several potential future directions via exploiting the big cancer panomics data [15] under the introduced network-aided drug repositioning infrastructure for the emerging development of precision oncology.

2 Materials: Hardware and Software

1. Computer requirements: Laptop computer, desktop computer, or computer workstations with Linux operating systems.
2. Text editors such as UltraEdit.
3. Molecular descriptor or substructure generators such as PaDEL-Descriptor [36] and Open Babel [37].
4. Drug-protein or drug-gene interaction databases (Table 1), such as DrugBank [38], ChEMBL [40], BindingDB [41], canSAR [50], and therapeutic target database (TTD) [39].
5. The human protein-protein interaction databases, such as human protein reference database (HPRD) [54].
6. Bioinformatics databases such as the Gene Oncology [55], National Center for Biotechnology Information [56], and UniProt [57].
7. Bioinformatics tools, such as BLAST [58].
8. Python and Java environment.

Table 1
Lists of chemoinformatics and bioinformatics resources and databases for constructing drug-target interaction networks and building the network-aided in silico models or tools

Name	URL	Refs.
DrugBank	http://drugbank.ca/	[38]
TTD	http://bidd.nus.edu.sg/group/cjttd/	[39]
ChEMBL	https://www.ebi.ac.uk/chembldb/	[40]
BindingDB	http://www.bindingdb.org/	[41]
SuperTarget	http://bioinf-apache.charite.de/supertarget_v2/	[42]
KEGG	http://www.genome.jp/kegg/	[43]
PharmGKB	https://www.pharmgkb.org/	[44]
STITCH	http://stitch.embl.de/	[45]
PubChem	http://pubchem.ncbi.nlm.nih.gov/	[46]
ChemProt	www.cbs.dtu.dk/services/ChemProt/	[47]
ChemBank	http://chembank.broadinstitute.org/	[48]
PROMISCUOUS	http://bioinformatics.charite.de/promiscuous	[49]
CanSAR	https://cansar.icr.ac.uk/	[50]
DGIdb	http://dgidb.genome.wustl.edu	[51]
CMap (v 2.0)	https://www.broadinstitute.org/cmap/	[52]
LINCSCLOUD	lincscloud.org	[53]

9. MATLAB package.
10. Network analysis tools such as Cytoscape [59], NetworkX (https://networkx.github.io), and Gephi (https://gephi.org).

3 Methods

In this chapter, we introduce a network-aided drug repositioning infrastructure (Fig. 2) for identification of new targets for old drugs, failed drugs in clinical trials, or NCEs. This network-aided drug repositioning infrastructure includes five steps: (1) building a comprehensive DTI network by integrating drug-protein binding profiles from various available data sources (Table 1), (2) generating chemical substructures for old drugs and NCEs to build a compound-substructure network, (3) building network-aided predictive models using weighted or non-weighted network-based inference algorithms, (4) evaluating performance of network-aided models via cross-validation and external validation and predicting new candidate DTIs for target-centric oncology drug repositioning on specific cancer targets of interest, and (5) experimentally verifying of new predictions using in vitro or in vivo experimental assays or using available patient data from electronic medical records or other healthcare databases. For predicting DTIs to old drugs, it only requires Step 1 and Steps 3–5. It will require all five steps to predict DTIs for failed drugs and NCEs. In general, this network-aided drug repositioning infrastructure could be applied for target-centric drug repositioning in various complex diseases of interest. Here, we mainly focus on introducing target-centric oncology drug repositioning to narrow the topics of this chapter.

3.1 Construction of Drug-Target Interaction Network

The DTI network can be described as a bipartite DT graph $G(D, T, E)$, where the drug is set as $D = \{d_1, d_2, \ldots, d_n\}$, target set as $T = \{t_1, t_2, \ldots, t_m\}$, and interaction set as $E = \{e_{ij} : d_i \in D, t_j \in T\}$. An interaction is drawn between d_i and t_j when the drug d_i binds with the target t_j with the binding affinity (such as IC_{50}, K_i, or K_d) less than a given threshold value such as 10 μM based on the curated data from variously public available databases, literatures, and high-throughput experimental assays (Table 1). Currently, several publically available drug-gene (protein or target) interaction databases provide large-scale quantitative drug-protein binding affinity information, such as DrugBank [38], TTD [39], ChEMBL [40], BindingDB [41], PharmGKB [44], STITCH [45], PubChem [46], PROMISCUOUS [49], canSAR [50], and DGIdb [51]. These data sources (Table 1) provide useful information for constructing the DTI networks.

Mathematically, a DTI bipartite network can be presented by an $n \times m$ adjacent matrix $\{a_{ij}\}$, where $a_{ij} = 1$ if the binding affinity between d_i and t_j is less than 10 μM, otherwise $a_{ij} = 0$, as described in Eq. 1.

$$a_{ij} = \begin{cases} 1 & \text{IC}_{50}(K_i) \leq 10\,\mu M \\ 0 & \text{IC}_{50}(K_i) > 10\,\mu M \end{cases} \quad (1)$$

3.2 Drug Similarity-Based Network Inference

The underlying hypothesis of drug similarity-based network inference asserts that if a drug interacts with a target, then other drugs similar to this drug will be inferred to the given target with high score [20] (Fig. 3a). An interaction between d_i and t_l is determined by the following predicted score:

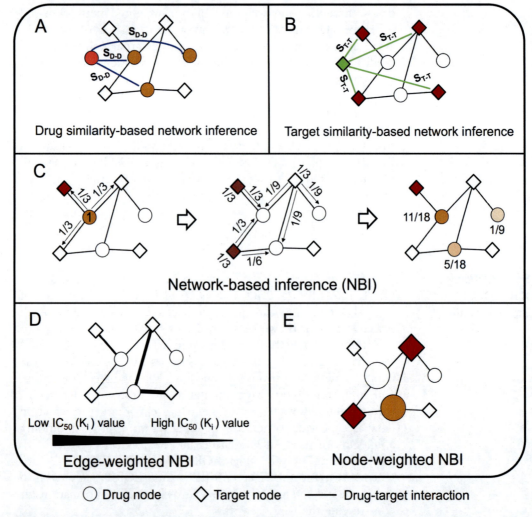

Fig. 3 Schematic diagram of illustrating three non-weighted (**a**–**c**) and two weighted (**d** and **e**) network-based inference approaches. The detailed descriptions of **a**–**e** are provided in Subheading 3.2–3.4

$$v_{il}^d = \frac{\sum_{i=1, i\neq j}^{n} S_x(d_i, d_j) a_{ij}}{\sum_{i=1, i\neq j}^{n} S_x(d_i, d_j)} \quad (2)$$

where $S_x(d_i, d_j)$ denotes similarity between drugs d_i and d_j, which can be measured by different approaches as briefly described as below.

3.2.1 Chemical Similarity

Chemical similarity $S_c(d_i, d_j)$ between drugs d_i and d_j is often measured by various chemo-physical descriptors or fingerprints [35]. For example, the Tanimoto similarity for drugs d_i and d_j can be calculated using various types of fingerprints (such as MACCS or FP4), freely available from Open Babel [37] or other tools [60].

$$S_c(d_i, d_j) = \frac{C_{ij}}{a_i + b_j - c_{ij}} \quad (3)$$

Where a_i and b_j denote the bit set in d_i and d_j fingerprint bit strings and c_{ij} represents these bits being set in both d_i and d_j. In addition to Tanimoto similarity, several other metrics, including Cosine, Hamming, Russell-Rao, and Forbes, are often used as described in a previous study [61].

3.2.2 Drug Side Effect Similarity

As described in a previous study, each drug is encoded by a given number of side effect bit vectors. Each bit denotes a side effect for a specific drug annotated in the public available databases [62]. If a side effect event is reported to associate with a given drug in clinic, the corresponding bit is set to "1"; otherwise, it is set to "0." Then, side effect similarity $S_{SE}(d_i, d_j)$ between drugs d_i and d_j can be measured by Tanimoto, Cosine, Hamming, Russell-Rao, or Forbes as discussed in the Subheading 3.2.1.

3.2.3 Drug Therapeutic Similarity

Drug therapeutic profiles, such as the Anatomical Therapeutic Chemical Classification System (ATC) codes, provide new dimension to explore drug similarity [61]. The drug ATC codes can be downloaded from some public databases, such as TTD and DrugBank (Table 1). Then the kth level drug therapeutic similarity (S_k) between d_i and d_j is calculated by the ATC codes as below:

$$S_k(d_i, d_j) = \frac{ATC_k(d_i) \cap ATC_k(d_j)}{ATC_k(d_i) \cap ATC_k(d_j)} \quad (4)$$

where $ATC_k(d)$ denotes all ATC codes at the kth level of drug d. Finally, a score $S_{ATC}(d_i, d_j)$ between d_i and d_j at all ATC codes is used to define the therapeutic similarity between d_i and d_j as below:

$$S_{ATC}(d_i, d_j) = \frac{\sum_{k=1}^{n} S_k(d_i, d_j)}{n} \quad (5)$$

where n denotes all five-level ATC codes (1 to 5). However, for some drugs with multiple ATC codes, the $S_{ATC}(d_i, d_j)$ is often calculated for each code, and the average therapeutic similarity is used for network building as described in Eq. 4.

3.3 Target Similarity-Based Network Inference

The biological hypothesis for target similarity-based network inference asserts that if a drug interacts with a target protein, then the drug will be inferred to other targets that share a similarly evolutionary distance (like protein sequence identity) or a closely functional similarity (like network topological similarity in the human protein-protein interaction network or the gene ontology [GO] similarity [63]) to a specific protein (Fig. 3b). An interaction between d_i and t_l is calculated by the following predicted score:

$$v_{il}^t = \frac{\sum_{i=1, i \neq j}^{m} S_x(t_i, t_j) a_{ij}}{\sum_{i=1, i \neq j}^{m} S_x(t_i, t_j)} \quad (6)$$

where $S_x(t_i, t_j)$ denotes the protein evolutionary distance or functional similarity between targets t_i and t_j as described as below.

3.3.1 Protein Sequence Identity

Protein evolutionary distances are often measured based on protein sequence alignment. For example, a normalized version of Smith-Waterman scores [64] is often used to calculate protein sequence identity between corresponding targets t_i and t_j as described in our previous studies [16, 20].

3.3.2 Network Topological Similarity in the Protein-Protein Interaction Network

The network distance $S_N(t_i, t_j)$ between corresponding targets t_i and t_j is calculated using all-pair network distances on the human protein-protein interaction network via the shortest path distance measure. Then, network distance is transformed to similarity measure using the below equation as described in a previous study [65]:

$$S_N(t_i, t_j) = A e^{-S(t_i, t_j)} \quad (7)$$

where A is often assigned an empirical value $0.9 \cdot e$ [65], and self-similarity is assigned a value of 1.

3.3.3 Biological or Functional Similarity Via Sharing the Terms of the Gene Ontology

The biological or functional similarity of drug corresponding targets is often measured by their shared gene ontology (GO) terms [63]. A functional similarity asserts that drug target-coding genes share very specific functions which are more similar to each other than those who only share generic GO terms. The biological or functional similarity $S_{GO}(t_i, t_j)$ between corresponding targets t_i and t_j is measured by the most specific GO terms they share:

$$S_{GO}(t_i, t_j) \equiv \frac{2}{\min(n_y)} \quad (8)$$

where n_y denotes the total number of genes annotated in the entire GO corpus. The value of $S_{GO}(t_i, t_j)$ ranges from 0 (no shared GO terms) to 1 (drug corresponding targets t_i and t_j are the only two according target-coding genes annotated to a specific GO term) [63].

3.4 Network-Based Inference

3.4.1 Unweighted Network-Based Inference

Considering the bipartite graph $G(D, T, E)$, a mass diffusion-based method can be used to generate the predicted list. For a given drug d_i, supposing that a kind of resource is initially located in the targets which are interacted with d_i, the resource will diffuse to all targets in the DTI network after the network-based resource allocation process as described in the previous studies [20, 21]. Each target node averagely distributes its resource to all neighboring drugs, and then each drug redistributes the received resource to all neighboring targets (Fig. 3c). The final resource on the targets that are not connected with the drug d_i in $G(D, T, E)$ could be considered as the predicted score for each target, and the targets with high scores are more likely to interact with d_i. Figure 3c gives a simple example to illustrate the network-based resource allocation process. It shows the initial resource of a_{ij} between d_i (cycle) and t_j (square) defined in Eq. 1.

Denoting $F_{0n \times m}$ as the initial resource and $F_{0ij} = a_{ij}$, $R_{n \times n}$ as the total resource (degree) for each drug:

$$R = \text{diag}\left(\sum_{j=1}^{m} a_{1j}, \sum_{j=1}^{m} a_{2j}, \ldots, \sum_{j=1}^{m} a_{nj}\right) \quad (9)$$

In addition, $H_{m \times m}$ as the total resource (degree) for each target:

$$H = \text{diag}\left(\sum_{i=1}^{n} a_{i1}, \sum_{i=1}^{n} a_{i2}, \ldots, \sum_{i=1}^{n} a_{im}\right) \quad (10)$$

Finally, the resource matrix (adjacency matrix) is obtained as

$$F_{1n \times m} : F_1 = F_0 W_{m \times m} \text{ or } F_1^T = F_0^T W_{n \times n} \quad (11)$$

where transfer matrix $W_{m \times m} = (F_0 H^{-1})^T (R^{-1} F_0)$ or $W_{n \times n} = (R^{-1} F_0)(F_0 H^{-1})^T$.

3.4.2 Edge-Weighted Network-Based Inference

Naturally, an edge between drug and target is weighted in the real biological systems, such as IC_{50} or K_i value. For the edge-weighted network-based inference (EWNBI) (Fig. 3d), each edge of DTI network is weighted by the drug-protein binding affinity $(x_{ij} = -\log_{10}(K_i \text{ (or } IC_{50})/100 \text{ μM}))$ between drug d_i and target t_j. The initial resource of a'_{ij} between d_i and t_j is defined as follows:

$$a'_{ij} = \begin{cases} x_{ij} & K_i(IC_{50}) \leq 10 \ \mu M \\ 0 & K_i(IC_{50}) > 10 \ \mu M \end{cases} \quad (12)$$

Denoting $F'_{0n \times m}$ as the initial resource and $F'_{0ij} = a_{ij}$, $R'_{n \times n}$ as the total resource of each drug:

$$R' = \text{diag}\left(\sum_{j=1}^{m} a'_{1j}, \sum_{j=1}^{m} a'_{2j}, \ldots, \sum_{j=1}^{m} a'_{nj}\right) \quad (13)$$

In addition, $H'_{m \times m}$ as the total resource for each target:

$$H' = \text{diag}\left(\sum_{i=1}^{n} a'_{i1}, \sum_{i=1}^{n} a'_{i2}, \ldots, \sum_{i=1}^{n} a'_{im}\right) \quad (14)$$

Finally, the resource matrix is obtained as $F'_{1n\times m}$, and $F'_1 = F'_0 W'_{m\times m}$ or $F'^T_1 = F'^T_0 W'_{n\times n}$, where transfer matrix $W'_{m\times m} = \left(F'_0 H'^{-1}\right)^T \left(R'^{-1} F'_0\right)$ or $W'_{n\times n} = \left(R'^{-1} F'_0\right)\left(F'_0 H'^{-1}\right)^T$.

3.4.3 Node-Weighted Network-Based Inference

In general, hub nodes with more receiving resources often tend to generate the higher predicted scores, which often lead to a potential risk of false positive rate. Compared to the unweighted NBI method, the node-weighted network-based inference (NWNBI, Fig. 3e) introduces a new expression of initial resource distribution by taking into account the influence of resources associated with the receiver nodes in DTI bipartite network as discussed in a previous study [21]. For the initial resource matrix, the resource for each drug and target node is the same to the unweighted NBI. The final resource matrices are calculated as $F''_{1n\times m}$, and $F''_{1D} = F_0 W''_{m\times m}$ for drugs and $F''_{1T} = F_0^T W''_{n\times n}$ for targets, where transfer matrix $W''_{m\times m} = (F_0 H^{-1})^T \left(R^{-1} F_0 H''^{-1}\right)$, where $H''_{ij} = H^\beta_{ij}$ for drug or $W''_{n\times n} = (R^{-1} F_0)\left(R''^{-1} F_0 H^{-1}\right)^T$ and where $R''_{ij} = R^\beta_{ij}$ for target, β as a tunable parameter to balance the influence. Compared with a uniform case ($\beta = 0$), a positive β value strengthens the influence of hub nodes, while a negative β value weakens the influence of hub nodes (*see* **Note 1**). The detailed descriptions are provided in the previous study [21].

3.5 Substructure-Drug-Target Network-Based Inference

The NBI method utilizing the naïve topology information cannot predict targets for NCEs or failed drugs that don't share the known targets in the existing DTI network [20, 21]. Recently, our group developed an integrated network and chemoinformatics tool, named substructure-drug-target network-based inference (SDTNBI), for large-scale DTI prediction to NCEs or failed drugs [66]. SDTNBI utilizes the chemical substructures, a defined series of features shared by different compounds, to bridge the gap between known drugs and NCEs (*see* **Note 2**). Specifically, SDTNBI integrates the known DTI network, drug-substructure linkages, and NCE-substructure linkages to infer new targets for old drugs, failed drugs, and NCEs (Fig. 4a) via five steps as briefly described as below.

3.5.1 Generation of Chemical Substructures

Several freely available chemoinformatics tools, such as PaDEL-Descriptor [36] and Open Babel [37], are commonly used to generate chemical substructures for old drugs or NCEs. For example, PaDEL-Descriptor (version 2.18) [36] includes seven commonly used substructures: substructure fingerprint (FP4), MACCS fingerprint (MACCS), CDK fingerprint, CDK extended fingerprint, CDK graph only fingerprint, PubChem fingerprint, and Klekota-Roth fingerprint. In addition, some commercial available

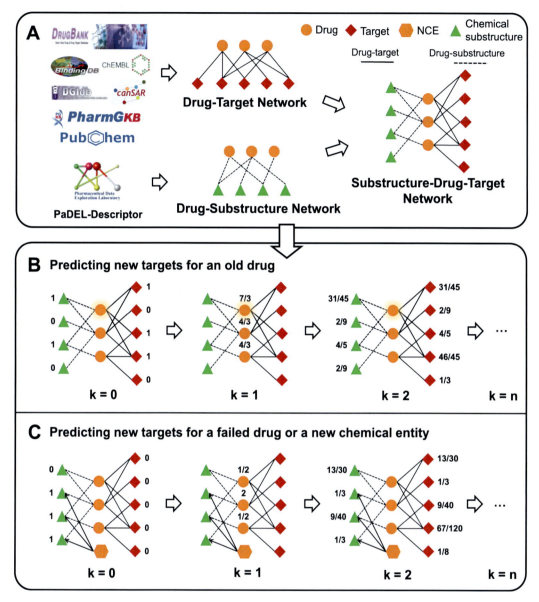

Fig. 4 Schematic diagram of showing substructure-drug-target network-based inference. (**a**) Construction of drug-substructure and drug-target interaction networks. (**b**) An example showing the process of predicting potential targets for old drugs. (**c**) An example representing the process of predicting potential targets for new chemical entities. The detailed descriptions of **a–c** are provided in Subheading 3.5

tools, such as Discovery Studio, including various extended connectivity fingerprints (like ECFP4) [67] are often employed for generating chemical substructures.

3.5.2 Construction of Substructure-Drug-Target Interaction Network

Denoting the drug set as $D = \{d_1, d_2, \ldots, d_n\}$, target set as $T = \{t_1, t_2, \ldots, t_m\}$, and chemical substructure set as $S = \{s_1, s_2, \ldots, s_s\}$, a substructure-drug-target network can be represented as a tripartite graph G(V, E), where $V = D \cap S \cap T$ is the set of its vertices and E is the set of its edges containing known drug-target interactions and drug-substructure linkages (Fig. 4a). Denoting the NCE set as $C = \{c_1, c_2, \ldots, c_m\}$, the substructure-NCE-target network can be extended as a new graph $G'(V', E')$, where $V' = V \cap C$ is the set of its vertices and E' is the set of its edges containing the known drug-target interactions, the drug-substructure linkages, and the new NCE-substructure linkages (Fig. 4a).

3.5.3 Predicting New Targets for Old Drugs via STDNBI

As shown in Fig. 4b, for each drug d_i in the network, it has initial resources located in its targets and its substructures (*see* Subheading 3.4.1). In the initial state ($k = 0$), scores located in the neighbor nodes of d_i are set as its initial resources. For each target node t_j, the score located in t_j is the score of d_i-t_j interaction after two resource spreading processes ($k = 2$), where the best score reveals a high probability that d_i potentially interacts with t_j.

3.5.4 Predicting New Targets for New Chemical Entities Via STDNBI

In the substructure-NCE-target network (Fig. 4c), namely, previously defined graph G', NCEs can be considered as special drugs with no known targets. For each NCE c_i in this network, its initial resources only located in its substructures. In the initial state ($k = 0$), scores located in the neighbor nodes of c_i are set as its initial resources. For each target node t_j, the score located in t_j is the score of c_i-t_j interaction after two resource spreading processes ($k = 2$), where a higher score implies a high probability that c_i interacts with t_j. The detailed theoretical description can be found in the recent study [66].

3.5.5 Guideline for a Command-Line Network Tool, NetInfer

Recently, our group developed a toolkit, called NetInfer: http://lmmd.ecust.edu.cn/methods/sdtnbi/, written in C++ programming language, for predicting new potential targets for known drugs, failed drugs, and NCEs (Fig. 5). NetInfer provides various useful network-based tools that we developed for target-centric drug repositioning for various complex diseases, including cancer. Both SDTNBI and previously developed NBI algorithms are implemented in NetInfer (*see* **Note 3**). Specifically, NetInfer is light weight and does not require the support of any third-party math libraries such as linear algebra libraries. To speed up the calculation and reduce the cost of memory space, different data structures are employed for the sparse and dense matrices. Figure 5 provides the detailed protocols to assist the researchers identify new cancer target of interest for old drugs, failed drugs, and NCEs by integrating public data or their in-house data using NetInfer for the development of molecularly targeted cancer therapies (*see* **Note 4**).

3.6 Measurements for Evaluation of Model Performance

Several indicators are commonly used to evaluate the performance and robustness of network-aided models according to individualized predicted scores (*see* **Note 5**), including precision (P),

❖ **Step 1**: Generating drug-target interaction networks as the first input file a tab-separated text format (e.g DT.tsv), where five columns denote:
  1. The type of drug node (e.g. 'DRUG')
  2. The identifier of drug node (e.g. 'D-0001')
  3. The type of target node(e.g. 'TARGET')
  4. The identifier of target node (e.g. 'P00374')
  5. The weighted value of edge (i.e. '1')

```
DRUG  D-0001  TARGET  P00374  1
DRUG  D-0002  TARGET  P08254  1
DRUG  D-0002  TARGET  P03956  1
DRUG  D-0003  TARGET  P00519  1
DRUG  D-0003  TARGET  P35968  1
...   ...     ...     ...     ...
```

❖ **Step 2**: Generating drug-substructure association network as the second input file (e.g DS.tsv). Canonical SMILES for all old drugs or new chemical entities (NCEs) are stored in a tab-separated text file (.smi). The CSV file is convert into a prepared input file of drug-substructure (or NCE-substructure) associations generated by PaDEL-Descriptor. The input file is a tab-separated text file, where five columns denote:
  1. The type of drug node (e.g. 'DRUG' or 'COMPOUND')
  2. The identifier of drug node (e.g. 'D-0001' or 'C-0001')
  3. The type of substructure node(e.g. 'SUB')
  4. The identifier of substructure node (e.g. 'MACCSFP22')
  5. The weighted value of edge (i.e. '1')

```
DRUG  D-0001  SUB  MACCSFP22  1
DRUG  D-0001  SUB  MACCSFP25  1
DRUG  D-0002  SUB  MACCSFP22  1
DRUG  D-0002  SUB  MACCSFP24  1
DRUG  D-0003  SUB  MACCSFP22  1
DRUG  D-0003  SUB  MACCSFP23  1
...   ...     ...  ...        ...
```

❖ **Step 3**: Predicting new targets for old drugs or NCEs via NetInfer as below:

  i. The known drug-target interactions and drug-substructure associations (e.g DT.tsv and DS.tsv generated from steps 1 and 2) were used as two input files for predicting potential targets for old drugs, failed drugs, or NCEs.

  ii. A command line is used to execute SDTNBI method for predicting new targets to old drugs via NetInfer:
  netinfer -method nbi -nbi_k 2 -command predict -node_type DRUG TARGET -length 20 -training_set DT.tsv+DS.tsv -output DT_OUT.tsv

  iii. A command line is used to execute SDTNBI method for predicting new targets to NCEs via NetInfer:
  netinfer -method nbi -nbi_k 2 -command predict -node_type COMPOUND TARGET -length 20 -training_set DT.tsv+DS.tsv CS.tsv -output CT_OUT.tsv

  iv. The output file 'DT_OUT.tsv' is a tab-separated text file containing the predicted DTIs and their scores. Six columns denote:
  1. The type of drug node (e.g. 'DRUG' or 'COMPOUND')
  2. The identifier of drug node (e.g. 'D-0001' or 'C-0001')
  3. The type of target node (e.g. 'TARGET')
  4. The identifier of target node (e.g. 'P00374')
  5. The score of DTI or NCE-target interaction
  6. The rank of DTI ('-' represents known DTI) or NCE-target interaction.

```
DRUG      D-0001  TARGET  P00374  0.05096  -
DRUG      D-0002  TARGET  Q12809  0.04989  1
DRUG      D-0001  TARGET  P28335  0.04894  2
DRUG      D-0003  TARGET  P08913  0.04883  3
...       ...     ...     ...     ...      ...
COMPOUND  C-0001  TARGET  Q12809  0.05981  1
COMPOUND  C-0002  TARGET  P28335  0.05878  2
COMPOUND  C-0003  TARGET  P08913  0.05804  3
...       ...     ...     ...     ...      ...
```

Fig. 5 A flowchart illustrating three steps of guideline for predicting potential targets to old drugs, failed drugs in clinical trials, and new chemical entities via a user-friendly tool, NetInfer (http:/lmmd.ecust.edu.cn/methods/sdtnbi/)

recall (R), precision enhancement (e_P), and recall enhancement (e_R), as briefly described below:

$$P(L) = \frac{1}{M} \cdot \sum_{i=1}^{M} \frac{X_i(L)}{L} \tag{15}$$

$$R(L) = \frac{1}{M} \cdot \sum_{i=1}^{M} \frac{X_i(L)}{X_i} \tag{16}$$

$$e_P(L) = P(L) \cdot \frac{M \cdot N}{X} \tag{17}$$

$$e_R(L) = R(L) \cdot \frac{N}{L} \qquad (18)$$

where M and N are the numbers of drugs and targets, respectively, in the model; X is the total number of missing DTIs (e.g., known DTIs in test set) for M drugs; X_i is the number of missing DTIs for drug d_i; $X_i(L)$ is the number of true positive predictions (e.g., known DTIs in test set are correctly recovered, see **Note 6**) ranked in the top L of the predicted target list to d_i; and L is the length of the predicted candidates of interest.

A receiver operating characteristic (ROC) curve is often generated by measuring a series of true positive rates and false positive rates under different L ($L = 1, 2, \ldots, N$). In addition, a precision-recall curve is also shown by measuring an array of $P(L)$ and $R(L)$ values under different L. Finally, the areas under these ROC curves or precision-recall curves will be yielded to show the performance of network-aided models.

3.6.1 N-Fold Cross-Validation

The N-fold cross-validation is often used for evaluating the performance of models, such as tenfold cross-validation and leave-one-out cross-validation. For a tenfold cross-validation, the entire DTI network is randomly divided into ten parts. One part is used as the test set in turn. The remnant network is used as the training set to build the network-aided model. For leave-one-out cross-validation, each drug or target (not a DTI link) in the entire DTI network is extracted to be the test set in turn. The remnant network containing N-1 drugs or N-1 targets is used as training set for building the network-aided models. Finally, different indicators, including P, R, e_B and e_R, and the areas under the ROC curves or precision-recall curves will be measured for evaluation of the performance of models.

3.6.2 External Validation

The N-fold cross-validation cannot measure the actual generalization ability for most computational models [68]. It is crucial that all computational models are recommended to pass the external validation (model performance is evaluated by an external validation set that is not used to develop the model) before applying for real research projects in practice.

3.6.3 Experimental Validation

In addition to cross-validation and external validation, experimental validation is the best solution to test the performance of computational models in practice (see **Note 7**). For network-aided oncology drug repositioning models, in vitro cell line assays and in vivo mouse models could assist to identify novel anticancer indications for old drug, failed drugs, and NCEs, through targeting specific cancer targets of interest, and would speed up the development of molecularly targeted cancer therapy.

3.7 Summary and Further Directions

In this chapter, we introduce a network-aided drug repositioning infrastructure under systems pharmacology framework for target-centric drug repositioning. Due to the advances of the high-throughput technologies, big cancer panomics data, including transcriptomics, genomics, epigenomics, proteomics, and radiomics, have shed the revolution of oncology drug discovery paradigm [15, 69–71]. For example, identifying the existing agents that target clinically relevant driver mutations or molecular features under systems biology framework would provide incredible opportunities for precision oncology. In the future, development of a novel network-based infrastructure by incorporating big cancer panomics data into various molecular networks, such as drug-target networks, gene regulatory network, signaling network, metabolic network, the human protein-protein interaction network, along with the network-based inference framework introduced in this chapter, would provide unexpected opportunities for oncology drug discovery and development by exploiting the promise of precision oncology [34, 72–78].

4 Notes

1. Although node-weighted and edge-weighted NBI approaches are introduced for prediction of DTIs in this chapter, only marginal improvement is yielded for both node-weighted and edge-weighted NBI approaches compared to the non-weighted NBI. The possible data noises, such as low reproducible rate for biological experiments and data incompleteness, may explain this marginal improvement.

2. The substructure-drug-target network-based inference (SDTNBI) can be used to predict DTIs for both old drugs and new chemical entities. However, the performance of predicting DTIs for old drugs via SDTNBI is lower than that of NBI. One possible reason is the information loss during building networks of drug target and drug substructures via chemical substructures comparing to the direct topological information of the known drug-target interaction network. Altogether, the researchers are suggested to perform the consensus prediction through combining multiple different network-based approaches introduced in this chapter, including drug similarity-based network inference, target similarity-based network inference, the weighted and non-weighted NBI, and STDNBI.

3. For STDNBI, the model performance decreases with the increasing of the number of resource spreading processes (symbolized as k) during both ten-fold and leave-one-out cross-validations. One possible reason for this phenomenon might

be that the resources will be located more dispersedly in the network as the increasing of k. This dispersion might lead to a worse performance. The researchers are suggested to use a default $k = 2$ when performing specific research projects in practice using STDNBI implemented in NetInfer.

4. Current network-based approaches introduced in this chapter mainly exploit topological information of drug-target interaction bipartite network. Potential experimental data noise or literature bias in public databases, such as incompleteness of network data and low reproducible rates for drug-protein binding affinity across different laboratories, may lead to a potential risk of false positive rate. Thus, the researchers are suggested to build a comprehensive drug-target interaction network with high-quality drug-protein binding affinity data that they could collect and add the complementary chemoinformatics or bioinformatics approaches or tools to reduce the risk of false positive rate.

5. All network-based inference algorithms introduced in this chapter are based on the personalized inference of new targets for a specific drug or new drugs for a specific target with individualizing scores as described in the previous studies [15, 20, 21, 31, 32]. Prioritizing drug-target pairs based on the global predicted scores generated from the aforementioned approaches (e.g., NBI and STDNBI) is not reasonable during the different initial resource for each target node or each drug node. Thus, the researchers are suggested to evaluate the performance of models for each drug or target with individualizing scores in turn, not the global predicted scores. In addition, the researchers are suggested to select the potential predictions for specific cancer targets of interest with individualizing scores for future experimental validation.

6. There is often a misunderstanding between "precision" and "recall." For a computational model, precision is only referred to as the positive predictive value that a description of a level of measurement yields consistent results when repeated, while recall is referred to the true positive rate (e.g., accuracy). Thus, the researchers are suggested to perform both receiver operating characteristic (ROC) curves and precision-recall curves analyses to check the performance and robustness of the constructed computational models.

7. Before the experimental validation, the researchers are suggested to perform both cross-validation and external validation to examine the actual generalization ability of network-aided models to increase success rates of experimental assays. Currently, most published network-aided models only pass the cross-validation with reasonable performance (e.g., accuracy

more than 80%), which have a high risk of "over-fitting" owing to lack of external validation and often lead to a low success rate for experimental validations in practice.

References

1. Lavecchia A, Cerchia C (2016) In silico methods to address polypharmacology: current status, applications and future perspectives. Drug Discov Today 21:288–298
2. Xie L, Xie L, Kinnings SL et al (2012) Novel computational approaches to polypharmacology as a means to define responses to individual drugs. Annu Rev Pharmacol Toxicol 52:361–379
3. Wang J, Hu K, Guo J et al (2016) Suppression of KRas-mutant cancer through the combined inhibition of KRAS with PLK1 and ROCK. Nat Commun 7:11363
4. Zhao Y, Hu Q, Cheng F et al (2015) SoNar, a highly responsive NAD+/NADH sensor, allows high-throughput metabolic screening of anti-tumor agents. Cell Metab 21:777–789
5. Cheng F, Zhao J, Zhao Z (2015) Advances in computational approaches for prioritizing driver mutations and significantly mutated genes in cancer genomes. Brief Bioinform 17:642–656
6. Cheng F, Liu C, Lin CC et al (2015) A gene gravity model for the evolution of cancer genomes: a study of 3,000 cancer genomes across 9 cancer types. PLoS Comput Biol 11:e1004497
7. Hudson TJ, Anderson W, Artez A et al (2010) International network of cancer genome projects. Nature 464:993–998
8. Chin L, Andersen JN, Futreal PA (2011) Cancer genomics: from discovery science to personalized medicine. Nat Med 17:297–303
9. Moses H 3rd, Matheson DH, Cairns-Smith S et al (2015) The anatomy of medical research: US and international comparisons. JAMA 313:174–189
10. DiMasi JA, Grabowski HG, Hansen RW (2015) The cost of drug development. N Engl J Med 372:1972
11. Cheng F, Murray JL, Zhao J et al (2016) Systems biology-based investigation of cellular antiviral drug targets identified by gene-trap insertional mutagenesis. PLoS Comput Biol 12:e1005074
12. Bertolini F, Sukhatme VP, Bouche G (2015) Drug repurposing in oncology--patient and health systems opportunities. Nat Rev Clin Oncol 12:732–742
13. Cheng F, Murray JL, Rubin DH (2016) Drug repurposing: new treatments for Zika virus infection? Trends Mol Med 22:919–921
14. Lu W, Yao X, Ouyang P et al (2017) Drug repurposing of histone deacetylase inhibitors that alleviate neutrophilic inflammation in acute lung injury and idiopathic pulmonary fibrosis via inhibiting leukotriene A4 hydrolase and blocking LTB4 biosynthesis. J Med Chem 60:1817–1828
15. Cheng F, Hong H, Yang S et al (2016) Individualized network-based drug repositioning infrastructure for precision oncology in the panomics era. Brief Bioinform 18:682–697
16. Cheng F, Zhou Y, Li J et al (2012) Prediction of chemical-protein interactions: multitarget-QSAR versus computational chemogenomic methods. Mol BioSyst 8:2373–2384
17. Cheng F, Xu Z, Liu G et al (2010) Insights into binding modes of adenosine A(2B) antagonists with ligand-based and receptor-based methods. Eur J Med Chem 45:3459–3471
18. Lu W, Cheng F, Jiang J et al (2015) FXR antagonism of NSAIDs contributes to drug-induced liver injury identified by systems pharmacology approach. Sci Rep 5:8114
19. Cheng F, Li W, Zhou Y et al (2013) Prediction of human genes and diseases targeted by xenobiotics using predictive toxicogenomic-derived models (PTDMs). Mol BioSyst 9:1316–1325
20. Cheng F, Liu C, Jiang J et al (2012) Prediction of drug-target interactions and drug repositioning via network-based inference. PLoS Comput Biol 8:e1002503
21. Cheng F, Zhou Y, Li W et al (2012) Prediction of chemical-protein interactions network with weighted network-based inference method. PLoS One 7:e41064
22. Li J, Wu Z, Cheng F et al (2014) Computational prediction of microRNA networks incorporating environmental toxicity and disease etiology. Sci Rep 4:5576
23. Cheng F, Li W, Liu G et al (2013) In silico ADMET prediction: recent advances, current challenges and future trends. Curr Top Med Chem 13:1273–1289
24. Cheng F, Zhao Z (2014) Machine learning-based prediction of drug-drug interactions by integrating drug phenotypic, therapeutic, chemical, and genomic properties. J Am Med Inform Assoc 21:e278–e286
25. Zheng MW, Zhang CH, Chen K et al (2016) Preclinical evaluation of a novel orally available SRC/Raf/VEGFR2 inhibitor, SKLB646, in

the treatment of triple-negative breast cancer. Mol Cancer Ther 15:366–378

26. Pan Y, Zheng M, Zhong L et al (2015) A preclinical evaluation of SKLB261, a multikinase inhibitor of EGFR/Src/VEGFR2, as a therapeutic agent against pancreatic cancer. Mol Cancer Ther 14:407–418

27. Wang Y, Cheng F, Yuan X et al (2016) Dihydropyrazole derivatives as telomerase inhibitors: structure-based design, synthesis, SAR and anticancer evaluation in vitro and in vivo. Eur J Med Chem 112:231–251

28. Zhao J, Cheng F, Wang Y et al (2016) Systematic prioritization of druggable mutations in approximately 5000 genomes across 16 cancer types using a structural genomics-based approach. Mol Cell Proteomics 15:642–656

29. Vuong H, Cheng F, Lin CC et al (2014) Functional consequences of somatic mutations in cancer using protein pocket-based prioritization approach. Genome Med 6:81

30. Wu Z, Lu W, Wu D et al (2016) In silico prediction of chemical mechanism-of-action via an improved network-based inference method. Br J Pharmacol 173:3372–3385

31. Cheng F, Jia P, Wang Q et al (2014) Quantitative network mapping of the human kinome interactome reveals new clues for rational kinase inhibitor discovery and individualized cancer therapy. Oncotarget 5:3697–3710

32. Cheng F, Zhao J, Fooksa M et al (2016) A network-based drug repositioning infrastructure for precision cancer medicine through targeting significantly mutated genes in the human cancer genomes. J Am Med Inform Assoc 23:681–691

33. Cheng F, Liu C, Shen B et al (2016) Investigating cellular network heterogeneity and modularity in cancer: a network entropy and unbalanced motif approach. BMC Syst Biol 10 (Suppl 3):65

34. Li J, Lei K, Wu Z et al (2016) Network-based identification of microRNAs as potential pharmacogenomic biomarkers for anticancer drugs. Oncotarget 7:45584–45596

35. Cheng F, Li W, Wu Z et al (2013) Prediction of polypharmacological profiles of drugs by the integration of chemical, side effect, and therapeutic space. J Chem Inf Model 53:753–762

36. Yap CW (2011) PaDEL-Descriptor: an open source software to calculate molecular descriptors and fingerprints. J Comput Chem 32:1466–1474

37. O'Boyle NM, Banck M, James CA et al (2011) Open babel: an open chemical toolbox. J Cheminform 3:33

38. Law V, Knox C, Djoumbou Y et al (2014) DrugBank 4.0: shedding new light on drug metabolism. Nucleic Acids Res 42: D1091–D1097

39. Yang H, Qin C, Li YH et al (2016) Therapeutic target database update 2016: enriched resource for bench to clinical drug target and targeted pathway information. Nucleic Acids Res 44: D1069–D1074

40. Gaulton A, Bellis LJ, Bento AP et al (2012) ChEMBL: a large-scale bioactivity database for drug discovery. Nucleic Acids Res 40: D1100–D1107

41. Liu T, Lin Y, Wen X et al (2007) BindingDB: a web-accessible database of experimentally determined protein-ligand binding affinities. Nucleic Acids Res 35:D198–D201

42. Gunther S, Kuhn M, Dunkel M et al (2008) SuperTarget and Matador: resources for exploring drug-target relationships. Nucleic Acids Res 36:D919–D922

43. Kanehisa M, Goto S, Sato Y et al (2014) Data, information, knowledge and principle: back to metabolism in KEGG. Nucleic Acids Res 42: D199–D205

44. Hewett M, Oliver DE, Rubin DL et al (2002) PharmGKB: the pharmacogenetics knowledge base. Nucleic Acids Res 30:163–165

45. Szklarczyk D, Santos A, von Mering C et al (2016) STITCH 5: augmenting protein-chemical interaction networks with tissue and affinity data. Nucleic Acids Res 44:D380–D384

46. Wang Y, Xiao J, Suzek TO et al (2009) PubChem: a public information system for analyzing bioactivities of small molecules. Nucleic Acids Res 37:W623–W633

47. Kim Kjaerulff S, Wich L, Kringelum J et al (2013) ChemProt-2.0: visual navigation in a disease chemical biology database. Nucleic Acids Res 41:D464–D469

48. Seiler KP, George GA, Happ MP et al (2008) ChemBank: a small-molecule screening and cheminformatics resource database. Nucleic Acids Res 36:D351–D359

49. von Eichborn J, Murgueitio MS, Dunkel M et al (2011) PROMISCUOUS: a database for network-based drug-repositioning. Nucleic Acids Res 39:D1060–D1066

50. Bulusu KC, Tym JE, Coker EA et al (2014) canSAR: updated cancer research and drug discovery knowledgebase. Nucleic Acids Res 42: D1040–D1047

51. Wagner AH, Coffman AC, Ainscough BJ et al (2016) DGIdb 2.0: mining clinically relevant drug-gene interactions. Nucleic Acids Res 44: D1036–D1044

52. Lamb J, Crawford ED, Peck D et al (2006) The connectivity map: using gene-expression signatures to connect small molecules, genes, and disease. Science 313:1929–1935
53. Duan Q, Flynn C, Niepel M et al (2014) LINCS canvas browser: interactive web app to query, browse and interrogate LINCS L1000 gene expression signatures. Nucleic Acids Res 42:W449–W460
54. Keshava Prasad TS, Goel R, Kandasamy K et al (2009) Human protein reference database – 2009 update. Nucleic Acids Res 37: D767–D772
55. Gene Ontology C (2015) Gene ontology consortium: going forward. Nucleic Acids Res 43: D1049–D1056
56. Coordinators NR (2016) Database resources of the national center for biotechnology information. Nucleic Acids Res 44:D7–D19
57. UniProt C (2015) UniProt: a hub for protein information. Nucleic Acids Res 43: D204–D212
58. Altschul SF, Madden TL, Schaffer AA et al (1997) Gapped BLAST and PSI-BLAST: a new generation of protein database search programs. Nucleic Acids Res 25:3389–3402
59. Shannon P, Markiel A, Ozier O et al (2003) Cytoscape: a software environment for integrated models of biomolecular interaction networks. Genome Res 13:2498–2504
60. Shen J, Cheng F, Xu Y et al (2010) Estimation of ADME properties with substructure pattern recognition. J Chem Inf Model 50:1034–1041
61. Willett P (2006) Similarity-based virtual screening using 2D fingerprints. Drug Discov Today 11:1046–1053
62. Cheng F, Li W, Wang X et al (2013) Adverse drug events: database construction and in silico prediction. J Chem Inf Model 53:744–752
63. Gene Ontology C, Blake JA, Dolan M et al (2013) Gene ontology annotations and resources. Nucleic Acids Res 41:D530–D535
64. Yamanishi Y, Araki M, Gutteridge A et al (2008) Prediction of drug-target interaction networks from the integration of chemical and genomic spaces. Bioinformatics 24:i232–i240
65. Perlman L, Gottlieb A, Atias N et al (2011) Combining drug and gene similarity measures for drug-target elucidation. J Comput Biol 18:133–145
66. Wu Z, Cheng F, Li J et al (2016) SDTNBI: an integrated network and chemoinformatics tool for systematic prediction of drug-target interactions and drug repositioning. Brief Bioinform 18:333–347
67. Rogers D, Hahn M (2010) Extended-connectivity fingerprints. J Chem Inf Model 50:742–754
68. Collins GS, de Groot JA, Dutton S et al (2014) External validation of multivariable prediction models: a systematic review of methodological conduct and reporting. BMC Med Res Methodol 14:40
69. Fang J, Wu Z, Cai C et al (2017) Quantitative and systems pharmacology. 1. In silico prediction of drug-target interactions of natural products enables new targeted cancer therapy. J Chem Inf Model. https://doi.org/10.1021/acs.jcim.7b00216 [Epub ahead of print]
70. Shen Q, Cheng F, Song H et al (2017) Proteome-scale investigation of protein allosteric regulation perturbed by somatic mutations in 7,000 cancer genomes. Am J Hum Genet 100:5–20
71. Fang J, Liu C, Wang Q et al (2017) In silico polypharmacology of natural products. Brief Bioinform. https://doi.org/10.1093/bib/bbx045 [Epub ahead of print]
72. Cheng F, Jia P, Wang Q et al (2014) Studying tumorigenesis through network evolution and somatic mutational perturbations in the cancer interactome. Mol Biol Evol 31:2156–2169
73. Zhang C, Hong H, Mendrick DL et al (2015) Biomarker-based drug safety assessment in the age of systems pharmacology: from foundational to regulatory science. Biomark Med 9:1241–1252
74. Baryshnikova A (2016) Systematic functional annotation and visualization of biological networks. Cell Syst 2:412–421
75. Fang J, Cai C, Wang Q et al (2017) Systems pharmacology-based discovery of natural products for precision oncology through targeting cancer mutated genes. CPT Pharmacometrics Syst Pharmacol 6:177–187
76. Fang JS, Gao L, Ma HL et al (2017) Quantitative and systems pharmacology 3. Network-based identification of new targets for natural products enables potential uses in aging-associated disorders. Front Pharmacol 8:747
77. Zhao J, Cheng F, Zhao Z (2017) Tissue-specific signaling networks rewired by major somatic mutations in human cancer revealed by proteome-wide discovery. Cancer Res 77:2810–2821
78. Lu W, Cheng F, Yan W et al (2017) Selective targeting p53WT lung cancer cells harboring homozygous p53 Arg72 by an inhibitor of CypA. Oncogene 36:4719–4731

Chapter 16

Modeling Growth of Tumors and Their Spreading Behavior Using Mathematical Functions

Bertin Hoffmann, Thorsten Frenzel, Rüdiger Schmitz, Udo Schumacher, and Gero Wedemann

Abstract

Computer simulations of the spread of malignant tumor cells in an entire organism provide important insights into the mechanisms of metastatic progression. Key elements for the usefulness of these models are the adequate selection of appropriate mathematical models describing the tumor growth and its parametrization as well as a proper choice of the fractal dimension of the blood vessels in the primary tumor. In addition, survival in the bloodstream and evasion into the connective spaces of the target organ of the future metastasis have to be modeled. Determination of these from experimental models is complicated by systematic and unsystematic experimental errors which are difficult to assess. In this chapter, we demonstrate how to select the best-suited mathematical function to describe tumor growth for experimental xenograft mouse tumor models and how to parametrize them. Common pitfalls and problems are described as well as methods to avoid them.

Key words Tumor growth, Metastatic progression, Spreading behavior, Mathematical model, Parametrization

1 Introduction

Despite the fact that more than 90% of cancer patients die from distant metastases and not from the primary tumor, the process of metastasis formation is still relatively little understood [1]. In particular, the biological importance of an individual step within the metastatic cascade is difficult to assess. Therefore, mathematical models of tumor growth are important not only to develop a fundamental understanding of both the dynamics of primary tumor growth and metastasis formation. In addition, these models can help to interpret clinical or experimental data in order to gain new insights into these processes and to develop new hypotheses. As a new field of application in the last years, these "classical" mathematical models were incorporated into several computer models of the metastatic progression which were developed to resolve important questions concerning fundamental mechanisms of the spread of malignant tumor cells in an entire organism, e.g., [2–6]. In these models, mathematical functions describe the growth of the primary tumor and its spreading behavior. An appropriate selection of the functions used and their appropriate parametrization is crucial for obtaining meaningful results. However, experimental and clinical data are prone to large and unsystematic errors resulting in unrealistic parameters which may cause misleading results of the simulations. As an example, we analyzed data from experiments with xenograft mouse tumor models where the size of the primary tumor was determined by palpation or weighing after sacrificing the animal. This procedure causes unsystematic errors and also depends on the experience of the experimenter who performs the measurements.

In the literature, many methods are described how to solve the problem of choosing the right functions and parameters for tumor growth. These approaches offer various types of mathematical formalisms considering their individual research objectives such as the stochastic [7], survival [8], or state space model which contains a combination of stochastic and statistical models [9]. Another approach is the observation of the carrying capacity of the tumor [10]. A further extension of this carrying capacity model allows the investigation of interactions and their influence on the behavior of tumor cells and its surrounding connective tissue [11]. All these methods face the same challenge of parameter estimation from limited data. Usually methods such as the regression or the maximum likelihood procedure can be used to estimate an unknown parameter. In fact, these methods require the knowledge of the maximum tumor size for parameter estimation.

Here we describe an approach to determine the best-suited functions to describe tumor growth from limited data. Also, the choice of other parameters of the model such as the growth rate constant or the fractal dimension from experiments using xenograft mouse tumor models are derived. The selection of the growth function and the parametrization of the model were first done using data from a control group of animals in which the growth and spreading behavior was not altered by treatment interventions. These parameters are then used as a starting point for the analysis of data from mice which received different treatments. With this knowledge, data from treated or untreated groups can be compared and quantified. With the help of the determined mathematical functions, it is also possible to analyze the individual tumor growth kinetics and to find out whether the individual growth is faster or slower in comparison with other tumors.

2 Materials

2.1 Growth Functions

The number of cells in a tumor at time t is denoted by the growth function $x(t)$. The change of $x(t)$ is described by the growth rate $g(x)$:

$$\frac{dx}{dt} = g(x), \quad N_0 := x(t=0), \tag{1}$$

where N_0 is the size of the tumor at time $t = 0$. In many models, the growth of a tumor is described by the exponential, power-law, or Gompertz growth function. Commonly, most tumors correspond to a Gompertz function [10, 12–14]. This function is a kind of sigmoid function, i.e., the growth is slowest both at the beginning of a time period and also at its end. The tumor growth is divided into the avascular and vascular phase. In the avascular phase, the tumor growth starts with an exponential pattern, but with the increased volume of the tumor, it will be limited due to the restricted nutrient supply due to the slow growth of the blood vessels. In contrast to the avascular phase, the tumor emits angiogenic signals to stimulate the growth of new (capillary) blood vessels from the surrounding tissue for further nutrient supply in the vascular phase. Therefore, the tumor growth behavior is not uniform, and due to the lack of nutrient supply, the tumor reaches a saturated level in the later life span after the initial exponential growth. The Gompertz growth rate is defined as

$$g(x) = a\, x\, \ln\left(\frac{b}{x}\right), \tag{2}$$

where a is the growth rate constant and b represents the maximum number of tumor cells, corresponding to a maximum tumor size. Integration yields a tumor size of

$$x(t) = b\left(\frac{b}{N_0}\right)^{-e^{-at}}. \tag{3}$$

In contrast to a Gompertz function, an exponential function has no saturated band. The exponential function is defined as

$$x(t) = N_0 e^{at}. \tag{4}$$

Figure 1 shows the Gompertz and the exponential function by fitting sample experimental data. In this case the Gompertz function covers all tumor data points thanks to its slow growth behavior at the end. For small t both growth functions give approximately the same values if parametrized accordingly. For larger t both functions diverge, since Eq. 3 is bounded by b and Eq. 4 is unbounded.

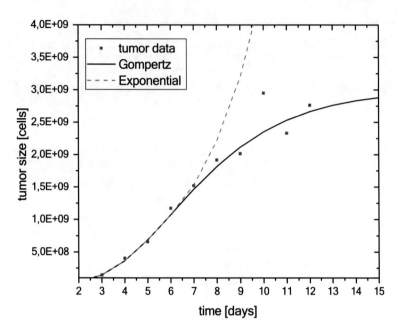

Fig. 1 A plot of sample tumor growth data with two different growth functions. In this case, the Gompertz function fits the data points better than exponential function. The exponential curve cannot fit the data at the end of tumor growth curve, respectively, at the saturated level

2.2 Colonization Rate

The primary tumor spreads malignant cells with a specific colonization rate $\beta(x)$. We assume an adopted form of the colonization rate from Iwata et al. [13]:

$$\beta(x) = mx^{\delta/3}, \qquad (5)$$

where m is the colonization coefficient and δ is the fractal dimension. This dimension describes how good the tumor is supplied with nutrients by the blood. With $\delta = 3$, the tumor is completely supplied with blood. $\delta = 2$ signifies that only the tumor's surface is supplied with blood. The reason why we assume this adopted form of the colonization rate will be explained more precisely in Subheading 4.

2.3 Experimental Setup

As an example setup, we analyzed data from experiments with mouse models where a reference group was untreated and other groups were subjected to different treatments. At the beginning one million cancer cells from the human small cell lung cancer line OH-1 were subcutaneously injected into immunodeficient mice to allow for the growth of a primary tumor. These untreated mice were sacrificed 28 days after the injection of the tumor cells. During the experiment, the tumor volumes were obtained by manual palpation. At the end of the experiment, the volume was determined by weighing of the extracted tumor. Furthermore, the number of metastases was determined in the bone marrow, brain, liver, and lung by Alu-PCR.

3 Methods

3.1 How to Select a Suitable Growth Function

The first step is to choose an appropriate growth function for the primary tumor. A common choice is the Gompertz growth function (Eq. 3). However, in mouse tumor models in many cases, the primary tumor does not have enough time to reach the saturated growth level, respectively, at the end of tumor growth (*see*, e.g., Fig. 4a). Thus, numerical fitting of a Gompertz function in order to estimate the parameters of the growth function is error prone. With this analytical method, we will first demonstrate the difference between all data points including the saturated level and the data points excluding the saturated level divided in three different cases with synthetic data:

1. Data points generated with Gompertz function.
2. Data points where only one point was arbitrary changed.
3. Data points affected by random noise (normal distribution with $\sigma = 10\%$ of the value). We generated and analyzed ten data sets each.

Case 3 was created to mimic data obtained from our mouse experiments. Synthetic data points for each day were generated using parameters: $a = 0.36$, $b = 3 \times 10^9$ and $N_0 = 0.4 \times 10^6$ for all four cases.

Figure 2a, b shows the results of two different fits for case 2 with the use of the Gompertz function using Origin software (OriginLab Corporation). In Fig. 2a, the range of data points

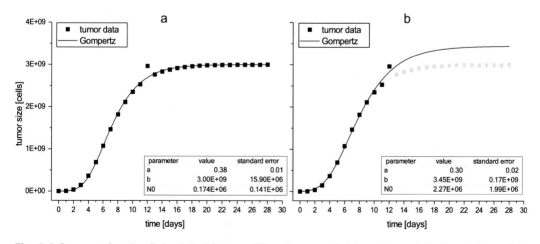

Fig. 2 A Gompertz function fit is plotted for two different cases: all data points and shortened data points excluding the saturated level. Sample date for this function is generated using parameters: $a = 0.36$, $b = 3 \times 10^9$ and $N_0 = 0.4 \times 10^6$. One data point (day 12) differs 0.3×10^9 from the original calculated points. (**a**) All data points are approximated with the Gompertz function. (**b**) Only data points up to day 12, which feature the exponential growth phase, are used for the fit. The resulting fit parameters are illustrated in the boxes

included in the fit includes the saturated level in contrast to in Fig. 2b where only the first 12 data points were included. Results from the fit with all data points correspond to the values of the growth function which was used to generate the data. If the data points from the saturated level were omitted as shown in b and only one point differs by 3×10^8 from the original calculated points, the results of the fit deviate significantly from the original values, especially N_0 differs by an order of magnitude. The results for all three cases are summarized in Table 1. For cases 1 and 2, the results of a fit with all data points are acceptable since parameters a, b, and N_0 are not much different from the original synthetic parameters. Only the parameters b and N_0 differ intensely from the original parameters in case 3 because the noise is too large in the selected example data. Concerning the fit with data excluding the saturated level, only the results in case 1 are acceptable. In case 2 and 3, the numerical fitting cannot compensate for the lack of the saturated data points for parameter estimation. The results for parameter N_0 differ by a one to two order of magnitudes from the original parameters. Please note that the results can considerably be affected by the choice of limits for each parameter in the fitting process. However, choosing these limits in order to improve the results might be difficult, if the restrict value range is not known from other sources.

Therefore, we conclude that in cases where no data points near the saturated level are available, no data about the saturation level can be determined by fitting. In this case the exponential growth (Eq. 4) should be used to avoid unrealistic results from the fitting process. The tumor data from the example discussed here include only data from the exponential growth stage. The saturated level would be reached, if the mice would have survived longer. We therefore recommend the usage of an exponential function for estimating experimental data where the saturated level is not available, since in its range, it describes the development over time in the time range of the experiment correctly and the possibility for errors is smaller. If the saturated level is available, the Gompertz function should be used.

3.2 Choosing a Suitable Fitting Process

To determine the parameters of a growth function, different procedures for fitting can be used. As described in the last section, a common useful choice is the exponential growth function $x(t) = N_0 e^{at}$, where N_0 is the start size of the tumor at time $t = 0$ and a is the growth rate constant. We investigated two possible fitting procedures: direct fit with an exponential function and the usage of linear regression with logarithmized x. For both of these methods, the software Origin was used to compute the parameters for two selected typical example mice data for each procedure. Table 2 shows the results for the parameters N_0 and a from a direct fit with an exponential function and results from linear function

Table 1
Results of a fit with the Gompertz function with synthetic data points. Four different cases were compared: (1) data points generated with Gompertz function, (2) only one data point at day 12 that was changed, and (3) all data points affected by a normal distribution noise ($\sigma = 10\%$ of the value). Minimum and maximum values of the fits to ten generated data sets are shown. The fits have been performed over all data points (4) and once just over the data points that show the exponential growth (5)

Case	All data points (4)				Shortened data points (5)			
	a	b	N_0	OK	a	b	N_0	OK
(1) Original data points (all)	0.36	3.00E+09	0.40E+06	X	0.36	3.00E+09	0.40E+06	X
(2) One point differs	0.38	3.00E+09	0.174E+06		0.30	3.45E+09	2.27E+06	
(3) Data points affected by noise $\binom{min}{max}$	0.37 $\binom{0.269}{0.446}$	3.02E+09 $\binom{2.93E+09}{3.18E+09}$	1.77E+06 $\binom{3.75E+03}{10.7E+06}$		0.34 $\binom{0.272}{0.442}$	3.24E+09 $\binom{2.73E+09}{4.09E+09}$	1.38E+06 $\binom{3.35E+03}{3.80E+06}$	

Table 2
Results of the comparison for the parameters *a* (growth rate constant) and N_0 (start size of the tumor at time t) between exponential fit and linear regression fit. In the second column, the results from the linear regression are shown

Parameter	Direct fit	Fit with linear regression
Mouse 1		
N_0	34.0E+03	43.9E+03
a	0.3689	0.3684
Mouse 2		
N_0	5.69E+06	5.25E+03
a	0.1630	0.4577

which are determined by linear regression for two different mice from the same untreated group.

To illustrate the results of both methods as an example, the fit of the exponential (a) and linear function (b) is shown in Fig. 3 for sample data of one tumor. The differences between the results from both methods are illustrated in the plot where both solutions are shown together (panel c). Data from another typical example is shown in panel d. In both samples, the curve, which parameters were computed with the values of the linear regression method (dashed lines), the relative errors of the later data points have less influence on the fitting process in comparison with the direct exponential fit. The dashed line fits closer to the original data points in the beginning of the tumor growth (days 13–21), whereas the solid line is influenced by the last data points and does not fit the data points at the beginning very well (*see* Fig. 3d). Thus, with the help of the linear regression method, outlier data points were better compensated compared with the direct exponential fit. This observation supports the assumption that the linear regression leads to more plausible results than the exponential fit method.

Both fitting methods differ in the results for the start size of the tumor N_0 (*see* Table 2). In the experiment, approximately 10^6 cells were implanted in the experiment (Subheading 2.3). Therefore, the range for N_0 can be restricted to $10^4 \leq N_0 \leq 1.5 \times 10^6$. All ~$1 \times 10^6$ implanted cells, which were injected at the beginning of the experiment in every mouse, would have to survive completely. This fact by itself is very unlikely, since many tumor cells undergo apoptosis and additionally the innate immune system kills many of the cells injected. Consequently, fit results for parameter N_0 over about 1.5×10^6 cells are not realistic. The primary tumor could not have more cells than the implanted at the beginning. While the

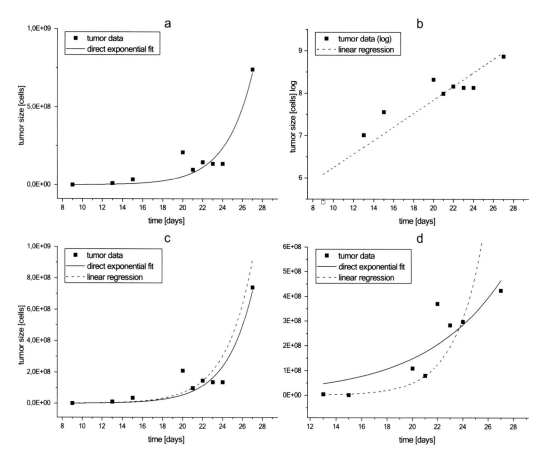

Fig. 3 Comparison between exponential fit and linear regression fit. The red lines show the exponential fit. The black lines show the exponential curve by using the linear regression values. The dots represent experimental data. In **a** a direct fit for the data of mouse 1 (*see* Table 2) was performed. In comparison **b** shows a fit where the data was logarithmized and a linear regression was executed. In **c** the fitted functions from **a** and **b** are shown together. In **d** the same process as in **c** is performed with mouse 2 (*see* Table 2)

linear regression for both samples delivers realistic values for N_0, the result from the direct exponential fit from mouse 2 (*see* Table 2) is above the limit of 1.5×10^6 cells for the start size of the tumor. (*See* also: Frenzel et al. [18]).

Overall, the linear regression method is less sensitive to data points with outlier data points and produces more realistic results for the parameters. We therefore recommend this approach for the analytical process to compare various groups of experimental data.

3.3 Joining Data from Different Experimental Methods

In many experiments, the size of the primary tumor is determined by variable methods with different systematic and unsystematic errors. In our example, the tumor size was obtained by palpation during the experiment and only the very last point by weighing when the animal was sacrificed. The data determined by palpation were measured by different persons which induces different

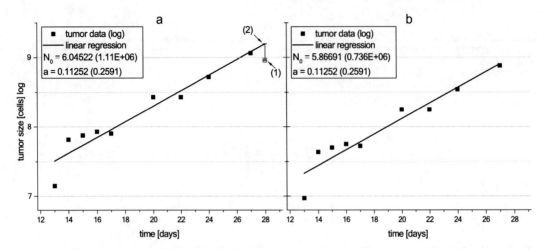

Fig. 4 A method for joining data from different experimental methods. (**a**) Shows the original data points with the linear regression method. (**b**) Shows the reduced data points by the mean value of the distance between (1) and (2). The values from parameter N_0 and *a* are in brackets

unsystematic and systematic errors by the experimentalists. The value obtained by weighing is expected to be more precise in general than the other data points. If, e.g., the value determined by weight is lower than the last value determined by palpation, the palpation values seem to be overestimated. Since the exact errors of both methods are not known, it is not possible to include the knowledge about the different reliability of the data into the fitting process. In order to cope with this problem, we developed the following procedure illustrated by experimental data in Fig. 4:

1. Execute a linear regression as described in the last paragraph including all data points excluding the data point obtained by weight.

2. Determine x_{end}^f the value from the function determined by fitting on the day where the data point by weight was obtained (in example day 28) for all samples.

3. Calculate the difference between x_{end}^f and x_{end}^s, the value determined by weight: $\Delta x_{end} = x_{end}^s - x_{end}^f$ (Fig. 4a (1) and (2)) for all samples.

4. Calculate the mean $\overline{\Delta x_{end}}$ of all Δx_{end} of the group.

5. Add $\overline{\Delta x_{end}}$ (positive or negative) to every data point from palpation in the group.

6. Perform a linear regression with the transformed data points.

In the example (Fig. 4), the data point determined by weight is lower than the last data point by palpation. Since there is only one sample in this example, the data points by palpation are overestimated; the mean value of the distance between (1) and (2) reduces the number of data points used for calculus.

3.4 Determination of the Spreading Behavior

The spreading behavior of the primary tumor is defined by the colonization rate $\beta(x)$ (Subheading 2.2) and cannot be measured directly in most experimental setups. We developed the following procedure to determine parameters of $\beta(x)$ by comparing the experimental data with results from computer simulations with our model [15] and adjusted the spreading parameters in the simulation until they fit to the experimental data.

1. For the fractal dimension, the tumor-bearing mouse was chosen, which had the largest tumor at the end of the experiment as measured by weight. The parameter δ is set on 2, which means that this primary tumor has a blood supply on the surface (*see* Subheading 4). We assume this, because a fast-growing tumor usually grows on the surface as most of the functional blood vessels are located around the surface. Thus, the biggest tumor should have the best blood supply, while smaller tumors might have a more limited blood supply.

2. Configure the simulation for this mouse with the previously determined parameters (growth rate, start size, etc.). For the colonization coefficient m, choose an arbitrary starting value, e.g., $m = 0.01$.

3. Perform the simulation, and adjust m until the number of metastases agrees with the simulated number of metastases.

4. With this determined colonization constant for other mice i in a group, an individual fractal dimension δ_i will be determined: perform simulations, and adjust δ_i until the number of metastases agrees with the simulated number of metastases.

5. After all simulation compute the mean value δ of the fractal dimensions δ_i.

The determined values can serve as parameters for simulations of other groups of mice which are affected by treatment interventions, e.g., chemotherapy or external beam radiation. In these groups, it might not be possible to determine the normal growth of the primary tumor or the blood supply because they are changed by therapy and not enough data from the untreated animals are available.

Please note that the assumption of the fractal dimension in **step 1** is not critically in most experimental setups where micrometastasis consists of single cells that are specifically termed disseminated tumor cells (DTCs). In this case possible inaccuracies of δ are balanced by the type of the determination of the colonization rate parameter m. However, in future experiments, experimentalists should include experimental analysis of the fractal dimensions of blood vessels, e.g., by the analysis of sectional images to increase the accuracy of the models and to prove the assumptions.

4 Notes

In the mathematical model for the growth and size of a tumor with multiple metastases introduced by Iwata et al., the spawning of new metastases is modeled by a colonization rate which "(...) mechanistically implies that the rate of metastasis from a tumor with size x is proportional to the number of tumor cells in contact with blood vessels, which provide channel for cell dispersal" [13]. Therein, it is written as

$$\beta(x) = mx^\delta, \qquad (6)$$

where x is the number of cells in the tumor, m is a coefficient, and δ is the fractal dimension [1].

We argue that the colonization rate, by the same reason, should instead be written as

$$\beta(x) = mx^{\delta/3}. \qquad (7)$$

The actual definition implied for the fractal dimension is not given in the original paper [13]. Here, we refer to the most common and, from a computational point of view, most handy form of a fractal dimension, the box-counting dimension. The same is also used by Gazit et al. [16] to which Iwata et al. [13] refer for their interpretation of the fractal dimension of a vessel system. The object is covered by a grid of nonoverlapping boxes with edge length ϵ which are then counted. The box-counting dimension of the object is defined to be

$$d_{bc} = \lim_{\epsilon \to 0} \frac{\log N(\epsilon)}{-\log(\epsilon)}, \qquad (8)$$

where $N(\epsilon)$ denotes the minimum number of boxes of size ϵ^3 required in order to fully cover the object.

As a trivial example, one may consider the object to be a box with volume V. The minimum number of small ϵ^3-boxes needed for covering the larger box is given by the ratio of their volumes; hence

$$N(\epsilon) = V/\epsilon^3 \propto \epsilon^{-3}. \qquad (9)$$

Inserting Eq. 9 in Eq. 8 yields a fractal (box-counting) dimension of 3. Even though this example may be somewhat trivial, it reflects an essential property of (any definition of) a fractal dimension. Being a generalization of the geometric dimension, i.e., the intuitive understanding of the term "dimension," the fractal dimension must agree with the geometric one, for any object which has a definite geometric definition.

The one-dimensional Cantor set (*see* Fig. 5), on the other hand, can be thought of as an object "somewhere between a point-set and a line," i.e., somewhere between $0d$ and $1d$. Continuing the scheme

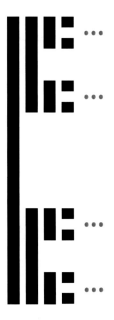

Fig. 5 Cantor's set. Adopted from: [17]

depicted in Fig. 5 to infinity, the one-dimensional Cantor set corresponds to the infinite step, i.e., "the last and infinite column" in this imaginary picture. In fact, it features a fractal dimension of 0.63.

Let us now consider a tumor blood vessel tree with a fractal dimension of d_{vasc} as the object of interest. One can then find a representation of the minimum number of boxes to fully cover the object that asymptotically approaches $N(\epsilon) \propto \epsilon^{-d_{\text{vasc}}}$. This is very similar to what we have already discussed in Eq. 9. Using that the volume of each box equals its length to the power of 3, it follows that, asymptotically,

$$N(x) \propto x^{-d_{\text{vasc}}/3}, \qquad (10)$$

where d_{vasc} denotes the fractal dimension of the vascular tree.

By virtue of the fact that $N(x)$, the minimum number of boxes to cover the vessel tree, is, up to a factor of proportionality, just the same as the number of cells contacted by these vessels, the number of these cells takes the same functional form as Eq. 10. Following the argument by Iwata et al. [13], the number of vessel-contacted cells exactly corresponds to the colonization rate, up to another factor of proportionality. Therefore, from Eq. 4 it follows that

$$\beta(x) = m \, x^{d_{\text{vasc}}/3}, \qquad (11)$$

with m as an appropriate factor of proportionality.

Considering the example of a ball-like tumor, which is vascularized only at its surface, the number of contacted cells grows with the total number of cells like $x^{2/3}$ [13]. Following our argument, this allows one to deduce a fractal dimension of the vasculature of 2 through Eq. 7, instead of 2/3 following from (Eq. 6). Recalling that exactly the surface of the tumor is assumed to be vascularized, that the surface of a ball has a geometric dimension of 2 and, finally, that the fractal dimension must recover the geometric one in case the latter exists, our reasoning presented here is supported by this example.

References

1. Valastyan S, Weinberg RA (2011) Tumor metastasis: molecular insights and evolving paradigms. Cell 147:275–292. https://doi.org/10.1016/j.cell.2011.09.024
2. Bethge A, Schumacher U, Wree A, Wedemann G (2012) Are metastases from metastases clinical relevant? Computer modelling of cancer spread in a case of hepatocellular carcinoma. PLoS One 7:e35689. https://doi.org/10.1371/journal.pone.0035689
3. Brodbeck T, Nehmann N, Bethge A, Wedemann G, Schumacher U (2014) Perforin-dependent direct cytotoxicity in natural killer cells induces considerable knockdown of spontaneous lung metastases and computer modelling-proven tumor cell dormancy in a HT29 human colon cancer xenograft mouse model. Mol Cancer 13:244. https://doi.org/10.1186/1476-4598-13-244
4. Bethge A, Schumacher U, Wedemann G (2015) Simulation of metastatic progression using a computer model including chemotherapy and radiation therapy. J Biomed Inform 57:74–87. https://doi.org/10.1016/j.jbi.2015.07.011
5. Benzekry S, Tracz A, Mastri M, Corbelli R, Barbolosi D, Ebos JML (2015) Modeling spontaneous metastasis following surgery: an in vivo-in silico approach. Cancer Res 76:535–547. https://doi.org/10.1158/0008-5472.CAN-15-1389
6. Newton PK, Mason J, Bethel K, Bazhenova L, Nieva J, Norton L, Kuhn P (2013) Spreaders and sponges define metastasis in lung cancer: a Markov chain mathematical model. Cancer Res 73:2760–2769. https://doi.org/10.1158/0008-5472.CAN-12-4488
7. Ferrante L, Bompadre S, Possati L, Leone L (2000) Parameter estimation in a Gompertzian stochastic model for tumor growth. Biometrics 56:1076–1081. https://doi.org/10.1111/j.0006-341X.2000.01076.x
8. Witten M, Satzer W (1992) Gompertz survival model parameters: estimation and sensitivity. Appl Math Lett 5:7–12. https://doi.org/10.1016/0893-9659(92)90125-S
9. Tan W-Y, Ke W, Webb G (2009) A stochastic and state space model for tumour growth and applications. Comput Math Methods Med 10:117–138. https://doi.org/10.1080/17486700802200784
10. Hahnfeldt P, Panigrahy D, Folkman J, Hlatky L (1999) Tumor development under angiogenic signaling: a dynamical theory of tumor growth, treatment response, and postvascular dormancy. Cancer Res 59:4770–4775
11. Benzekry S, Lamont C, Beheshti A, Tracz A, Ebos JML, Hlatky L, Hahnfeldt P (2014) Classical mathematical models for description and prediction of experimental tumor growth. PLoS Comput Biol 10:e1003800. https://doi.org/10.1371/journal.pcbi.1003800
12. Barbolosi D, Benabdallah A, Hubert F, Verga F (2009) Mathematical and numerical analysis for a model of growing metastatic tumors. Math Biosci 218:1–14. https://doi.org/10.1016/j.mbs.2008.11.008
13. Iwata K, Kawasaki K, Shigesada N (2000) A dynamical model for the growth and size distribution of multiple metastatic tumors. J Theor Biol 203:177–186. https://doi.org/10.1006/jtbi.2000.1075
14. Kozusko F, Bajzer Ž (2003) Combining Gompertzian growth and cell population dynamics. Math Biosci 185:153–167. https://doi.org/10.1016/S0025-5564(03)00094-4
15. Bethge A, Wedemann G (2014) CaTSiT - Computer simulation of metastatic progression and treatments. In: CaTSiT - Computer simulation of metastatic progression and treatments. http://bioinformatics.hochschule-stralsund.de/catsit/. Accessed 12 Nov 2015
16. Gazit Y, Baish JW, Safabakhsh N, Leuning M, Baxter LT, Jain RK (1997) Fractal characteristics of tumor vascular architecture during tumor growth and regression, microcirculation, Informa healthcare. Microcirculation

4:395–402. https://doi.org/10.3109/10739689709146803

17. Jurczyszyn K, Osiecka BJ, Ziółkowski P (2012) The use of fractal dimension analysis in estimation of blood vessels shape in transplantable mammary adenocarcinoma in Wistar rats after photodynamic therapy combined with cysteine protease inhibitors. Comput Math Methods Med 2012:793291. https://doi.org/10.1155/2012/793291

18. Frenzel T, Hoffmann B, Schmitz R, Bethge A, Schumacher U, Wedemann G (2017) Radiotherapy and chemotherapy change vessel tree geometry and metastatic spread in a small cell lung cancer xenograft mouse tumor model. PLOS ONE 12(11):e0187144. https://doi.org/10.1371/journal.pone.0187144

Correction to: Computational Analysis of Structural Variation in Cancer Genomes

Matthew Hayes

Correction to:
Chapter 3 in: Alexander Krasnitz (ed.),
Cancer Bioinformatics, Methods in Molecular Biology, vol. 1878,
https://doi.org/10.1007/978-1-4939-8868-6_3

The author originally had the wrong programming command and the chapter was inadvertently published with error. The same has been updated later as below

```
samtools view -b -F 14 alignment.sorted.nodup.bam \
> alignment.sorted.nodup.nocon.bam
```

The updated online version of this chapter can be found at
https://doi.org/10.1007/978-1-4939-8868-6_3

Index

A

Alignability 103–105
Allele 96, 100, 102–107,
    109, 111–115, 117–121, 125–127, 129, 132,
    133, 162, 164–167, 177–179, 218, 219, 223, 224
Area under the curve (AUC) 163–165, 232

B

Binding affinity 164–166, 247,
    248, 251, 258
Breakpoint 67, 69, 70, 76
Breast cancer
    basal-like 197
    HER2+ 197
    luminal 197, 198
    triple-negative 197

C

Cancer cell fraction (CCF) 218–224
Cancer immunotherapy 157, 165, 169
Cancer ontology 23, 33
Cancer stratification 201–203
Cantor set 274, 275
Clonal evolution 217
Cloud computing 19, 45
Colonization rate 266, 273–275
Common Workflow Language (CWL) 40, 60
Computing cluster 90
Copy-number alteration (CNA) 85–92,
    127, 134, 202, 205, 218, 222
    somatic 85, 87,
    128, 134, 218
Cox model 143–145, 147–149, 197

D

Depth-of-coverage (DOC) 69, 70, 74, 77
Dissimilarity 210, 211
Distribution
    null 86, 211, 212
    Pareto 212
DNA methylation 125, 173–188
Docker 17, 18, 40–47,
    57, 58, 60, 62
    container 17, 40, 42–46, 57, 58, 60, 62

Dockerfile 42, 43,
    45, 57, 58
Driver genes 95–107
Drug
    repositioning 243–259
    target interactions 244, 246–248,
    251, 253–254, 256–258

E

Epitope prediction 163, 164
Exon 96, 99, 101,
    102, 106, 112, 132, 162, 184
Expression 23, 24, 29,
    41, 42, 47, 51, 59–63, 75, 95, 96, 107, 120, 121,
    125–135, 139–144, 147, 149, 150, 152, 158,
    165–168, 173, 181, 184, 193–200, 205, 206,
    210, 212, 227, 228, 230–232, 238, 252
    allele-specific 125–135, 175
Extreme-value theory 211

F

Feature selection 184, 229,
    232–234
Fractal dimension 264, 266,
    273–276

G

Gene expression quantification 47
Germline variant 80, 97,
    98, 103–105, 113, 115, 122, 161
Growth function 265–268

H

Heat map 179, 181, 202, 209
Hierarchical clustering (HC) 102,
    106, 179–181, 195, 209–211

I

IC_{50} 164, 165, 247, 251
Immunodeficient mouse 266
Immunoediting 167
Immunogenicity 162–163, 165
Intratumor heterogeneity 217
Inversion 65, 66, 70

L

Lasso method 144, 147–148, 151
Linear regression 55, 56, 135, 228, 229, 234, 235, 238, 266, 270–272
Long noncoding RNAs (lncRNAs) 25, 139–152

M

Machine learning 184, 195, 197, 244, 245
Maximum likelihood (ML) 41, 212, 264
Metadata 10, 11, 46, 48–51, 53, 59, 61, 62
Metastatic progression 263
Missing value estimation 231–232

N

Naïve Bayes classifier 196
Neoepitope 157–169
Network-based inference 248, 251–253, 257, 258
Non-synonymous mutation 168

P

Panomics 245, 257
Parallelization 89, 91, 212
PCR duplicates 81, 100, 103, 105
Permutation test 198
Phylogenetic tree 220, 222–223
Phylogeny 225
Plugin 40
Polypharmacology 243–259
Precision oncology 245, 257

R

Random forests 141, 184, 185, 228, 229, 232–235, 238, 239
Receiver operating characteristics (ROC) 163, 195, 256, 258
Regression model 135, 143, 145, 148, 182, 228, 229, 234–235

Reproducibility 39, 40, 57, 195
R language 86, 210

S

Self-tolerance 166
Sequence dataset
  paired-end 66, 69
  single-end 66, 67, 70, 75
Sequencing
  high-throughput 1, 3–20, 66, 95, 99, 143, 150, 158, 162
  next-generation 66–71, 76–78, 80, 90, 125–135, 157, 158, 175, 217, 244
  whole-exome 95, 96, 110, 112, 119, 127–132, 134, 158, 166, 217
Single-nucleotide polymorphism (SNP) 65, 87, 97, 102, 127, 129–135, 177, 179, 225, 227, 228, 230
Structural variation 65–81
Subclone 217, 219–220, 225
Systems biology 257
Systems pharmacology 245, 257

T

Targeted therapy 34
Transcriptome 47, 95, 96, 99, 103, 104, 126, 127, 129, 135, 158, 229, 230
Translocation 65, 70
Tumor subtype 175, 194, 195, 197, 200, 209–216

U

Unsupervised learning 209

V

Variant calling 73, 97, 99, 101–103, 107, 161–162, 166, 168

W

Whole-exome sequencing (WES) 95, 96, 110, 112, 119, 127–132, 134, 158, 166

Printed in the United States
By Bookmasters